Relational Spirituality in Psychotherapy

Relational Spirituality in Psychotherapy

Healing Suffering and Promoting Growth

Steven J. Sandage, David Rupert, George S. Stavros, and Nancy G. Devor

AMERICAN PSYCHOLOGICAL ASSOCIATION
Washington, DC

The opinions and statements published are the responsibility of the authors, and
such opinions and statements do not necessarily represent the policies of the American
Psychological Association.

Published by
American Psychological Association
750 First Street, NE
Washington, DC 20002
https://www.apa.org

Order Department
https://www.apa.org/pubs/books
order@apa.org

In the U.K., Europe, Africa, and the Middle East, copies may be ordered from Eurospan
https://www.eurospanbookstore.com/apa
info@eurospangroup.com

Typeset in Meridien and Ortodoxa by Circle Graphics, Inc., Reisterstown, MD

Printer: Sheridan Books, Chelsea, MI
Cover Designer: Nicci Falcone, Potomac, MD

Library of Congress Cataloging-in-Publication Data

Names: Sandage, Steven J., author. | Rupert, David (David Alan), author. |
  Stavros, George, author. | Devor, Nancy G., author.
Title: Relational spirituality in psychotherapy : healing suffering and promoting growth /
  by Steven J. Sandage, David Rupert, George S. Stavros, Nancy G. Devor.
Description: Washington, DC : American Psychological Association, [2020] |
  Includes bibliographical references and index.
Identifiers: LCCN 2019034528 (print) | LCCN 2019034529 (ebook) |
  ISBN 9781433831669 (paperback) | ISBN 9781433831782 (ebook)
Subjects: LCSH: Psychotherapy—Religious aspects. | Interpersonal
  relations—Religious aspects. | Spirituality—Psychology.
Classification: LCC RC489.S676 S26 2020 (print) | LCC RC489.S676 (ebook) |
  DDC 616.89/14—dc23
LC record available at https://lccn.loc.gov/2019034528
LC ebook record available at https://lccn.loc.gov/201903

http://dx.doi.org/10.1037/0000174-000

Printed in the United States of America

10 9 8 7 6 5 4 3 2 1

To Jim Maddock and Noel Larson, my key clinical mentors,
who transformed my understanding of relational psychotherapy
through their teaching, all the while embodying such vital existential
and spiritual traits—compassion, wisdom, courage, humility, and humor;
and to Danielle Sandage, my life partner in spiritual dwelling and seeking.

—STEVEN J. SANDAGE

To Holden, who lived so bravely, with heart and soul.

—DAVID RUPERT

To my beloved mentors, Fr. Costas Sitaras, Dr. Kyriaki Fitzgerald,
and Dr. Joseph Shay, each of whom embodies the healing power
of hospitality; and to Despina Stavros, my dearest friend and
fellow pilgrim in a journey of love.

—GEORGE S. STAVROS

In memory of Ward Cromer, PhD, my clinical mentor,
whose unflinching honesty and challenge was matched only
by his commitment, compassion, and presence;
and to Dick Devor, whose love and humor heal me daily.

—NANCY G. DEVOR

CONTENTS

PREFACE AND ACKNOWLEDGMENTS

While working on this volume on relational spirituality in psychotherapy, we were surprised and delighted to discover a convergence of approaches between the Albert and Jessie Danielsen Institute at Boston University (the current professional home of all the authors) and Bethel Seminary, where Steve began the research leading to the relational spiritual model (RSM). Leland Eliason was the dean at Bethel Seminary (St. Paul, Minnesota) when he encouraged Steve and Carla Dahl to start a program of research on the spiritual and personal formation of seminary students drawing on social science and theology. Eliason had received his doctorate in pastoral psychology from Boston University, where he studied with Merle Jordan, the former executive director of the Danielsen Institute, whose teaching career spanned four decades and included Nancy and George among his students. Merle was masterful at conveying his passion for interdisciplinary clinical integration that combined scholarly depth and tremendous heart. These converging streams of influence of relational and systemic perspectives on spirituality and psychotherapy have brought us to the place from where we write today.

Steve's initial conceptual and empirical work on the RSM while in Minnesota benefited greatly from learning in dialogue with many colleagues, students, and therapy clients. In addition to Carla, key scholarly collaborators have included Peter Jankowski, LeRon Shults, Mary Jensen, Everett Worthington, Sarah Crabtree, Maria Schweer-Collins, Ian Williamson, and Dan Jass. Through their teaching and consultation, Jim Maddock and Noel Larson also shaped many of the clinical perspectives behind the RSM. The early research work on the RSM was supported by grants from the Lilly Endowment, the John Templeton Foundation (JTF), and the Fetzer Institute.

This current version of the RSM has also been influenced by two research grants from JTF: "Mental Healthcare, Virtue, and Human Flourishing" (No. 61245) and "Developing Humility in Leadership" (No. 60622). We also appreciate the contributions from many team members working with us on various relational spirituality projects in the research center at the Danielsen Institute in recent years, including David Paine, Chance Bell, Elizabeth Ruffing, Sarah Moon, Hee An Choi, Claire Wolfteich, and James Tomlinson. Dean Mary Elizabeth Moore has enthusiastically supported the interdisciplinary research on the RSM.

The vision of the founders, Jesse and Albert Danielsen, is also a guiding inspiration behind this book—to bring the resources of spirituality, religion, and psychology to alleviate suffering and promote healing and growth through psychotherapy, training, and research. Their vision for the Danielsen Institute was born out of the personal pain of Albert, an orphan who had suffered loss and cruelty and whose resiliency originated in loving relationships. It is a constant reminder to us of how relational spirituality and psychotherapy can help us move through experiences of suffering and trauma to lives of hope, meaning, and generativity.

The fabric of the Institute's daily, relational rhythms of clinical service, teaching, training, supervision, and research is woven deeply into this volume. We are immeasurably grateful for the opportunity to work with one another and with our Danielsen Institute colleagues—Brooke Amendola, Miriam Bronstein, Nicolae Dumitrascu, Lauren Kehoe, Michele Klau, Christopher O'Rourke, Loveleen Saini, Marina Williams, and Mary Wilson. We are indebted to the many courageous clients and thoughtful training fellows who have accompanied and taught us, both before and during the writing of this book. Your presence and wisdom have been invaluable in our lives and work. Alongside each of you, we experience a warm and vibrant professional ecosystem that provides the necessary support and challenge to articulate our most deeply held beliefs about and approaches to psychotherapy.

Relational Spirituality in Psychotherapy

Introduction

Relational Model of Spiritually Integrative Psychotherapy

A growing interest and receptivity to acknowledging the importance of spiritual and religious dynamics in mental health treatment and psychotherapy has developed over the past few decades. While some skepticism or antagonism toward spirituality and religion can still readily be found among mental health providers, all the major mental health fields have called for spiritual and religious sensitivity and competence among practitioners. Empirical research has demonstrated that spiritual and religious factors can often be positively associated with mental health (Koenig, 2018), and there is also empirical evidence that a majority of psychotherapy clients hold important religious and spiritual beliefs and prefer to have these considered as part of their psychotherapeutic treatment (Post & Wade, 2009; Rose, Westefeld, & Ansley, 2008).

It is now widely recognized that ethical clinical service involves treating the religious and spiritual practices and beliefs of clients with respect, cultural sensitivity, and openness (e.g., American Psychological Association [APA], 2017). Additionally, it is also crucial to ethical practice that mental health professionals be aware of potential personal biases they may have regarding religion and spirituality in order to minimize any negative impact their bias may have in treating their clients (Bartoli, 2007; Vieten et al., 2016). Moreover, research shows that clinical outcomes can be at stake, given evidence that highly religious or spiritually committed clients tend to show superior outcomes when treatment involves explicit integration of religion or spirituality

http://dx.doi.org/10.1037/0000174-001
Relational Spirituality in Psychotherapy: Healing Suffering and Promoting Growth,
by S. J. Sandage, D. Rupert, G. S. Stavros, and N. G. Devor

(Hook, Worthington, & Davis, 2012; Worthington, Hook, Davis, & McDaniel, 2011). These clients can also report negative experiences in psychotherapy if they perceive that their therapist opposes their religious views or avoids discussing spiritual and religious issues with them (Cragun & Friedlander, 2012). Therefore, it is imperative for clinicians to understand respectful and effective ways to engage the sacred in psychotherapy with sensitivity to clients' diverse perspectives and preferences in this regard.

SPIRITUALLY INTEGRATIVE PSYCHOTHERAPIES

The growing clinical and research literature and the wider professional discussion on spirituality and religion in psychotherapy have focused considerable attention on ways of incorporating certain spiritual or religious practices (e.g., mindfulness meditation, prayer, forgiveness, yoga, gratitude; see Aten, McMinn, & Worthington, 2011) into treatment. This focus on practices or techniques has been a helpful development to provide ways of efficiently engaging spiritual and religious dynamics in established treatment models. However, in our opinion, the field of spirituality and religion in psychotherapy has reached a point where there is a need to move beyond a focus on specific techniques or practices to also articulate different theoretical approaches to *spiritually integrative psychotherapy.* By using this term, we are referencing a broad range of clinical approaches that intentionally engage spiritual and religious dynamics in psychotherapy in ways that are theoretically and clinically coherent. Pargament and Saunders (2007) similarly referred to spiritually integrative psychotherapies as therapies "whose component parts work together in synchrony with one another" (p. 34).

Several models of what we consider to be spiritually integrative psychotherapy are now available and are based on different theoretical orientations and spiritual traditions (e.g., Al-Karam, 2018; Cashwell & Young, 2014; Frankel, 2003; Jennings, 2010; R. Johnson, 2013; Linehan, 1993, 2015; McMinn & Campbell, 2007; Pargament, 2007; Park, Currier, Harris, & Slattery, 2017; Peteet, 2010; Richards & Bergin, 2005; Sorenson, 2004b; Sperry, 2012; Starr, 2008; Worthington & Sandage, 2016). We suggest that spiritual and religious integration into psychotherapy will be more effective in models where the understanding of spiritual and religious dynamics is conceptually and clinically consistent with the theoretical orientation and overall clinical strategies of a particular model of psychotherapy. Therefore, we developed the relational spirituality model (RSM) described in this book to integrate our theory and research on relational spirituality (i.e., "ways of relating to the sacred"; Worthington & Sandage, 2016, p. 38) with our preference for relational models of psychotherapy (e.g., Wampold & Imel, 2015, and their contextual model). We do not view relational dynamics as a kind of add-on topic for individualistic conceptualizations of either psychotherapy or spirituality; rather, we understand relationality to be constitutive of human experience, spirituality, and therapeutic growth (see Chapter 1, this volume, for the clinical implications of this relational worldview). There is some evidence that clients' relational dynamics with God or the sacred can shift in constructive ways over the course of psychotherapy (Cheston, Piedmont, Eanes, & Lavin, 2003; Tisdale et al., 1997); therefore, we have been seeking to understand therapeutic processes involving relational spirituality and transformation (Worthington & Sandage, 2016).

BACKGROUND OF THE RELATIONAL SPIRITUALITY MODEL

In 2001, I (SJS) started a program of quantitative research on the spiritual and psychological development of seminary students at Bethel Seminary (Minnesota, United States), along with colleagues Carla Dahl and Mary Jensen in the marriage and family therapy department and the Center for Spiritual and Personal Formation (Sandage & Jensen, 2013; see also Porter, Sandage, Wang, & Hill, 2019). This initial project was supported by a grant from the Lilly Endowment, and we received subsequent funding from the Fetzer Institute and the John Templeton Foundation. Simultaneously, I was trying to understand the relational dynamics of change in my clinical practice and working on interdisciplinary research and clinical applications of forgiveness and spirituality with theologian F. LeRon Shults (Shults & Sandage, 2003, 2006). Each of these projects contributed to initial formulations of the RSM as a model to describe spiritual development and transformation from a relational, dialectical, and systemic perspective (Sandage, Jensen, & Jass, 2008; Sandage & Shults, 2007). To date, we have published 30 empirical studies on the RSM, and this research has informed three books on clinical practice (Sandage & Brown, 2018; Stavros & Sandage, 2014; Worthington & Sandage, 2016).

The current book project emerged after I came to the Albert and Jessie Danielsen Institute at Boston University, which is a community mental health training clinic and research center with a long history of engaging spiritual, existential, religious, and theological (SERT) dynamics in depth-oriented psychotherapy from diverse and pluralistic perspectives. By *depth psychotherapy*, we mean approaches informed by psychoanalytic and existential traditions that emphasize both conscious and unconscious dynamics and the potential constructive role of destabilization in nonlinear patterns of change. We utilize contemporary relational models of depth psychotherapy that are increasingly informed by interpersonal neurobiology and the developmental influence of nonverbal and emotion-laden right-brain functioning (Schore, 2018), although we have also been collaborating with clinicians applying the RSM to cognitive behavior therapies (Boettscher, Sandage, Latin, & Barlow, 2019; Correa & Sandage, 2018).

The Danielsen Institute trains psychologists, social workers, marriage and family therapists, and psychiatry residents. The training program includes an APA-accredited internship in a community setting serving a range of client populations, though focusing primarily on adults. We have found that a majority of our clients view religious, spiritual, and/or existential issues as important parts of their treatment (Sandage, Paine, et al., 2017; discussed in Chapter 1). Within our diverse client population, there are also many who have no stated interest in SERT dynamics. Therefore, clinician flexibility and diversity sensitivity that go beyond surface identifiers such as "religious" and "nonreligious" is critical. We seek to attend to the worldviews, beliefs, and values of all of our clients.

The RSM emphases on (a) relational development, (b) empirically supported relational dynamics in psychotherapy, (c) systemic and nonlinear views of change, (d) respect for diversity, (e) depth understandings of suffering and meaningful growth, and (f) self of the therapist formation represent values, frameworks, and practices the four of us share. We brought together our clinical and training experience and ongoing research to frame this new formulation of the RSM, building on a core conceptual and experiential dialectic of spiritual dwelling and seeking. By *dialectic*, we mean that both dimensions (in this case, dwelling and seeking) are usually present; neither dimension exists independently; neither can be collapsed or fully explained by the other; and they may have greater or lesser salience in different situations. Dialectical theories of human development suggest that the opposing tensions between these kinds of polarities (e.g., dwelling and seeking, acceptance and change, safety and risk, forgiveness and justice, relational security and exploration) actually help generate change. The RSM frame also consists of three central relational development systems—attachment, differentiation, and intersubjectivity—that integrate within the process of psychotherapy. These developmental systems overlap in functioning to some extent, but each offers unique features that are relevant to mental health, relational psychotherapy, and spirituality and religion (see Chapters 2, 5, 6, and 7). Integrating these three developmental systems also offers points of connection with differing disciplines or subfields within social science and psychotherapy, including contemporary relational psychoanalysis, couple and family therapy, human development, cognitive science and interpersonal neurobiology, common factors in psychotherapy research, religious and spirituality studies, intercultural communication, and relational models in philosophy and theology.

Diversity and Traditions

We locate the RSM within the context of a growing awareness in the mental health field of the need for more inclusive and sensitive consideration of spiritual and religious diversity in treatment (McGoldrick & Hardy, 2019; Richards & Bergin, 2014; Walsh, 2010), as well as intersections between spirituality, religion, and other diversity dynamics. Regrettably, some evidence indicates that clinicians get less training in spiritual and religious diversity than they do in many other areas of diversity training (Vogel, McMinn, Peterson, & Gathercoal, 2013). We are also concerned that some of the clinical literature on spirituality and religion seems to take a rather thin approach that is overly psychologized and decontextualized from the thickness of spiritual and religious traditions that offer depth and grounding. We recognize this as another kind of diversity problem (Dueck & Reimer, 2009; Geertz, 1973). There is a risk in simply trying to appropriate or assimilate certain spiritual and religious ideas or practices into the dominant health treatment paradigms; namely, that doing so can reduce the richness of spiritual and religious traditions and dynamics to clinical categories of biopsychosocial functioning.

Therefore, in our own context of RSM-based clinical practice, training, and research at the Danielsen Institute, we place an emphasis on relational strategies for intentional appreciation of both diversity and traditions. The Danielsen Institute has a 67-year history as a spiritually and religiously diverse and pluralistic context of treatment, training, and research where we value depth engagement with the particularities of various spiritual and religious traditions without seeking to privilege one tradition or community over others.

We also believe it is important to cultivate relational spaces where clinicians can gain self-awareness and support through reflecting upon and locating themselves in relation to any SERT traditions that inform and support their clinical work (Rupert, Moon, & Sandage, 2018). Many have told us this clinical combination of valuing both diversity and rich engagement with spiritual and religious traditions seems uncommon, let alone including an emphasis on therapist formation. In this book, we describe our relational and developmental approach to spiritual and religious diversity dynamics in clinical practice, training, and research. Our RSM prioritizes a differentiated style of relating to spiritual and religious diversity and the traditions of clients, which is consistent with research in the areas of intercultural/multicultural competence, cultural humility, and social justice. We view diversity competence as more than a professional skill set; we see it as a central part of healthy relational and spiritual development that is ultimately relevant for both clinicians and clients.

Existential and Empirical

The RSM is also based on valuing both existential and empirical orientations to clinical practice. Despite the popularity of Yalom's (1980) classic existential contributions to psychotherapy, existential perspectives have not been especially prominent recently in the mental health fields of the United States (this is somewhat different in other parts of the world). This is probably due, in part, to the fact that many existential approaches to psychotherapy have not been well integrated with empirical research. However, a growing body of empirical research is beginning to bridge this gap, including terror management theory, which is based on existential psychology (Routledge & Vess, 2018; Sullivan, 2016), along with the wider literature on meaning-making in positive psychology and the psychology of religion (Park, Currier, Harris, & Slattery, 2017; Van Tongeren, Davis, Hook, & Johnson, 2016; Wong, 2011).

Researchers in each of these areas are contributing relevant insights about existential themes related to trauma, suffering, and meaning-making that are highly relevant to psychotherapy.

In our description of the RSM we discuss key existential themes (e.g., death, freedom, tragedy, isolation, estrangement, meaninglessness, alterity) that often generate anxiety and that regularly emerge in psychotherapy. Our RSM suggests these specific existential themes can be both challenging and meaningful for exploration at "ordinary" levels of suffering but that extremes of emotional suffering or trauma often activate severe levels of anxiety about these existential themes that can inhibit or "freeze" relational processes of spiritual and psychological development. We go on to describe ways in which relational processes in psychotherapy can provide attachment and limbic regulation to reduce clients' preoccupation with security functions and reactivate processes of meaning-making and spiritual and existential development that can contribute to healing and growth.

Throughout the book, we engage both existential and empirical perspectives on suffering, growth, and psychotherapy. We make use of empirical research on human development and psychotherapy, and we also provide interdisciplinary formulations drawing on disciplines such as philosophy and theology that offer reflections on the complexities of human existence. This fits with our valuing of both embodiment and ultimate concerns, and accountability to scientific data on effective psychotherapy and respect for the ambiguities of human change.

Suffering and Growth

This book also suggests we should give greater consideration to both suffering and growth in psychotherapy. We argue that deeper and more diverse understandings of the variety of views of suffering that can emerge across different clients are needed. We make considerable use of the multifaceted clinical literature on trauma, but we also suggest that trauma is always existential and that there is danger in an overly medicalized view of treatment that misses some of the important differences in how clients may understand their suffering across various spiritual and religious traditions. In fact, there is no spiritually or culturally neutral understanding of suffering, so if psychotherapy is aimed at alleviating suffering, then clinicians will need to learn about various worldviews related to suffering.

The same point can be raised about positive psychological definitions of meaningful growth. Our RSM is a developmental model and targets clinically relevant developmental processes that can help clients move toward more meaningful lives of well-being and flourishing. This stands in contrast with the dominant model in mental health care focused purely on the lower bar of symptom alleviation. However, like the topic of suffering, definitions of meaningful growth and well-being are diverse and value laden (Boettscher et al., 2019; Wong, 2011), so this too requires our RSM emphasis on seeking to assess and understand clients' diverse frameworks and goals related to meaning in life.

Our RSM also proposes a view of relational spirituality as a potential source of suffering or growth. In contrast to definitions of spirituality and religion as either all good or all bad, our relational perspective opens conceptual space to consider the many relational dynamics that can be in play across individual differences in spiritual experience. Our clinical case studies explore a wide range of human expressions of spirituality that include the salutary and the pathological.

Relational Dynamics Inside and Outside of Treatment

We are also interested in the various relational dynamics that unfold both inside and outside of treatment. Inside the treatment space, we prioritize the therapeutic alliance as a major source of gain in effective psychotherapy (Wampold & Imel, 2015), but we also recognize alliance dynamics can be complex with rupture and repair processes and the negotiation of client–therapist differences holding great importance (Doran, Safran, & Muran, 2016, 2017). Moreover, clients are often working with multiple providers and also engaging in relational dynamics with administrative staff in many treatment settings, so we give attention in our RSM approach to the larger systemic dynamics that shape relational ecologies of treatment (Kehoe, Hassen, & Sandage, 2016; Sandage, Moon, et al., 2017) and describe our theory and research on this under-considered clinical dynamic.

Yet relational change needs to happen for clients both inside and outside of treatment settings. Practice-based outcome research at our clinic has found that clients' reports of reduced interpersonal conflict over time have predicted improved life satisfaction, and these effects have been mediated by improved affect regulation (Jankowski et al., 2019). Latent trajectories of change also showed differing patterns, with some clients showing curvilinear patterns (i.e., getting worse before getting better). These initial findings need further replication but offer support for the basic framework of many contemporary relational models of psychotherapy (DeYoung, 2015; Huang, Hill, Strauss, Heyman, & Hussain, 2016; Schore, 2018; Wampold & Imel, 2015) that high-light the importance of relational changes in clients' lives and nonlinear patterns of change as relatively common trajectories (Frankfurt, Frazier, Syed, & Jung, 2016; Hayes, Laurenceau, Feldman, Strauss, & Cardaciotto, 2007; Owen et al., 2015). The RSM attention to the relational lives outside of treatment for clients is also consistent with our concern about ways clients can build natural support systems to sustain their progress of growth in and beyond psychotherapy.

Therapist Formation and Accountability

Finally, our RSM promotes the valuing of therapist formation and account-ability. Our attention to therapist formation is consistent with psychodynamic, family systems, and humanistic therapy traditions and the importance of the personal development or self of the therapist. We take this to be true for us as therapists not just during training, but throughout our careers. Healthy and mature formation over time is not a given just because we do clinical practice. In fact, chronic exposure to suffering and trauma is deleterious to a person's formation without ongoing sources of processing, support, and growth. From our relational spirituality framework, we are particularly interested in relational and SERT dynamics in training and ongoing clinical consultation for therapist formation, and integrate these considerations throughout the book (but particularly in Chapter 11).

In addition to this formation emphasis, we believe that relational accountability is an important part of clinical practice. This fits with our concern for empirical accountability, and we describe our relational understanding of clinical research at Danielsen and its importance from an RSM perspective. We also consider the importance of deliberate practice strategies for training and consultation to sustain growth in effectiveness and counter myopic risks among clinicians (Rousmaniere, 2016, 2019). The impetus to write this book is a step of our own accountability, albeit one that comes with various existential anxieties (!), and this process has helped us engage in our own critical reflection and submit our clinical understandings for professional dialogue and critique.

AN OVERVIEW OF THE BOOK

Part I (Chapters 1–4) outlines the RSM contours of our theoretical model of relational spirituality. Chapter 1 explains our definition of relational spirituality and related concepts (e.g., religion, theology, existential concerns) and distinguishes our RSM from more reductionistic forms of the medical model of mental health treatment. Chapter 2 provides a summary review of how various meanings and conceptualizations of "relational spirituality" in the social science literature compare and contrast with our RSM. We also connect the RSM to the three relational development systems of attachment, differentiation, and intersubjectivity and relational spirituality emphases on dialectics, diversity competence, and relational selfhood. Finally, we introduce a relational integrative framework for coherence in understanding spirituality, psychotherapy, training, and research as they work in concert to heal suffering and promote growth. Chapter 3 takes an interdisciplinary approach to elucidating the key RSM constructs of spiritual dwelling, spiritual seeking, spiritual struggles, and crucibles of transformation as they emerge in psychotherapy. The developmental process of balancing dwelling and seeking is proposed as central to our RSM understanding of therapeutic change. Chapter 4 argues for an existential understanding of anxiety, trauma, and suffering in formulating the concept of the suffering–trauma matrix. Diverse existential themes and views of suffering are considered to offer greater diversity sensitivity and existential nuance to RSM-based treatment.

Part II (Chapters 5–7) considers the clinical relevance of the three core relational developmental systems engaged in the RSM. These chapters highlight developmental dynamics that unfold across the life span; however, our treatment focus largely applies to adult populations, with some consideration of adolescence. Chapter 5 focuses on the attachment development system in its promotion of emotional security, exploration, trust, and relational regulation. Attachment theory has also had a major influence on empirical research in the psychology of religion and spirituality, and that literature factors into the RSM clinical process. Chapter 6 describes the interdisciplinary contours of the differentiation developmental system and its relation to self-regulation, self-identity, interpersonal flexibility, and relating across differences. Many of our RSM studies have investigated associations between differentiation of self and various aspects of spiritual development, relational virtue, and diversity competence, and this literature is used in this chapter along with a description of some key clinical strategies. Chapter 7 presents and discusses the multidimensional intersubjectivity system also in relation to human development, culture, relational spirituality, and clinical strategies. Human interactions can have profoundly enlivening or disruptive effects, and this chapter explores ways that healthy intersubjectivity may promote vital living and intimacy.

Part III (Chapters 8–12) applies the RSM to clinical practice by considering assessment, diversity considerations, treatment planning, and clinical intervention strategies. Chapter 8 applies the RSM to a case study of individual therapy that also includes family therapy. Chapters 9 and 10 do the same with couple therapy and group therapy, respectively. And Chapter 11 offers some of our key RSM ideas about the role of relational spirituality in therapist formation, including training, ongoing consultation, and self-care. Chapter 12 concludes with a summary of core themes and ideas of the RSM and outlines future research directions based on this model.

Throughout the book we make liberal use of case material to illustrate key clinical dilemmas and our tips for working through them. In all case examples in the book, we have altered identifying information to protect confidentiality, and the examples represent either composites of actual cases or constructions of clinical examples.

For clinicians whose training has lacked a thicker, more diverse view of spirituality and religion, especially in dialogue with the key concepts of relationally oriented depth psychotherapy, we hope that this volume offers some ways to expand clinical practice to be more attentive to and inclusive of the suffering, growth, and meaning of clients' experiences. It is our hope that our colleagues will find, with us, new ways of seeking and dwelling in the rich terrain of spirituality and religion that infuses the struggles and triumphs of our clients—and our own.

THEORETICAL FRAMEWORK OF RELATIONAL SPIRITUALITY

1

Relational Spirituality After the Medical Gaze

Spirituality is the practice of addressing ontological suffering by relating to something more authentic and larger than the egoistic self. It is informed by suffering on the one hand . . . and love on the other.

—j. a. powell, *RACING TO JUSTICE* (2012, P. 208)

In this opening chapter, we outline our definition of *relational spirituality* to locate it within the growing and diverse literature on the topic and to explain our framework for differentiating spirituality, existential concerns, religion, and theology as they relate to psychotherapy. However, we first want to offer some historical background to situate our relational spirituality model (RSM) after the *medical gaze* (Foucault, 1963/1994) of modern medical reductionism as exemplified in the biomedical disease model. In resonance with powell's (2012) statement above, we connect the RSM to our overall clinical strategy of treating persons who are suffering, in contrast to the purely biomedical goal of seeking to alleviate symptoms of mental disorders or diseases. Yet our integrative intention is to retain the valuable resources and tools of modern empirical science in combination with the deep wisdom offered by existential, sociocultural, spiritual, and religious traditions regarding suffering and healing. We start by considering a case study that surfaces some of the key dilemmas related to existential meaning, relational spirituality, trauma, and suffering that we will explore throughout this book.[1]

---

[1] All case examples in this book involve altered identifying information to protect confidentiality and represent either composites of actual cases or constructions of clinical examples.

http://dx.doi.org/10.1037/0000174-002
Relational Spirituality in Psychotherapy: Healing Suffering and Promoting Growth,
by S. J. Sandage, D. Rupert, G. S. Stavros, and N. G. Devor

Sofia (age 22; Mexican American) is a young adult who is living with cystic fibrosis (CF). CF is a genetically inherited chronic pulmonary disease that typically leads to a shortened life span of approximately 37 years (MacKenzie et al., 2014), and Sofia was diagnosed at birth. Her lung functioning had been relatively stable during her adolescent years, but over the previous 3 years she had been hospitalized five times with pulmonary exacerbations (serious difficulty clearing mucus from her lungs). When not in the hospital, her daily care regimen still takes about 2 hours, including nebulizer treatments, wearing a vest to facilitate airway clearance, and taking various medications. Earlier this year, she became malnourished due to difficulties absorbing nutrients and needed a g-tube in her stomach for several months. She started college 3 years ago but dropped out after one semester following a tragic car accident in which she sustained mild physical injuries but a close friend (the driver) was killed. Sofia has not been working or going to school since that time and mostly stays home doing chores or preparing meals for her parents, who both work full-time.

Sofia's parents, Renata (age 43) and Jorge (age 44), are both first-generation Mexican Americans whose parents immigrated to the United States when they were young. They are devout Catholics who seek to be very involved in Sofia's health care, and they each pray for her regularly. As an only child, Sofia has typically been quite close with her parents throughout her life; however, she has been much more agitated and closed off to them over the past 2 years. She has been inconsistent with her daily medical self-care, which has stoked her parents' anxiety and frustration and has turned into a considerable power struggle, with both parents "nagging" her (by her report), though with no obvious effect.

The team of health care professionals treating Sofia in the hospital has also grown frustrated with her inconsistent daily treatment self-care and her lack of motivation to pursue goals they deem "developmentally appropriate." Here is a discussion from an interdisciplinary staff meeting to review Sofia's case during her most recent hospitalization:

DR. GORDON (PULMONOLOGIST):	Eric (doctoral-level psychology intern), you met with Sofia yesterday, right? What is her mind-set about the psychiatric eval and Dr. Winters's (psychiatrist) recommendation of an antidepressant and psychotherapy?
ERIC:	I think she may be open to it. At first, she seemed fairly defensive, but I guess the big surprise was that when I pressed the need for her to get outpatient treatment given the depression diagnosis from Winters, she actually broke down crying. I was really taken aback after how shut down and adversarial she has been with me . . . or really, all of us. We just sat there

	for a while, and she finally said she's afraid she's going to die and she "doesn't see the point."
CECILIA (NURSE):	The point of what? (sounding agitated)
ERIC:	I gathered she meant . . . the point of life. But maybe she just meant the point of treatment.
DR. GORDON:	(shaking his head) I've talked with her about how the medications are improving and there is more and more reason to be optimistic about future treatment advances. This confirms that we need to push the SSRI and outpatient treatment.
CECILIA:	And can we try again to get her working or moving toward returning to college? I'm sure she will get even more depressed if she doesn't have anything going on besides sitting around her parents' house. What do you think, Adeline?
ADELINE (SOCIAL WORKER):	She has not been open to those ideas, but we can try again. Dr. Winters said we need to find her an outpatient therapist for cognitive restructuring, so if she goes along with this recommendation it might finally help get her moving forward.

Sofia did agree to start antidepressant medication and also began seeing an outpatient psychotherapist, a woman in her 60s whose unusual combination of warm presence and irreverent humor proved to be a good fit. In her 14th session of psychotherapy, Sofia really opened an existential vein and shared a powerful example of relational spirituality by lamenting:

> I really believe God is sentencing me to an early death for something . . . I'm not sure for what exactly . . . I really wish I knew. . . . Not even a trial . . . I guess just for being a disappointment . . . or somehow not being worthy of a good life. Or not being worthy of surviving the accident. It's like He's decided to make a point out of me, that no matter how hard I try I will keep coming up short, keep getting sicker, and so I must just deserve to be sick and unhappy and die young. . . . Why even try? When God is against you, you are really fucked.

This disclosure offers a window into one expression of what we mean by relational spirituality or "ways of relating to the sacred" (Shults & Sandage, 2006, p. 161; Worthington & Sandage, 2016). We can see that Sofia has an intense relational conflict in her experience of God, which is wrapped around deep existential questions and a tragic narrative of divine punishment for ambiguous reasons. Despite their concern for her health, the medical team described in this case study does not show evidence of a framework to help them constructively engage Sofia's stated existential concerns about her mortality or explore *her* sense of meaning in life. Instead, her existential concerns were reduced to medical issues that necessitated medication and cognitive restructuring, for the purpose of "[getting] her working or moving toward returning to college." The team assumed that working or going back to college should be goals for Sofia. In contrast, the concerns Sofia expressed to her therapist are much deeper, needing to be taken seriously before she is ready to "move forward" with other life goals.

We could understand an argument for holistic approaches to cognitive behavior therapy (CBT) in a case such as this even if it is not our primary therapeutic approach (for an excellent contemporary CBT approach grounded in emotion regulation and mindfulness, see Barlow & Farchione, 2018); however, the specific sequence of assessment, diagnosis, and treatment planning among the hospital team was at risk of implying Sofia was irrational or crazy for having her existential concerns and impending despair. Existential questions about death, loss, guilt, and meaning in life in the face of losses and serious threats to one's being and survival do not usually "snap into place" with cognitive restructuring interventions alone. The latter is based on rational logic and neocortical processes, whereas existential concerns like Sofia's engage limbic-based neurobiological processes involving the search for ultimate security and a sense of purpose despite awareness of threats to one's existence (E. B. Davis, Granqvist, & Sharp, 2018). We suggest that there is a crucial *relational* dimension to the construction and reconstruction of existential meaning, and this is particularly important in cases like Sofia's where she had a hard time finding people whom she could trust to "sit with her" in the traumatic darkness of her real feelings and raw questions.

Trauma is always existential and involves ruptures in meaning (see Chapter 4, this volume). We believe that healing the ruptures of trauma and other forms of suffering involves relational processes that bring anxiety to manageable levels. Paradoxically, once anxiety is manageable it allows us to move into deeper existential terrain (or ontological anxieties) and coconstruct transformed meaning. Sofia's rejection of the primary prosocial goals for young adults (i.e., paid work or college) in the dominant systems of American society was interpreted reductively by the health care providers in the hospital through the medical power–knowledge label of *depression*. Receiving a diagnosis of depression can make clients feel weak or that they have a character flaw; moreover, it can potentially reinforce the doctor–patient power imbalance, where doctors have more knowledge or more specialized knowledge than patients, and the prerogative of assigning a reductive label to their patients' suffering in ways that do not do justice to spiritual and religious diversity. We likely would have concurred with the clinical diagnosis, but in a case such as this we also would entertain the possibility that it signals existential strength, as Sofia questions the meaning of such pursuits within the life context of chronic suffering and death before midlife. Therefore, we concur with clinical scholars who have offered holistic, multidimensional assessment approaches with psychotherapy clients that include attention to the highly interrelated biological, sociocultural, relational, existential, and spiritual dimensions (Peteet, 2010; Richards & Bergin, 2005; Sperry, 2012).

REDUCTIONISM AND THE MEDICAL GAZE

Before describing our understanding of relational spirituality, we want to briefly consider historical shifts that led to the biomedical reductionism we are critiquing in the case description above. In his book *The Birth of the Clinic: An Archaeology of Medical Perception*, philosopher Michel Foucault (1963/1994) traced a paradigm shift in European medicine during the 18th and 19th centuries toward a decontextualized and reductionistic focus (or *medical gaze*) on the physical body of a patient dualistically separated from their personal narrative. His interest in the post-Enlightenment rise of "clinics" or teaching hospitals was an investigation of the expansion of the modern medical technology beyond the confines of more socially separate institutional settings into wider community settings:

> The appearance of the clinic as a historical fact must be identified with the system of these reorganizations. This new structure is indicated—but not, of course, exhausted—by the minute but decisive change, whereby the question: "What is the matter with you?", with which the eighteenth-century dialogue between doctor and patient began (a dialogue possessing its own grammar and style), was replaced by that other question: "Where does it hurt?", in which we recognize the operation of the clinic and the principle of its entire discourse. From then on, the whole relationship of signifier to signified, at every level of medical experience, is redistributed: between the symptoms that signify and the disease that is signified, between the description and what is described, between the event and what it prognosticates, between the lesion and the pain that it indicates, etc. The clinic—constantly praised for its empiricism, the modesty of its attention, and the care with which it silently lets things surface to the observing gaze without disturbing them with discourse—owes its real importance to the fact that it is a reorganization in depth, not only of medical discourse, but of the very possibility of a discourse about disease. The *restraint* of clinical discourse (its rejection of theory, its abandonment of systems, its lack of philosophy; all so proudly proclaimed by doctors) reflects the non-verbal conditions on the basis of which it can speak: the common structure that carves up and articulates what is seen and what is said. (pp. xviii–xix)

Foucault went on to suggest that this shift from a meaningful dialogue between doctor and patient involving interpretations of suffering was replaced by a biological reductionism that gave medical doctors tremendous power, through the presumption of objective knowledge, to heal. Through advances in surgery, doctors were able to enter into their patients' bodies. These technological advancements combined with the focus on bodily symptoms (medical gaze) conveyed an almost mystical ability of doctors to see below the bodily surface into the depths of disease, making them the new modern sages to supplant the powerful roles of clergy, shamans, and other spiritual healers. This also led to modern attempts at objective classifications of various diseases, including mental illnesses.

We would agree with those who critique Foucault as too negative about the empirical sciences, and we are certainly grateful for the advances of modern medicine. Biological reductionism served a historical purpose in the development of medical science and technology. And we also have no desire to idealize the past or gloss over the reality that spiritual and philosophical narratives about illnesses have frequently been far more stigmatizing than healing. Susan Sontag (2001) argued quite poignantly that cultural metaphors and myths about cancer, AIDS, and many other illnesses historically have been harmful to those afflicted and that demystifying diseases as simply biological could, in some cases, be helpful for promoting treatment and social acceptance. However, we see advantages in bridging empirical and existential perspectives (Ghaemi, 2010). Attention to biological factors and empirical science can be integrated with attention to psychological, sociocultural, and spiritual dimensions.

Consider the comparison offered in Table 1.1. The column on the left offers some of the relational spirituality language Sofia uses to voice her particular existential, moral, and spiritual questions about her suffering. The column on the right includes the diagnostic categories from the *Diagnostic and Statistical Manual of Mental Disorders* (5th ed.; *DSM–5*; American Psychiatric Association, 2013) required by her insurance company to reimburse psychotherapy services, which fits Foucault's depiction of the medical gaze. We utilize the spiritual and religious problem v-code in the *DSM–5* when appropriate, but our impression is that it is rarely used by clinicians relative to the frequency of spiritual and religious struggles. Moreover, diagnosing Sofia with a "spiritual or religious problem" implies a pathologizing of her spiritual and existential struggle in ways that could overshadow the strengths she is showing in authentically wrestling with a search for meaning.

We affirm the responsible use of diagnostic categories in mental health care and research and recognize that treatment studies would be impossible without them. But we also think it is worth considering what is lost in a case like Sofia's if the "thin" and universalizing medical gaze is allowed to overshadow the "thick" phenomenological description of suffering through individual voices (on thick and thin, see Geertz, 1973; see also Dueck & Reimer, 2009). Sofia's voice in the left column offers access to her unique narrative and

TABLE 1.1. Relational Spirituality and Medical Gaze Interpretations of Suffering

Interpretations of suffering	
Relational spirituality	**Medical gaze**
"I really believe God is sentencing me for something . . . I'm not sure for what exactly . . . I really wish I knew. . . . Not even a trial . . . I guess just for being a disappointment . . . or somehow not being worthy of His attention or approval. It's like He's decided to make point out of me, that no matter how hard I try I will come up short, and therefore I deserve to be unhappy and alone. . . . When God is against you, you are really fucked."	*DSM–5* codes: F33.2—Major Depressive Disorder, Recurrent, Severe Without Psychotic Features Z65.8—Spiritual or Religious Problem Rule out F43.10—Posttraumatic Stress Disorder

the relational spirituality shaped by her existential anxieties and concerns. It thickens our particular understanding of her worldview and her personal experience of suffering.

DISEASE, ILLNESS, AND SUFFERING

The way we define a problem actually shapes the kinds of solutions we imagine (Thibodeau & Boroditsky, 2013). As Foucault argued, modern Western medicine set in place the biomedical disease model as the dominant framework for mental health treatment, which focused on bodily symptoms. Kiesler (2000) traced the modern ascension of the biomedical disease model of psychopathology and called it the "American way of understanding mental disorders" (p. 15) because of a preference in the United States for the use of medicines and medical technologies to solve problems. In his critique of the biomedical disease model, Kiesler is among those marshalling empirical evidence to show that mental disorders often have multiple causal factors, including psychosocial and environmental causes (see, e.g., Maddux & Winstead, 2015).

In his book *Illness Narratives*, psychiatrist and anthropologist Arthur Kleinman (1988) provided a powerful sociocultural and existential critique of the biomedical model with his differentiation of *disease* and *illness*. Kleinman said, "Disease is the problem from the practitioner's perspective. In the narrow biological terms of the biomedical model, this means that disease is reconfigured only as an alteration in biological functioning or structure" (p. 5). This parallels Foucault's point that employing the disease model offers the apparent efficiency of not needing to understand the patient's worldview (i.e., "What is the matter with you?") to make a diagnosis. As Foucault explained, "one must subtract the individual, with his [sic] particular qualities" (p. 14). In contrast, Kleinman explained:

> By invoking the term illness, I mean to conjure up the innately human experience of symptoms and suffering. Illness refers to how the sick person and members of the family or wider social network perceive, live with, and respond to symptoms and disability. (p. 3)

Illness is "polysemic" and generates multiple layers of meaning. Illness narratives engage culturally shaped questions and answers about the meaning of suffering. Kleinman clarified "the problem of illness as suffering raises two fundamental questions for the sick person and the social group: Why me? (the question of bafflement) and what can be done? (the question of order and control)" (p. 29). He noted that modern biomedical science avoids the question of what he called *bafflement*, which is one of the key existential questions Sofia was asking. *Bafflement* is an odd word choice, but it implies confusion, puzzlement, bewilderment, and feeling dizzy from an absence of meaning in the face of very powerful human predicaments. These bafflement synonyms signify some of the puzzling *dis*-order of meaning that can be part of illness but may not convey the traumatic levels of shock, the violent emotional pain, and the disorientation that can come with some experiences of suffering in cases like Sofia's. Traditional societies have drawn upon cultural, moral, and spiritual narratives and practices to shape meaningful contexts for understanding and dealing with suffering, but contemporary Western health care systems struggle to construct anything comparable on this side of medical reductionism. It could be critical in cases like Sofia's to attempt to dialogue with her about the sociocultural, spiritual, religious, and other narrative perspectives that inform her sense of illness narrative and suffering.

Cassell (2004) offered an influential definition of *suffering* as "the state of severe distress associated with events that threaten the intactness of person" (p. 32). According to Cassell, "suffering is experienced by persons" (p. 32) and not just bodies; thus, suffering extends beyond the physical and includes distress over impending personal disintegration. He underscored existential and temporal aspects of suffering:

> People in pain frequently report suffering from pain when they feel out of control, when the pain is overwhelming, when the source of pain is unknown, when the meaning of the pain is dire, or when the pain is apparently without end. (p. 35)

Cassell rejected mind–body dualism and argued that assigning suffering to only the body and bodily pain is depersonalizing and becomes its own source of suffering. He also noted the uncomfortable point for health care providers that treatments can at times actually cause suffering, and he highlighted the web of relationships that influence personal experiences of suffering.

Our relational spirituality model of psychotherapy is oriented toward the treatment of suffering. Concretely, we have found it makes a positive difference toward a more holistic perspective to actually use the term *suffering* in our dialogues with clients and clinical colleagues. As we develop later, we affirm the importance of embodiment and attention to biological and genetic influences and the appropriate use of medications and other medical technologies. But we resonate with the frameworks on suffering offered by Kleinman and Cassell that highlight the crucial sociocultural, existential, relational, and spiritual dimensions of illness and suffering, and we give these dimensions prominence in our model.

KEY INFLUENCES ON RELATIONAL SPIRITUALITY

Spirituality can be very complicated to define. In a comprehensive historical review of definitions of spirituality, Bregman (2014) noted that the term is "deeply and irrevocably ambiguous" (p.3). By 2002, occupational therapists Unruh and colleagues were able to document 92 different definitions of spirituality just in health literatures, and definitions have continued to proliferate since then (Unruh, Versnel, & Kerr, 2002). We will not resolve all this complexity, but we want to start by framing what we mean by *spirituality* and *relational spirituality*.

DEFINITIONS

Several key influences have contributed to our definition of relational spirituality. Eliade's (1959) classic work, *The Sacred and Profane: The Nature of Religion*, integrated scholarship in the history of religion with existential and depth psychology perspectives in describing the sacred as "saturated with *being*," power, and reality in many traditional religious worldviews (p. 12, emphasis in original). Sacred and profane are taken to be opposing existential situations in the worldview of many with the sacred dimension being *wholly other* and more real than the "homogenous and neutral" profane space of everyday life (p. 22). Communal definitions of sacred space and sacred objects reveal an ontology or a fixed point of orientation amid the surrounding anxiety and chaos of life. The sacred objects offer an "opening to the transcendent" (p. 34) that allows relational spirituality dynamics of "living as close as possible to the gods" (p. 91) and offers "an absolute point of support" (p. 28). Eliade could be critiqued for making certain generalizations across religious traditions, but we accept his overall thesis that an important part of spirituality and religion is to sanctify certain aspects of human life in response to existential and relational needs for orientation and closeness to sacred objects, groundedness in a sense of *being*, and a recapitulation of cosmic meaning. Sofia's question—"What is the point?"—combined with her conflicted relational experiences of God, revealed her existential struggles with orientation, meaning, and security.

P. C. Hill and Pargament (2003) drew on Elide and developed an inclusive psychological definition of spirituality as related to "a search for the sacred." They used the term *sacred* to signify "a person, object, principle, or concept that transcends the self" (p. 65). The sacred can include "a divine being, divine object, Ultimate Reality, or Ultimate Truth" that is "set apart" as holy and beyond the ordinary (p. 65). The term *search* implies seeking or active questing toward sacred meaning, and they noted that for many devout persons this engagement with sacredness is not restricted to special times or occasions but can be part of everyday life (see also Ammerman, 2013, p. 9). Sofia's case is also an example of how the sacred and the profane (as signified by profanity) can seem to collide in confusing or distressing ways.

Our phenomenological orientation toward defining spirituality in relation to whatever a person considers sacred allows for individual differences and broad diversity in understandings of the sacred (Rizzuto, 1979). Clinically, this involves trying to understand clients' ultimate values and ideals or whatever may be deeply important or grounding to them. Schnarch (1991) described this as seeking to know what is "near and dear" to clients' hearts (p. 352). It is important to note that some clients do not consider themselves "spiritual" and do not believe in a "sacred" dimension of life but nevertheless hold ideals or values they consider ultimate or deeply important. While some have suggested everyone is "spiritual" (Baird, 2016; Faver, 2004; Lepherd, 2015; Walter, 1997), we do not impose the language of spirituality or the sacred on clients because of our commitment to valuing diversity, self-definition, and autonomy.

Shults and Sandage (2006; Sandage & Shults, 2007; Worthington & Sandage, 2016) adapted the definition of spirituality offered by P. C. Hill and colleagues (2000) to fit a relational theoretical orientation by defining *relational spirituality* broadly as "ways of relating to the sacred" (p. 161).[2] In this sense, people can relate to the sacred in a variety of ways, including fear, surrender, complaint, love, attention-seeking, avoidance, playfulness, questioning, sacrificial service, rage, and many other relational styles. Lack of interest, avoidance, or cutoff in relation to the sacred can also be signature themes in the relational spiritualities of some individuals, so we are interested in the broad array of relational stances.

It might seem obvious to apply a relational spirituality framework when individuals believe in personal divine beings, angels, and spirits (E. B. Davis, Granqvist, & Sharp, 2018). For example, the Islamic Sage Imām al-Haddād (2010) wrote, "To love God the Exalted is for the servant to feel inclination in his [sic] heart, attachment, and passion for that holiest and loftiest of presences" (p. 250). Many traditions also promote ancestor veneration or the sacralization of animals, plants and the natural world, and various inanimate objects, and individuals can have various forms of relational spirituality with these sacred objects. Spiritual traditions that are not theistic also offer rituals and practices for relating with the sacred, and thus can be viewed through a relational framework. For example, in his work on anger, Buddhist teacher Thich Nhat Hanh (2001) invoked relational imagery by suggesting that we are "mothers of our anger, and we have to help our baby, our anger" (p. 165). He suggested, "the mother is the living Buddha," an "internal figure that is a source of mindfulness energy that one needs to recognize and keep alive" (p. 169). Buddhist teacher and psychotherapist John Welwood promoted the integration of Buddhism and attachment theory, explaining,

> We are not just humans learning to become buddhas, but also buddhas waking up in human form, learning to become fully human. And these two tracks of development can mutually enrich each other. . . . The great paradox of being both human and buddha is that we are both dependent and not dependent. (Fossella, 2011, p. 45)

In many Buddhist traditions, relationships are "the central vehicle" for spiritual development (Jennings, 2010, p. 214), and this point could be extended to many (perhaps most) spiritual and religious traditions.

Our understanding of relational spirituality also builds on the classic phenomenological work of William James (1902/1958) in his book *The Varieties of Religious Experience*. In recounting many personal narratives, James came to define personal religion as the "feelings, acts, and experiences of individual men [sic] in their solitude, so far as they apprehend themselves to stand in relation to whatever they may consider divine" (p. 42). The second part of

---

[2]It is worth noting the term *spirituality* does not always translate very clearly from English into other languages and cultural contexts, and terms like *faith* or *religion* might be closer to this meaning of spirituality in the U.S. context.

that definition ("to stand in relation to") refers to the relational dynamics of what we mean by spirituality. We would say that the "varieties" of relational spirituality emerge as we relate to the developmental and existential challenges of making meaning in the midst of the ambiguity of life (Fowler, 1981; Kegan, 1980; Sperry, 2012), and relational representations of the sacred can be complex, ambiguous, and unstable over time (Silverman, Johnson, & Cohen, 2016). We also agree with those who critique James for an individualistic bias and a neglect of attention to sociocultural, communal, institutional, and historical influences on spiritual experience (Taylor, 2002; Wulff, 1997). As Ammerman (2013) put it,

> Sacred stories also imply audiences—what I call "spiritual tribes"—who listen and co-create each tale. Each story is situated in a context, with circles of listeners who play a role, sacred or otherwise. It is important then to pay attention to the role of religious communities themselves. To what extent do those religious settings provide relationships, practices, and ways of thinking that show up in the stories people tell? (p. 10)

RELATIONAL SYSTEMS AND SPIRITUALITY

Expanding on Ammerman's point about the influential role of "spiritual tribes," we look beyond religious communities to the surrounding influence of family systems, communities, traditions, and wider ecological and systemic influences on the relational spirituality of persons such as Sofia. We would want to assess the roles of Sofia's relational network and spiritual communities in both her struggles and her strengths, particularly her parents, who are deeply involved in her experience of suffering. This relational, ecological, and contextual emphasis on spirituality also facilitates moving beyond the individualistic construals of spirituality that do not fit well with many collectivistic cultural or religious traditions. For example, Paris (1995) described a communal spirituality of African peoples as rooted in four fully interdependent spheres of existence—God, family, community, and person. He explained that links with both living and ancestral communities are essential to relational spirituality and the cultivation of virtue from an African worldview. Explicitly "relational" contemporary movements have been heralded across numerous religious traditions (e.g., on Relational Buddhism, see Kwee, 2010; on Relational Judaism, see Wolfson, 2013; on Relational Christianity, see Montgomery, Oord, & Winslow, 2012), which move beyond a focus on specific beliefs and ritual practices to emphasize the importance of relational dynamics and communities in those traditions.

In a case like Sofia's, with a client speaking of feeling like a disappointment to God and possibly deserving punishment, our relational spirituality model might lead a clinician to dialogue with the client about other "voices" or social or systemic influences that might be merging into her experience of the sacred. This leads us to two other important points about the RSM. First, various forms of social injustice, oppression, and bigotry (e.g., racism, sexism, homophobia, classism) can negatively impact the relational spirituality of persons from nondominant groups, and this is particularly relevant to connections between spirituality and suffering. As powell (2012) argued, "if spirituality is to engage suffering and its causes, it must also be concerned with how institutions and structures function in society" (p. 199). We return to this point throughout the book. Second, some definitions of spirituality are rooted in dualistic frameworks that tend to view spirituality as "all good" (e.g., transcendence) and as a kind of singular substance of which individuals have a certain quantitative amount (e.g., "She is a very spiritual person"). Our relational model draws attention to the varieties of ways people relate to the sacred and how those relational dynamics may change over time—not just in quantity but in quality. We find that exploring relational dynamics in spirituality can deepen our understanding of the complex and conflicting motivations people bring in relating to the sacred, including both healthy and destructive motivations. Pargament and colleagues referred to this as the "multiple valences of religion and spirituality," which can include a wide range of helpful and harmful effects (Pargament, Mahoney, Exline, Jones, & Shafranske, 2013, p. 7; see also Griffith, 2011; Peteet, 2010).

Sofia's relational spirituality at the start of therapy was sincere, conflictual, and fraught with both shame and longing for acceptance. Her struggle was not that she was not "spiritual enough" but that she was relating to the sacred in painful and anxiety-provoking ways that intensified and perpetuated her suffering. Exline and colleagues have generated a body of research on these kinds of spiritual and religious struggles that can impact mental health (Exline, Pargament, Grubbs, & Yali, 2014; see also Chapter 3, this volume). Sofia showed the courage to authentically face her spiritual struggles and despair and voice this to her therapist, which, paradoxically, could be viewed as a healthy act of relational spirituality even if it did not immediately enhance her sense of spiritual well-being.

SPIRITUAL–EXISTENTIAL–RELIGIOUS–THEOLOGICAL FRAMEWORK

Definitions and models of spirituality also need to differentiate related concepts, such as religion, meaning, and theology. We use a spiritual–existential–religious–theological (SERT) framework in our training program and clinical practice (Rupert, Moon, & Sandage, 2018; a SERT training video is available for free viewing on our Danielsen Institute website: http://www.bu.edu/Danielsen/). The SERT acronym reminds us of the multidimensionality and diversity of approaches to the sacred and ultimate meaning, and the various sources of what we call *deep wisdom* about suffering and healing. As mentioned above, spirituality can be defined in various ways, and we use the relational framework above (i.e., "ways of relating to the sacred") and informed by core relational themes tied to attachment, differentiation, and intersubjectivity (introduced in Chapters 5, 6, and 7). By *existential*, we reference Yalom's (1980) definition of existential conflicts as "a conflict that flows from the individual's confrontation with the givens of existence" (p. 8), which include human predicaments about death, isolation, freedom and responsibility, and meaning/ meaninglessness, among others. Existential dynamics figure prominently in the RSM; we explore such themes in depth in Chapter 4. We consider existential issues of meaning relevant to all clinical cases, and we find this highly inclusive dimension of SERT to be particularly helpful for clients who do not believe in the sacred per se and may not resonate with spiritual, religious, or theological perspectives.

There are many approaches to the differentiation of *spirituality* and *religion*. We prefer the approach of P. C. Hill and Pargament (2003; Pargament, 2007), as they defined both religion and spirituality as involving the "search for the sacred" (P. C. Hill & Pargament, p. 65). They argued that the "polarization of religion and spirituality into institutional and individual domains ignores the fact that all forms of spiritual expression unfold in a social context" (p. 64), and they made spirituality the broader construct that can potentially be expressed through religious (social and institutional systems) or other social contexts. Pargament (2007) suggested "we cannot decontextualize spirituality. This dimension of life does not unfold in a vacuum, but rather in a larger religious context, even if it is a context that has been rejected" (p. 31). Thus, for most people influenced in some ways by religious traditions, contexts, and rituals, spiritual and religious development can be broadly understood as interactive and overlapping (Hay, Reich, & Utsch, 2006). However, by framing religion as connected to social, communal, and institutional systems and rituals, we also need to remain mindful that individual experiences with religion are diverse and range from positive to abusive. While many identify as both "religious and spiritual," some individuals identify as "spiritual but not religious," some as "religious but not spiritual," and some as "none of the above" (Pargament, 2007).

A Pew (2017) national survey in the United States found that about 48% of adults considered themselves religious and spiritual; 27%, spiritual but not religious; 18%, neither spiritual nor religious; and 6%, religious but not spiritual. However, we cannot assume that if we know a client's spiritual or religious demographics we will know their preferences for engaging SERT issues in psychotherapy. At our clinic in Boston, which is a significantly less spiritual and religious regional context compared to national data, we surveyed clients ($N = 110$) with separate items about whether, in order to resolve the concerns that brought them to therapy, it would be important for them to discuss (a) spiritual issues (70.9% said *yes*), (b) religious issues (52.7% said *yes*), and (c) issues of meaning and purpose (82.7% said *yes*). Thus, a majority of clients agreed that discussing religious, spiritual, and existential issues was important in their therapy, and these findings are similar to other surveys of client preferences (Rose, Westefeld, & Ansley, 2008). Not surprisingly, in our study client ratings of the personal importance of spirituality and religion was positively correlated with feeling the need to discuss spiritual, religious, and meaning/purpose issues in psychotherapy, and this also fits with a larger body of literature (Hook, Worthington, & Davis, 2012). Yet when we disaggregated the data based on individual spiritual and religious demographics in our study, it was intriguing to notice cases of atheist or agnostic clients who felt it was important to them to discuss spiritual or religious issues, as well as highly religious clients who did not think it was important to discuss those issues. Moreover, 23.6% of clients indicated multiple religious orientations (e.g., Hindu and agnostic; Jewish, Unitarian, and atheist; Christian and Buddhist), which shows nearly a quarter of our sample held a hybrid of multiple religious/nonreligious identities. Therefore, clinicians need to assess client preferences for engagement of SERT issues in therapy rather than rely on assumptions related to demographics or the clinicians' own SERT perspectives.

Theology represents the fourth major dimension of our SERT framework. Theology has often been framed as discourse about God in theistic traditions. However, David Tracy (2005) defined *theology* more broadly as "intellectual reflection . . . within a religious tradition" (p. 9126). Although Buddhism is typically nontheistic, some Buddhists have argued for the legitimacy of Buddhist theology as critical reflection within a tradition similar to Tracy's definition (Jackson & Makransky, 2000). Neville (2006, 2013) defined *theology* as symbolic engagement with ultimate concerns and is among those who argue for a public theology or theology "without walls," meaning that theology does not need to be restively located within religious traditions as Tracy suggested, and may include cultural or philosophical perspectives on ultimate concerns. We endorse this broader and more inclusive understanding of theology across and outside various traditions and find Neville's symbolic and existential orientation to fit nicely with our relational and depth orientations for psychotherapy. We also believe the "intellectual" aspects of theology, as with all disciplines, are shaped by conscious and unconscious relational influences and semantic, episodic, and procedural memory (see E. B. Davis, Granqvist, & Sharp, 2018). Thus, it is important to surface our "unconscious theologies" (Duvall, 2000) and to practice self-awareness about personal dimensions of beliefs and ultimate concerns.

In a model that merges spirituality and theology, Jewish theologian Michael Fishbane (2008) said theology is a spiritual practice of "attunement" and "not merely a type of thinking but also a type of living" (p. xii) aimed at "spiritual consciousness and self-transformation" (p. xiv). In some traditions, the content of theological belief can be less important than ethical action and communal involvement (Silverman et al., 2016). Given her invocation of theological themes, it is likely critical to dialogue with a client like Sofia about possible relational influences on her theology and how her theology influences her current experiences of living and anticipation of dying. We might ask, for example, "How did you learn that God punishes people?" "What do you consider the purpose of that kind of spiritual punishment?" "When you say that 'if God is against you, you are really fucked,' what do you mean by 'fucked' in this case?" This last question reflects back Sofia's relationally provocative mixing of the sacred and the profane with a nonanxious willingness by the therapist to enter that complicated space. We have found clients who present such charged expressions of spirituality often appreciate therapists offering nonreactive and sincere curiosity, which can be a corrective relational experience in contrast to other experiences of judgment for raw expressions of spiritual conflict.

We are struck that spirituality and religion have become mainstream topics in the field of psychotherapy, but the discipline of theology has been largely neglected (Dein, Cook, & Koenig, 2012; Sandage & Brown, 2018). Many approaches to psychotherapy are highly pragmatic and focus on "doing what works." However, some clients deeply value the truths and questions they find in certain theological beliefs, and it is important to be aware of the influence of differing theological and religious traditions on clients' worldviews and treatment perspectives (Strawn, Wright, & Jones, 2014; Wright, Jones, & Strawn, 2014). Our clinical experience has been that many clients will voice particular explicit or implicit theological beliefs, especially in relation to interpretations of suffering and other human predicaments, ethical norms and ideals, and understandings of healing. Those who are conversant with theology may recognize that Sofia is voicing poignant theological themes and perspectives on the nature of suffering (or theodicy) that have riddled human beings throughout time, and without help in first attuning to these perspectives and questions we might wonder about the effects of the prescribed cognitive restructuring interventions on her beliefs and her relational spirituality. For instance, minimizing or avoiding Sofia's spiritual and theological concerns might imply they are "irrational" and miss significant connections between her beliefs and relational themes in her life experience that serve to maintain the problems (e.g., disappointment, personal worth and agency, deserving punishment). When emotional struggles are embedded in limbic-based internal working models of attachment (see Chapter 5), as they seem to be for Sofia, cognitive interventions may be less effective without clinical attention to sources of relational insecurity (Castonguay, 2013). Sofia's stated attachment dynamics with God sound highly conflictual and insecure, and yet it seems to be a relationship that is vitally important to her. Clinicians will likely be justifiably concerned that her spiritual beliefs are contributing to her psychological distress, and yet her attribution of her suffering to moral and spiritual failure is also relatively common at a global level (see Chapter 4). A relational stance of respectful curiosity and interest by a clinician, at least prior to exploring change and belief restructuring, represents a more hospitable approach to clients' theologies. It would be important for the clinician to try to invite conversation about the history of her relationship with God and other dynamics within her spiritual and existential development to gain a broader understanding of how this traumatic rupture unfolded and whether there are other aspects of her relational spirituality not immediately apparent in her comments above. This process of exploration could help strengthen the working alliance with a client such as Sofia, who may need to know her therapist will not only respect her belief system but is resilient enough to move into some of the deep and painful existential terrain of conflicts within her relational spirituality. This can potentially restore a sense of agency to Sofia in the process of meaning construction/reconstruction that could be compromised in highly directive interventions by a therapist.

The SERT framework invites clinicians to attend to what is deeply important to their clients, how they make sense of their suffering, and what might motivate them or catalyze hope toward healing and growth. We start with seeking to understand client worldviews rather than imposing the therapists' SERT assumptions, in contrast to the medical gaze Sofia encountered with the health care professionals in the hospital. Since all clinicians will have personal views on SERT dynamics and some orientation toward relational spirituality (even if not considering oneself "spiritual"), we also place a strong emphasis in the RSM on clinician self-awareness, encouraged and developed within relational ecologies that support this kind of awareness of countertransference and ongoing consultation and learning (see Chapter 11).

CONCLUSION

Studies to date have shown most clients prefer to discuss SERT issues in therapy, and most therapists report they are open to discussing those kinds of issues with clients (Post & Wade, 2009). We have not seen data on the frequency with which SERT dynamics are actually assessed in clinical practice or factored into a clinical conceptualization and treatment plan, but our own clinical experiences suggest it may be relatively uncommon. Perhaps many clinicians struggle to formulate a coherent integration of these kinds of SERT factors into their working models of psychotherapy. Given the powerful medical gaze orientation described by Foucault, it makes sense that clinicians' attention may often be pushed toward concrete symptoms of biopsychosocial functioning. For decades, there have been calls in the mental health fields for broader and deeper understandings of cultural, spiritual, existential, relational, and systemic dynamics that shape clients' illness narratives and interpretations of their own suffering and their visions of a meaningful life. In recent years, we have been seeing some conceptual models in clinical practice that facilitate this kind of assessment and therapeutic contextualization, and our RSM is one contribution in this direction based on relational development theories of psychotherapy and relational understandings of spirituality. In Chapter 2, we summarize various meanings and expressions of *relational spirituality* in the growing literature on this topic and consider how they interface with the RSM.

2

Varieties of Relational Spirituality

Oh, how I was changed, and everything became new. My horses and hogs and even everybody seemed changed.
—Testimony from a farmer converted at a tent meeting
—W. JAMES, *VARIETIES OF RELIGIOUS EXPERIENCE* (1902/1958, P. 200)

The quote above by the converted farmer describes the all-encompassing positive relational impact of his own spiritual transformation experience in an interview recorded in William James's classic book on the psychology of religion, *Varieties of Religious Experience*. It speaks to the potential for systemic or holistic effects of spiritual experience to enhance relational dynamics in constructive ways. In this chapter, we consider a variety of possible meanings and dimensions of relational spirituality, including some that are less positive or salutary than that of James's farmer. In Chapter 1, we defined *relational spirituality* as "ways of relating with the sacred" and offered some initial framing of our relational spirituality model (RSM) as an empirically informed, holistic alternative to medical reductionism that takes a depth orientation toward suffering and healing. We also briefly outlined differing dimensions and definitions within the spiritual–existential–religious–theological (SERT; Rupert, Moon, & Sandage, 2018) framework as they can inform clinical practice from our relational spirituality perspective. The use of the term *relational spirituality* has grown in psychological literatures in recent years with a variety of meanings and dimensions grounded in different theoretical or philosophical

http://dx.doi.org/10.1037/0000174-003
Relational Spirituality in Psychotherapy: Healing Suffering and Promoting Growth,
by S. J. Sandage, D. Rupert, G. S. Stavros, and N. G. Devor

traditions. Here we locate our RSM in relation to these other traditions and consider the clinical implications, as well as positive and negative valences, of the "relational" in relational spirituality.

UNDERSTANDINGS OF RELATIONAL SPIRITUALITY

Tomlinson and colleagues (Tomlinson, Glenn, Paine, & Sandage, 2016) offered a conceptual review of literature using the term *relational spirituality* and identified five categories of usage (see Table 2.1). The first approach focuses on relational spirituality as part of *cognitive appraisals of stress and coping* (e.g., D. E. Davis, Hook, Van Tongeren, Gartner, & Worthington, 2012; D. E. Davis et al., 2014). This led to a series of empirical studies on interpersonal forgiveness with relational spirituality conceptualized as a dynamic within "cognitive systems" (D. E. Davis et al., 2012, p. 254) that can impact the appraisal and coping processes related to interpersonal transgressions or how we interpret and respond to offensive actions by others. For example, a spouse forgetting to follow through on a promised chore might be interpreted as an innocent human mistake that is automatically forgiven or a passive–aggressive failure based on a character flaw that reinforces the felt need for judgement and unforgiveness. D. E. Davis and colleagues (2014) noted that individual differences in relational spirituality might impact these differing appraisal and coping processes in ways that make forgiveness either more or less likely. While not explicitly stated by these authors, this approach to relational spirituality emphasizes individual differences in cognitive processes of appraisal that impact coping with stress both positively and negatively, an approach that easily integrates with cognitive behavioral approaches to psychotherapy and the vast literature on spiritual and religious coping (Pargament, 2007).

A second approach focuses on relational spirituality as part of *implicit relational development*. While the stress and coping researchers focus on the explicit dimensions of relational spirituality in cognitive appraisal processes, some relational psychoanalytic researchers emphasize "implicit" aspects of the construct that are strongly shaped by developmental experiences that may not be consciously learned or processed (Hall, 2007, p. 29; see also E. B. Davis,

TABLE 2.1. Categories of Relational Spirituality

Category	Example references
Cognitive appraisals of stress and coping	D. E. Davis et al. (2012)
Implicit relational development	Hall (2004); E. B. Davis, Granqvist, & Sharp (2018)
Couple, family, and community contexts	Mahoney & Cano (2014)
Social interconnection	Lahood (2010a, 2010b)
Differentiation-based model	Shults & Sandage (2006)

Note: Data from Tomlinson, Glenn, Paine, and Sandage (2016).

Granqvist, & Sharp, 2018). Hall (2004) offered one of the first implicit concep-tualizations of relational spirituality grounded in attachment theory and other relational psychoanalytic theories. His conception of relational spirituality involves what he termed *implicit relational representations* (Hall, 2004, p. 67). Implicit relational representations may be understood as intrapsychic templates formed through relational experiences that shape knowledge of self, knowl-edge of others, and emotional appraisals of meaning in relationships, including relationship with the sacred (Hall & Fujikawa, 2013). For example, a person whose early attachment experiences involved parents who were rarely supportive and frequently disapproving may develop a limbic-based internal working model of relationships that activates similar relational assumptions about the sacred (i.e., God or the sacred as typically unhelpful/uncaring and regularly disapproving). E. B. Davis, Granqvist, and Sharp (2018) similarly offered a sophisticated model of theistic relational spirituality drawing on attachment theory, dual-process theories of social cognition, and interpersonal neurobiology. Some empirical studies have also emerged from this frame-work (e.g., Augustyn, Hall, Wang, & Hill, 2017; Bailey et al., 2016; Hall, Fujikawa, Halcrow, Hill, & Delaney, 2009; Olson, 2011; Simpson, Newman, & Fuqua, 2008). Theorists from this approach extend the influence of relational spirituality well beyond coping with interpersonal transgressions, and yet the contributions explicitly using the term *relational spirituality* in this category appear to be largely focused on individual development and interpersonal experience rather than broader social systemic influences on spirituality (e.g., coping with systemic racism or religious bigotry). Implicit relational development models of relational spirituality have also tended to focus on theistic god images, since most of the related psychology of religion research on attachment has been in theistic (and predominantly Christian) contexts, although there are some emerging extensions to other spiritual and religious orientations (for an overview, see E. B. Davis et al., 2016; Mikulincer & Shaver, 2016).

A third approach to the topic of relational spirituality references *couple, family, or community contexts*. For example, Mahoney and Cano (2014) called the field of relational spirituality an "emerging subfield" of marriage and family research (p. 585). For Mahoney, relational spirituality refers to how particular aspects of spirituality can affect the discovery, maintenance, and transforma-tion dynamics within family relationships. Drawing upon Pargament's view of spirituality as a search for the sacred, Mahoney (2013) identified three tiers or ways by which relational spirituality may become incorporated into family relationships: "(a) one or more family members' relationship with the divine, (b) one or more family relationships invested with spiritual properties, and (c) one or more family members' relationships with religious communities" (p. 369). These three tiers of relational spirituality can each generate particu-lar resources and struggles in family relationships. Several other teams of researchers in this grouping have studied various facets of relational spiritual-ity in the context of adolescent development and highlight the reciprocal relational influences from friends, family, community and cultural contexts, and personal experiences of the sacred (Desrosiers, Kelley, & Miller, 2011; Desrosiers & Miller, 2007; S. Kim, Miles-Mason, Kim, & Esquivel, 2013; King, Carr, & Boitor, 2011; L. Miller, 2015, 2016). Theorists in this grouping have drawn attention beyond the individual to the spiritual influences from the surrounding family and community relationships, with L. Miller (2016) estimating about 70% of individual differences in relational spirituality being due to environmental factors or "formation that comes largely through socialization" (p. 131; leaving 30% due to genetic influences). L. Miller (2015) described the relational influences of the "intergenerational transmission of spiritual attunement" (p. 79) from parents to children. Mahoney's work, in particular, also highlighted the fact that certain relationships (e.g., marriage) are sanctified (i.e., considered sacred) by some spiritual and religious communities, calling attention to ways that communal contexts and traditions may impact relational spirituality. This group of theorists does not focus on individual differences in implicit relational development like Hall and Davis et al.; they instead focus on individuals in relation to systemic experiences and resources within their wider social ecologies in ways that could resonate with family systems approaches to spirituality and religion (e.g., Walsh, 2013). Clinically, this can focus attention on the impact of relational spirituality dynamics in an intergenerational family system, such as the stress and anxiety that might be experienced by a person who is the first to marry outside the family religious tradition or personally converts to a different spiritual orientation. This suggests the clinical benefit of considering spiritual and religious dynamics when doing family genogram work with clients (see Hodge, 2001, 2005).

A fourth approach considers relational spirituality as an alternative to individualistic notions of spirituality and grounded in a broader web of *social interconnection*. Faver (2004) drew on the feminist philosopher Carol Ochs's (1997) definition of spirituality as "the process of coming into relationship with reality" (p. 10) in her qualitative study exploring the sources of vitality that sustain social workers and other social caregivers in their work. For Faver, spirituality is an intrinsically relational process that includes any connection to someone or something beyond the self, a definition which she says could include atheists and nontheists. Relatedness is an important sustaining factor because of human finitude and the reality that we all have limited perspectives, thus helping "complete, challenge, or expand" our own understanding (p. 242).

Like Faver (2004), Lahood (2010a, 2010b) drew on Martin Buber's I–Thou relational philosophy to affirm the importance of immanent forms of relational spirituality with others through social connection and to offer an alternative to the narcissistic individualism he saw in certain New Age and transpersonal spirituality movements. However, Lahood focused on group experiences that cocreate charismatic spiritual events through creative rituals rather than the broader relationality of Faver. Notably, both Faver and Lahood advanced a philosophy of what spirituality *is* (ontology) rather than starting with social science categories. They also seemed to view relational spirituality as inherently constructive and did not consider dysfunctional or harmful expressions of relational spirituality. We resonate with Faver's point about the need among caregivers for supportive relational connections (and discuss this below). Certainly, some clients will resonate with this general view of spirituality as "connections between things." However, many other clients will have more specific and transcendent understandings of spirituality, and her thesis that everyone could be considered "spiritual" also conflicts with the self-definition of some individuals who do not consider themselves "spiritual," as mentioned above.

The fifth approach in the Tomlinson et al. (2016) review was the differentiation-based model of relational spirituality developed and empirically tested by Sandage and colleagues, which now integrates three primary relational development systems (attachment, differentiation, and intersubjectivity) within the RSM (Sandage, Jensen, & Jass, 2008; Shults & Sandage, 2006; Worthington & Sandage, 2016). This approach combines several features from the other relational approaches above and adds some innovations. Like category one (cognitive appraisals of stress and coping), this model suggests relational spirituality templates in the brain are often activated by stressors and interpersonal conflicts and involve cognitive processes of appraisal or interpretation, but the RSM also seeks to understand relational spirituality in a variety of situations and contexts and gives greater primacy to emotion and processes of affect regulation. Like category two (implicit relational development), the RSM employs attachment and other relational psychoanalytic theories to identify ways that implicit relational development or limbic-based unconscious influences strongly impact relational spirituality via affect regulation, leading to both healthy and pathological forms of spiritual development (Granqvist & Kirkpatrick, 2016; Tung, Ruffing, Paine, Jankowski, & Sandage, 2018). At the same time, the RSM extends beyond Christian theologies and theistic worldviews to engage a variety of spiritual and religious traditions. Like category three (couple, family, and community systems), our RSM attempts an integrated multilevel systemic understanding of relational spirituality as part of individual development nested within various family, social, and cultural ecologies. Thus, our current RSM incorporates particular concepts from categories two and three but with greater theoretical specificity. This integration of individual relational development theories with the broader ecological understanding of systems theories is psychologically and spiritually challenging but also potentially transformative toward a kind of humility. In *Steps to an Ecology of Mind*, Bateson (2000) described it in this way:

> Freudian psychology expanded the concept of mind inwards to include the whole communication system within the body—the automatic, the habitual, and the vast range of unconscious process. What I am saying expands the mind outwards. And both of these changes expand the scope of the conscious self. A certain humility becomes appropriate, tempered by the dignity or joy of being part of something much bigger. (pp. 462–463)

Like Bateson, category four (social interconnection) theorists seem to hold a philosophical belief in some form of relational ontology, which means that "relations between entities are ontologically more fundamental than the entities themselves" (Wildman, 2010, p. 55; see also Shults, 2003). We also draw on relational feminist theories (e.g., Benjamin, 2018; Jordan, 2018) and prefer a relational ontology over substance-dualist ontologies, and these relational commitments are consistent with our primary theoretical allegiances (i.e., attachment theory, family systems and ecological theories, and relational psychoanalysis). In some individualistic or Cartesian models of psychotherapy, relationships are added to the experience of individual subjects, whereas thoroughly relational models view persons as constituted through relationality. Kenneth Gergen (2009) countered Descartes' cogito ("I think, therefore I am") with a parallel statement of relational ontology—"I am linked, therefore I am." However, in contrast to category four theorists above we prefer a *differentiated* relational ontology that views both relations and entities as real, meaning differentiated entities in relation. We believe differences or differentiated entities exist within a relational matrix, and yet relations are basic to *being*. Stated another way, personhood is experienced by distinct persons in relation with one another. This has important implications for diversity-sensitive psychotherapy, training, and research, which we discuss later. Obviously, clients will often hold differing assumptions about spirituality and the nature of reality, and as clinicians we value the importance of working respectfully with clients within their worldview frameworks. But we think diversity-sensitive practice is facilitated when clinicians are self-aware of their own theoretical, ethical, and philosophical assumptions, and ways those might differ from clients and other clinicians (Tummala-Narra, 2016).

THREE KEY DEVELOPMENTAL SYSTEMS

Our RSM is a developmental approach, but there are many aspects of relational development that can be helpful to consider. We have chosen to focus on the integration of three overlapping yet distinct developmental systems— attachment, differentiation, and intersubjectivity—each of which is important for healthy relational development, constructive spiritual development, and effectiveness in relational psychotherapies (see Figure 2.1).[1] Our conceptualization of a developmental system is similar to Bowlby's (1969/1982; see Mikulincer & Shaver, 2016) concept of a behavioral system, which he borrowed from the field of ethology to apply to attachment. This led Bowlby to investigate the ways the attachment and other innate behavioral systems (e.g., caregiving, sexuality, affiliation) had evolved into adaptive, cybernetic systems

---

[1]Mitchell (2000) and Blaustein and Kinniburgh (2010) are two helpful examples of other theorists who have offered models highlighting differing aspects of relational development, and each model partially overlaps with our own.

FIGURE 2.1. Relational Development Systems

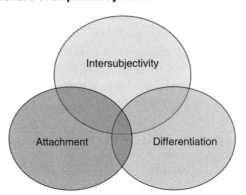

with specific neurobiological processes of activation and deactivation in relation to certain contexts and motivations for "set-goals." This cybernetic understanding of behavioral systems suggests a level of complexity among interrelated, goal-corrected functions of the system that goes beyond what is typically implied by terms like *trait* or *need*. We prefer the term *developmental system* to reference the ways attachment, differentiation, and intersubjectivity each involve complex motivational systems of developmental behaviors and capacities which influence subsequent developmental potentialities and not simply the equilibrium of the person. Attachment, differentiation, and intersubjectivity are somewhat overlapping and inter-related constructs, but each is also unique in meaning with differing scholarly and clinical traditions that have influenced those meanings. We also recognize that sociocultural contexts may shape the expression and development of attachment, differentiation, and intersubjectivity, so we do not hold a universal but rather a contextual model of these interacting developmental systems. We devote a chapter to each of these developmental systems (Chapters 5, 6, and 7) but offer a summary here.

The developmental systems of attachment, differentiation, and intersubjectivity share a deeply relational focus, and enrich each other by highlighting particular facets of relational experience. These systems also highlight important possibilities for integrating developmental and clinical research for understanding both spiritual development and psychotherapy.

The attachment system attends to safety and exploration, emphasizing the adaptive impact of felt security through dependable connection. Secure attachment relationships offer refuge and support in times of difficulty (referred to as the *safe haven function*) and encourage exploration and expansion in contexts of relational security and safety (referred to as the *secure base function*). Insecure attachments promote inflexible working models and narrow developmental and relational possibilities in ways that often impair personal, relational, and spiritual functioning over time (Tung et al., 2018).

The differentiation system focuses on the identity aspects of self and other and intrapsychic engagement of emotion and thought, with particular attention to how people balance their interpersonal stance in given situations and manage anxiety related to difference. Relationships offer connection and comfort but also present challenges such as differences that evoke anxiety and struggles for power and control (Maddock & Larson, 1995, 2004). A flexible, differentiated stance facilitates healthy connection and negotiation of differences. Persons with low differentiation may resort to problematic interpersonal stances such as fusion or disengagement, and/or problematic intrapersonal functioning such as overreliance on thinking or feeling (neglecting the non-preferred mode).

The intersubjectivity system attends to the developmental forces of self and other(s) in close or even intimate interactions, with particular attention to how constructive interactions may be enlivening and facilitate growth. Subjectivity emerges in and through relationship. Interactions promote connection, intimacy, and self-expansion when people experience recognition and responsiveness; interactions often produce disruption, distress, and even violence when intersubjectivity collapses. Misattunements and ruptures occur in all relationships, and thus acknowledgment and repair are critical aspects of healthy intersubjectivity. Serious and ongoing failure of mutual recognition may have destructive psychological and social consequences ranging from constricted development to social oppression.

RELATIONAL DIALECTICS

Another unique facet of the RSM within the broader relational spirituality literature is the emphasis on *dialectics*, as defined in the Introduction to this volume: the systemic notion that relational tensions between two opposing dynamics can be useful for generating change and that developmental growth often involves transcending polarities and appreciating paradox (Shults & Sandage, 2006). Our process-oriented and systemic understanding of relational spirituality is not just "relational" as interpersonally shaped but relational also through the dialectical nature of human development. Spiritual development is conceptualized in the RSM as unfolding through dialectical processes of spiritual *dwelling* and *seeking* (drawing on the sociological work of Wuthnow, 1998), which we describe in-depth along with other related dialectical themes in Chapter 3. Spiritual dwelling refers to stable patterns of relational dynamics with the sacred often embedded within a particular spiritual or religious tradition or familiar context, while spiritual seeking involves exploring existential questions or new spiritual experiences and understandings. But numerous other dialectics are also part of the RSM, including hope and humility, emotion processing and emotional regulation, autonomy and connection, forgiveness and justice, among others (see Worthington & Sandage, 2016). The wisdom of dialectical thinking has been a centerpiece of Linehan's (1993; Swenson, 2016) dialectical behavior therapy, as demonstrated in the value she places on emphasizing both acceptance and change or wise mind that integrates reason and emotion (among other dialectics). Various other dialectical models of human development and/or psychotherapy emphasize how the synthesis or integration of dialectical tensions can potentiate growth and transformation (e.g., Almagor, 2011; Bakan, 1966; Basseches & Mascolo, 2010; Gelo & Salvatore, 2016; Kegan, 1994; Kegan & Lahey, 2009; Sameroff, 2010). Like Linehan, Maddock and Larson (2004) suggested dialectical thinking is central to systemic or ecological approaches to psychotherapy that seek to understand relations between form and movement or various subsystems (e.g., family members) within a larger ecosystem (e.g., larger family processes over time). We believe human relational dynamics are inherently dialectical, and growth often requires achieving a new synthesis of opposing tensions.

ALTERITY, INTERSECTIONALITIES, AND DIVERSITY COMPETENCE

The RSM also emphasizes spiritual *alterity* or ways of relating to *otherness*, to differences present through diversity and intersectionality (i.e., ways differing aspects of identity, such as religion and sexual orientation, may interact in complex ways). *Alterity* has been defined as "developmental forms of relating to the *differentness* of others" (Sandage, Jensen, & Jass, 2008, p. 183; Sandage, Paine, & Morgan, 2019). In our view, these connections between relational spirituality and diversity have been underemphasized in social science and clinical literatures. In some cases, experiences of alterity and diversity can prompt empathic perspective-taking, respect for shared humanity, appreciation for the value of human differences, deepened self-awareness and learning, and even positive spiritual transformations (Sandage & Brown, 2018). In other cases, encountering spiritual or religious diversity may prompt fear, angry judgment and hateful behaviors, idealistic projections, or profound estrangement depending upon how alterity is processed (Morgan & Sandage, 2016). "Othering" is also used for sociopolitical purposes of exclusion and oppression in ways that may traumatize those who are deemed outsiders to the in-group. These different ways of relating to otherness are due in large measure to implicit self-other templates arising from developmental experiences and from contextual and systemic factors that may lead to differences being perceived either as negative and threatening or as relationally sustaining and life enhancing (Sandage & Brown, 2018; Sandage, Paine, & Morgan, 2019). The range of possible outcomes from encounters with spiritual and religious diversity is staggering and can powerfully impact the mental health and overall well-being of those involved.

We suggest in Chapter 6 that mature alterity involves differentiated relational capacities for (a) diversity competence and (b) a commitment to social justice. Empirical studies show significant individual differences in connections between spirituality and these aspects of alterity. In our developmental view of relational spirituality, diversity competence and social justice commitment are important aspects of spiritual maturity and spiritual responses to the realities of suffering in the world (see powell, 2012). We also advance the understanding that humility and a positive social identity are important correlates of mature alterity, similar to related ideas in the cultural humility and intercultural competence literatures (D. E. Davis, DeBlaere, et al., 2018; Hook, Davis, Owen, & DeBlaere, 2017; Paine, Jankowski, & Sandage, 2016; Sandage & Brown, 2018).

Relational dynamics of spiritual alterity have important implications for psychotherapy, including the therapeutic alliance, as well as mental health implications for clients beyond the therapy setting, because negative experiences of alterity through prejudice, discrimination, and violence can induce trauma and related mental health symptoms. Clinical attention to diversity and alterity can also draw focus toward some of the systemic challenges for clients who are spiritual or religious minorities in their social contexts and clients who are struggling with intersectional identities in domains that have often proven historically challenging to integrate (e.g., transgender identity and religious identity). We are particularly interested in relational dynamics that may be either helpful or harmful for clients in navigating existential experiences of otherness and identity conflicts. From an evolutionary psychology perspective, it has been argued that the dominant function of most spiritual and religious communities to date has been to promote in-group or kinship bonding rather than cooperative relations with out-groups (Griffith, 2011; Kirkpatrick, 2005), so mature expressions of spiritual alterity remain the minority.

RELATIONAL SELFHOOD

Relational spirituality also involves how we relate to ourselves. The topic of selfhood is exceedingly complex and requires intercultural contextualization, but the main point here is that we take a relational approach to selfhood and self–other configurations and consider capacities for healthy self-reflexivity important for the psychological and spiritual development of adult clients in the increasingly diverse, global contexts where psychotherapy is practiced. *Self-reflexivity* is the capacity to reflect on the role of one's subjectivity and social context in the process of interpreting life experience, which is an important part of the ability to mentalize (Allen, Fonagy, & Bateman, 2008). Kierkegaard (1849/1980b) defined the self as follows: "the self is a relation that relates itself to itself or is the relation's relating itself to itself in the relation; the self is not the relation but it is the relation's relating itself to itself" (p. 13). One of our clients demonstrated this connection between relating to oneself and mentalization by reporting in session an insight they had come to in a moment of loneliness: "Why am I so afraid of being alone? I'm not alone. I'm here with myself."

Kierkegaard (1849/1980b) went on to note that the dialectical tensions between human freedom or agency and the necessities of human finitude and embodiment are central to the formation of the self. His famous description of the self as a relational synthesis of "infinitude and finitude" offers another helpful dialectic for self-development within relational spirituality (p. 29). According to Kierkegaard (1849/1980b), by balancing or integrating infinitude and finitude we might (in his words) avoid both "the fantastic" and "reductionism" (pp. 32–33).

Kierkegaard's (1849/1980b) notion of the fantastic represents an over-spiritualized, narcissistic desire to actually become infinite or unlimited and to transcend human embodiment in a kind of spiritual dissociation. Several clinical theorists and researchers have referred to this tendency among some psychotherapy clients as *spiritual bypass*, or the tendency to use spiritual ideas and practices in an attempt to avoid dealing with psychological pain or unresolved developmental tasks (Cashwell, Myers, & Shurts, 2004; Fox, Cashwell, & Picciotto, 2017; Welwood, 2000). Spiritualized versions of consumerism prevalent in the United States can promote idealistic visions of spirituality, which prove contrary to the embodied processes of human development. For example, in certain spiritual or religious communities, leaders convey a simplistic message that followers will be happy and prosperous if they simply practice certain spiritual principles. This notion of spirituality as a kind of happiness product fits within a consumeristic culture of bypassing suffering through obtaining products and services. Yet it distorts the existential wisdom of most spiritual and religious traditions that, in differing ways, hold out hope for eventual liberation from suffering and growth in well-being through a challenging (and sometimes painful) process of spiritual development. Consumeristic spirituality also tends to stigmatize those experiencing ongoing suffering rather than cultivating compassion, and the chronic reliance on spiritual bypass will leave important gaps in a person's relational development (Fossella, 2011; Welwood, 2000).

Reductionism is the opposite dialectical tendency from the fantastic and moves toward a restriction of life purpose and becoming absorbed in temporal concerns. Kierkegaard (1980b) suggested that this diminishes the uniqueness of selfhood and the need for existential commitments. Traumatic and other experiences of extreme suffering can sometimes generate these kinds of reductionism of existential and spiritual meaning, as a person's psychological focus understandably moves defensively to self-protection and survival. In addition to intrapsychic and interpersonal etiological factors, our RSM also invites awareness of systemic dynamics that can press for reductionism of relational selfhood and self-identity (e.g., poverty, prejudice, discrimination, marginalization). This is a particular risk among oppressed, nondominant groups who may internalize relational dynamics of oppression and nonrecognition in self-negating (Fanon, 1963) or self-silencing ways (Jack & Ali, 2010) and may lack systemic resources for pursuing broader life purpose and fulfillment.

We relate these dynamics of self-reflexivity to the dialectical tensions between hope and humility (Worthington & Sandage, 2016; see also Pieper, 1986) or the trust in benevolent future possibilities (hope) and constructive engagement with human limitations (humility). Clinicians are probably more familiar with the therapeutic effects of hope (Wampold & Imel, 2015) than humility, but healthy forms of humility involving accurate self-awareness of one's strengths and limitations involves a kind of psychological "middle way" between grandiosity and shame. In a study of clients at our clinic indicating religion held some level of importance to them, the relationship between individual differences in religious salience or commitment and psychosocial functioning was moderated by humility (Paine, Sandage, Ruffing, & Hill, 2018). That is, clients needed a moderate or higher level of humility for religiosity to be conducive to healthy psychosocial functioning. At low levels of humility, religiosity was negatively related to healthy psychosocial functioning, as humility may be a key virtue within relational spirituality that facilitates the ability to be in community with others and temper the risk of grandiosity or spiritual bypass that could result from overidentification with the sacred (Jankowski, Sandage, Bell, Ruffing, & Adams, 2018).

Kierkegaard's (1849/1980b) complicated definition of relational self-hood essentially speaks to the developmental need to relate to oneself and one's existential and/or spiritual dilemmas with self-reflexivity or reflective ability. This is consistent with insights from contemporary theories of mind, mentalization-based approaches to psychotherapy, and developmental models of intersubjectivity (Allen, 2013; Allen, Fonagy, & Bateman, 2008; Bateman & Fonagy, 2019; Benjamin, 2018; Stern, 2004). We will suggest that the dynamics of relational spirituality facilitate self-reflexivity for some, while others relate to the sacred in ways that inhibit, obstruct, or overpower self-reflexivity. Mental health involves, among other things, an ability to balance hope and humility or possibility and necessity. Certain forms of relational spirituality involve high levels of grandiosity or shame (or both), and this can be contrasted with forms of relational spirituality across many traditions that facilitate healthy, balanced versions of hope and humility.

These issues of relational selfhood also become clinically relevant when considering the use of spiritual and other self-care practices as interventions in psychotherapy. For example, practices such as mindfulness meditation, self-compassion, yoga, prayer, forgiveness, and others could be psychologically and spiritually helpful for many clients, yet some clients relate to themselves in hostile, shame-ridden, or dissociative ways based on internalized introjects formed through relational development. An approach to spiritually integrative psychotherapy that focuses on practices or structured interventions alone might miss an important relational dimension of the healing process and underestimate the anxiety, conflict, shame, and guilt some clients have in trying to relate to themselves in constructive and caring ways. In some cases, corrective relational experiences in psychotherapy and the cultivation of a strong working alliance may be necessary precursors for clients forming capacities for mentalization, self-reflexivity, and healthier forms of relational selfhood and constructive spiritual practices. E. B. Davis et al. (2016) referred to these positive therapeutic effects on relational spirituality and relational selfhood as "security-based self-representations . . . that are derived from the internalization of security-enhancing interactions with attachment figures" (p. 11), which might result from corrective experiences in the client–therapist relationship. We also affirm the increasing attention to relational forms of spiritual practice that move beyond the isolated individual subject, such as relational mindfulness (Falb & Pargament, 2012; Surrey & Kramer, 2013), which may also facilitate the development of relational selfhood. In the chapters that follow, we will consider strategies that can help clients overcome these kinds of struggles with healthy relational selfhood.

RELATIONAL INTEGRATION OF SPIRITUALITY, PSYCHOTHERAPY, TRAINING, AND RESEARCH

Relationality also serves as an *integrative motif* in our RSM in an effort to be coherent across our understanding of spirituality, our theoretical orientation in psychotherapy, our approach to training and ongoing professional consultation, and our practice of engaging research for ongoing learning and growth. As stated in the introduction, we utilize relational approaches to psychotherapy building upon the vast empirical literature showing that (a) relational factors (e.g., therapeutic alliance dynamics) are among the strongest predictors of outcomes (Wampold & Imel, 2015) and (b) improvements in clients' relational functioning at our clinic have strongly predicted improvements in affect regulation, clinical symptoms, and life satisfaction (Jankowski et al., 2019). Aspects of our relational spirituality framework have been used within other theoretical approaches to psychotherapy (e.g., cognitive behavior therapy; Correa & Sandage, 2018), and we affirm the value of psychotherapy integration. However, defining spirituality in relational terms is consistent with our clinical orientation and RSM view of change, and we consider this consistency to be an important dimension of a cohesive approach to spiritually integrative psychotherapy. Our own personal worldviews also lead each of us to view the therapeutic alliance as sacred, consistent with the teachings on relational dynamics in healing in many spiritual and religious traditions. We also find that it is common for clients to experience similar relational dynamics with their therapist as they experience in relating to the sacred or ultimate. For example, a client whose relational spirituality is characterized by narcissism, emotional detachment, and superiority in relation to others will likely manifest this same relational style toward their therapist in the early phase of treatment. Conversely, a highly shame-prone client with dependent personality traits who primarily seeks guidance and rescue from the sacred might tend to initially expect the same from their therapist. Attachment researchers of spirituality and religion have built on the work of earlier psychoanalytic theorists of relational influences on god images (e.g., Rizzuto, 1979; Rizzuto & Shafranske, 2013) to demonstrate considerable empirical evidence of this *correspondence effect* based on internal working models of relationship that can apply to other humans *and* the sacred (Granqvist & Kirkpatrick, 2013). This parallel relational process can potentially double the effects of corrective relational experiences in psychotherapy, as when "default" relational expectations are countered by a new and constructive relational experience with a therapist.

Relational Modalities of Treatment

As we described in Chapter 1, the dominant health care system in the United States is highly individualistic, with a focus on symptoms, diagnoses, and functioning of individual patients. This typically translates into practices where the primary "unit" of treatment is the individual, and relational modalities of therapy (e.g., couple therapy, family therapy, group therapy) might be added in a secondary fashion on top of individual treatment. Based on a relational ontology consistent with systems and ecological frameworks, we prefer to orient ourselves toward persons in a web of relations. Clinically, this means we often prefer to work with relational units if possible, or at least bring individual clients' family members or significant others into a session (or more) for assessment purposes. Even individual psychotherapy can be conducted in a way that regularly attends to and references the significant web of our clients' relationships. Our working assumption is to view relational modalities as a potential "treatment of choice" at least as often as individual modalities.

Relational Ecologies of Treatment

Our RSM also directs attention to the multifaceted relational ecology of psychotherapy. The literature on relational factors in psychotherapy largely assumes relational dynamics occur exclusively within a therapist–individual client dyad, with an exception being group therapy and couple and family therapy literatures. However, many outpatient clinics clients have an array of relational encounters with administrative staff involving sensitive relational or attachment issues, such as initial entry into the clinic, finances, insurance, scheduling, therapist availability, crises, transitions between sessions, transitions between providers, and termination among others (Kehoe, Hassen, & Sandage, 2016). At our clinic, administrative staff are viewed as transitional objects whom clients typically engage during their "coming and going" in the spaces between the therapist's private office and the "outside world." In our relational model of psychotherapy, transitions at the micro level (e.g., between sessions) or macro level (e.g., between therapists or therapies) are often important *liminal spaces* (Turner, 1969) that activate limbic-based attachment templates and the associated dynamics of relational spirituality. It is interesting to reflect upon possible reasons these "betwixt and between" processes and the roles of administrative staff have been understudied in field of psychotherapy, perhaps reflecting some modernistic bias that it is the "professionals" who carry all the treatment effects. An initial study at our clinic found client ratings of their alliance dynamics with administrative staff predicted their ratings of therapy outcomes above and beyond the effects of their alliance with their therapists (Sandage, Moon et al., 2017). These findings offer preliminary support for our relational ecology hypothesis that the larger relational dynamics within a clinic may influence treatment, which builds upon earlier theories of milieu treatment effects in inpatient settings and work on relational models of health care (Maunder & Hunter, 2015; McArdle, 2008; Raia & Deng, 2015). This suggests the potential value of clinicians and clinic administrators regularly reflecting on the relational dynamics of their organization and how that might impact clinical care (for better or for worse).

Relational Formation and Clinical Training

We view relational dynamics as central to effective clinical training and ongoing consultation for therapists over the course of their career, which we discuss further with practical strategies in Chapter 11. Given the personal sensitivity of SERT dynamics in therapy and the importance of diversity competence, we believe it is vital for therapists to have healthy relational spaces during training and throughout their career that offer opportunities to process (a) their own spiritual and religious histories, perspectives, values, and attitudes; and (b) their own ways of making and struggling with meaning as they work with clients facing intense and complicated forms of trauma and suffering. Pargament (2007) highlighted the need for self-awareness among clinicians on these matters, suggesting

> Knowingly or unknowingly, the spirituality of the therapist permeates his or her understanding of people, problems, and change. Spiritually integrated psychotherapy makes explicit the importance of the therapist's own orientation to spirituality. (p. 187)

This call to self-awareness regarding SERT dynamics can be described as "managing countertransference" or, more broadly and constructively, "self of therapist" awareness and formation (see Chapter 11). The limited available research on clinical training related to spirituality and religion suggests the importance of (a) spiritual self-awareness of the therapist; (b) relational dynamics with faculty, in supervision, and in the therapist's own support system; and (c) opportunities for trainees to process and relationally construct an understanding of their own spiritual journey (M. M. Miller, Korinek, & Ivey, 2006; Sorenson, 2004b; Stavros & Sandage, 2014; Tillman, Dinsmore, Hof, & Chasek, 2013). Sorenson's (Sorenson, Derflinger, Bufford, & McMinn, 2004) research on the process of integrating spirituality and psychology among clinical doctoral trainees across four religiously affiliated clinical psychology programs is noteworthy as the only real programmatic body of research in this area. Across these different training programs, trainees tended to show a pattern of trying to integrate psychology and spirituality relationally by forming implicit, sometimes unspoken, relationships or attachments with faculty and using whatever those faculty modeled in terms of their own attempted integration. It was not a particular approach to integration that trainees seemed to be seeking, but rather some level of authentic access to the personhood of the faculty and their own ways of holding together psychology and spirituality. From a relational development perspective, this suggests trainees were often implicitly trying to connect with faculty and borrow, experiment with, internalize, or even differentiate from their examples of integration. If generalized beyond Sorenson's samples, this might be somewhat intimidating to those of us in faculty and clinical supervision roles. On the other hand, it could also be relieving and clarifying to recognize that quantity of knowledge and technical skill may be less important than formative qualities of personhood and relational dynamics for effectiveness in both psychotherapy and clinical training.

Relational Collaboration and Consultation

It might be easy to understand the importance of relational factors during the formative period of graduate training, but what about relational dynamics of collaboration and consultation among professionals throughout their careers? We are suggesting that practicing psychotherapy, as with many other helping professions, involves vastly disproportionate exposure to tragedy, human suffering, and a multitude of complex existential issues. At times, clinicians will feel *existentially dysregulated* or confused as to how to find meaning in their work and fend off burnout and despair. At a milder level, it is natural for clinicians to sometimes feel confused, discouraged, or uninformed about how to approach certain cases. As mentioned above, our RSM places a premium on cultivating healthy and diverse relational ecologies for clinical training and consultation. Helpful ecologies or holding environments provide consistent times of connection to foster self-awareness, open dialogue, metabolizing of countertransference, and gaining fresh inputs regarding clinical strategies from trusted colleagues. Even though we are clinical educators who write books (like this one) and articles and engage in formal continuing education, in our view it is not books, classes, or continuing education seminars that make the greatest impact on clinical effectiveness and clinician development, but rather relational experiences with healthy professional communities that, like good psychotherapy, balance challenge and support amidst diverse perspectives. This kind of authentic relational connection is not always present in formal clinical staff meetings; it comes from sharing our stories with colleagues who know us and our clinical work over time. We find this is just as true for seasoned clinicians as it is for novices. Throughout our professional journeys, we can benefit from the wisdom, clarity, and limbic recalibration that comes from community with colleagues who are also engaged in seeking to stretch toward personal and professional growth.

Relational Dynamics in Research

Finally, we view clinical research as relational. Research is frequently defined as: "the systematic, rigorous investigation of a situation or problem in order to generate new knowledge or validate existing knowledge" (J. A. Cooper & McNair, 2015, p. 209). This definition suggests research involves organized and systematic approaches to knowledge construction. If we also consider a more expansive *clinical practice* view of research as "accessing and reflecting upon scientific and professional data," there are probably multiple points in every workday when clinicians informally engage research or research-related considerations at some level. This could include considering choices in assessment tools, interpreting assessment data, arriving at diagnoses, developing or reformulating treatment plans among the various alternatives, reflecting on diversity considerations, forming administrative strategies for clinical management, considering ways to responsibly integrate SERT resources and traditions into treatment, selecting among supervision and training models, or choosing self-care strategies to avoid burnout and cultivate well-being.

A commitment to ongoing learning and growth is relational in the systems dynamic of remaining open to new inputs, seeking fresh information, and experimenting with innovations in practice. There is empirical evidence that clinician openness to empirical research is positively correlated with their openness to innovations or new approaches to their clinical work (Aarons, 2004). If a clinician or clinic were not open to new insights or new clinical strategies, it would represent a closed system attitude and there would be no need for research. When we read and make use of research conducted outside our system, present our research at professional conferences or submit our research to peer review with journals, or consult or collaborate with researchers in other contexts, we are opening our system to outside inputs, influences, and critique. This requires humility and serves as a *differentiating process* (i.e., cultivating differentiation in the system) and allows us to see our ideas, theoretical assumptions, and practice strategies from other perspectives and with critical refinement. This parallels what we typically ask of clients—to be open to new inputs, look at things from new perspectives, and be receptive to feedback in a spirit of humility. This kind of research engagement is also part of the seeking system in relational spirituality, which we discuss further in Chapter 3.

From a relational perspective, research offers a boundaried way of listening to client voices and sharing the power of knowledge construction and treatment evaluation. Quantitative data points in clinical research are symbolic representations of client experiences, which can reveal important patterns and exceptions to patterns. Qualitative data offer access to the unique perspectives and experiences voiced by individual clients and the possibility of discovering themes for greater understanding. These kinds of research projects allow clients to speak back into the clinical process with the appropriate boundaries and confidentiality that can allow complete candor. Ultimately, this can be empowering of clients and the overall politics of clinical practice. Certainly, clinical research can be misused and exploitive of clients, and there are important epistemological issues to negotiate related to the strengths and limitations of any research methodology and the complexities of clinical practice. But to not engage research at all would imply clinicians unilaterally know what is best for clients, and this could reflect authoritarian hegemony related to the power dynamics involved (Sandage & Brown, 2018).

For many busy clinicians, the most common formal engagement with research probably comes as a consumer of research "products" or knowledge generated by others. It is an even greater challenge and systemic shift to seek to participate or contribute as constructors of research ourselves. When possible, this systemic shift changes the subject–object relationship we have with the process of research toward intersubjectivity; that is, from a unidirectional relationship of using research as consumers to a bidirectional relationship of coconstructing new knowledge. When we engage in research, collaborate with others, or share our ideas with colleagues (including those outside our own clinical setting), we are opening ourselves to new learning, feedback, and expanded social networks. In our experience, participating in relational discovery and construction of new knowledge is often formative in part because it is existentially anxiety-provoking and forces us to engage relational dialectics of selfhood. For example, in teaching, presenting, researching, or writing, we might grapple with questions such as, "Do I have anything original to contribute or should I safely and compulsively overcite the work of others? On the other hand, whom *should* I cite and give credit out of gratitude for their generativity even if I am taking their ideas in new directions? Are my ideas ridiculous, revolutionary, or 'good enough'? How should I treat persons with competing theories and perspectives? Can I take in feedback and refine my perspective, or will I be defensively stubborn? How can I metabolize the 'bipolar' reactions from others, ranging from projected idealization to hostile denigration? How should I handle the diversity dynamics of my research and attend to the limits of what I can claim? Can I make constructive use of what clients are teaching me with ethical integrity to their rights to privacy? In collaborative research, how will we share the work, the successes, the setbacks? How will we negotiate differences and power dynamics often embedded in roles and disciplines?" If you have not thought about these kinds of relational dynamics of research, we might suggest you do a bit of ethnography at your next professional conference to see what you might notice among the presenters and attendees and the relational dynamics that manifest.

CONCLUSION

In this chapter, we summarized differing conceptualizations of relational spirituality in the social science literature in comparison with our RSM approach to defining spirituality and related dynamics. This led to introducing three relational development systems we target in the RSM—attachment, differentiation, and intersubjectivity—which will be the focus of Chapters 5–7. We also considered some unique relational spirituality emphases in the RSM, including dialectics; alterity, intersectionalities, and diversity competence; and relational selfhood. Finally, we introduced our relationally integrative framework for seeking to understand spirituality, psychotherapy, training, and research through a relational development lens. In Chapter 3, we focus on the central theoretical and clinical dialectic of the RSM: dwelling and seeking.

3

Balancing Spiritual Dwelling and Seeking

Place is security; space is freedom: we are attached to the one and long for the other.
—Y.-F. TUAN, *SPACE AND PLACE* (1977, P. 3)

The existential reflection above by Tuan (1977) is from his book *Space and Place: The Perspective of Experience*, which helped establish the field of human geography. Tuan noted that the relations between space and place form a dialectic and that "the ideas of 'space' and 'place' require each other for definition. From the security and stability of place we are aware of the openness, freedom, and threat of space, and vice versa" (p. 6). What does this have to do with relational spirituality? In this chapter, we suggest that relational spirituality involves dialectical processes of spiritual *dwelling* and *seeking* that roughly approximate the metaphors offered by several spiritual and psychological depth theorists across other disciplines, including Tuan's complex insights about human needs for place and space. Like Tuan, we suggest humans can have both longings for and existential ambivalence about spiritual dwelling and seeking, places and spaces, and that attending to these dialectical relational processes can be helpful for understanding spiritual and psychological changes over time.

http://dx.doi.org/10.1037/0000174-004
Relational Spirituality in Psychotherapy: Healing Suffering and Promoting Growth,
by S. J. Sandage, D. Rupert, G. S. Stavros, and N. G. Devor

WUTHNOW'S SOCIOLOGY OF SPIRITUAL DWELLING AND SEEKING

The language of spiritual dwelling and seeking used in the relational spiritual model (RSM) was originally adapted from sociologist of religion Robert Wuthnow's (1998) research on important shifts in the spirituality and religion in North America in the last half of the 20th century (see Shults & Sandage, 2006; Worthington & Sandage, 2016). Wuthnow described a changing spiritual and religious landscape where many people were moving from the prior predominant orientation of spiritual dwelling, or relating to the sacred through particular religious communities and congregations, toward a sharp increase in spiritual seekers who sought more "portable" and personal expressions of spirituality beyond the physical and theological boundaries of religious institutions. In Tuan's terms, Wuthnow described something of a reduced emphasis on religious *place* and more emphasis on spiritual *space*. In fact, many sociologists of religion have noted a rising demographic of those who self-define as "spiritual but not religious" in recent decades as well as more multiple or hybrid spiritual and religious identifications (Ammerman, 2013). However, Wuthnow was careful to note that orientations toward spiritual dwelling and seeking are not mutually exclusive and that some persons seek to integrate the two. Wuthnow's contribution highlights the important roles that historical and systemic dynamics—what Bronfenbrenner (1979) called the macrosystemic level—can play in shaping of spirituality. Our RSM applies these dialectical themes of spiritual dwelling and seeking at the level of individual development while attempting to remain cognizant of multiple levels of systemic context and influence.

DYNAMICS OF SPIRITUAL DWELLING

In the RSM, spiritual dwelling references archetypal themes related to a sense of *home* or *refuge*, the consecration of an *abode* or *habitat*, and an existential need for continuity of *place* (Eliade, 1959; Kegan, 1982; Tuan, 1977). Eliade (1959) generalized that "habitation always undergoes a process of sanctification" (p. 52), and spiritual dwelling or taking refuge for security and guidance is a theme across many spiritual teachings and traditions. More specifically, *spiritual dwelling* refers to a variety of ways of relating to the sacred that can potentially facilitate spiritual grounding or commitment, self-regulation, community, and intimacy (see Table 3.1). Spiritual dwelling is a multidimensional construct, and certain dimensions may be more prominent than others within certain spiritual and religious traditions and across individual differences.

Healthy forms of spiritual dwelling can contribute to high levels of spiritual well-being (E. B. Davis, Granqvist, & Sharp, 2018). For example, persons may relate to the sacred in harmonious and meaningful ways that generate feelings of happiness, fulfillment, life satisfaction, and personal integration

TABLE 3.1. Attachment Functions and Developmental Outcomes of Spiritual Dwelling and Seeking

Relational spirituality dimension	Attachment system function	Key developmental outcome

Spiritual dwelling
   Commitment
   Self-regulation
   Community
   Awareness
	Safe haven	Well-being

Spiritual seeking
   Exploration
   Tolerating ambiguity
   Openness
   Complexity
	Secure base	Growth

(Pargament, 2007). A. B. Cohen and Johnson's (2017; see also Van Tongeren, Davis, Hook, & Johnson, 2016) review of research suggested that many indices of religion and spirituality are positively associated with measures of well-being, and these often appear to be mediated by spiritual or religious influences on factors such as self-control and other virtues, a sense of meaning or purpose in life, and a sense of community to provide support and alleviate loneliness. However, they also noted, consistent with our RSM framework, that differing expressions of religion and spirituality can sometimes diminish well-being by generating distress (e.g., perfectionistic expectations and pathological guilt). Norms of spiritual and religious dwelling are diverse and must be understood in differing social contexts with differing mental health correlates.

Personal Commitment and Grounding

Some spiritual dwellers hold strong personal commitments to their relational spirituality, which can contribute to a sense of existential grounding and an orienting meaning framework for interpreting life events. Pargament (2007) referred to this as the *conserving* function of spiritual and religious coping, a kind of "holding on" to and enhancing one's relationship with the sacred. Kegan (1982) also described the lifelong developmental need to hold on to people, places, and meanings in dialectical tension with letting go. Studies have shown that clients who are high in spiritual or religious commitment may have different preferences or expectations about integrating spiritual and religious issues into psychotherapy than those with lower commitment, and the neglect or diminishment of spiritual and religious issues can lead to poorer outcomes with highly committed clients (Hook, Worthington, & Davis, 2012).

A large body of empirical research in the psychology of religion has also investigated individual differences in intrinsic versus extrinsic spiritual and religious motivations as an important distinction in (what we are calling) spiritual dwelling, with *intrinsic motivation* referring to internalized commitments to spirituality or religion as "an end in itself" while *extrinsic motivations* approach spirituality and religion as a means to other ends (Hood, Hill, & Spilka, 2018). The research suggests that intrinsic spiritual and religious commitments tend to be associated with positive indicators of mental health and well-being, whereas extrinsic commitments do not, although these findings might reflect some level of individualistic bias; also, extrinsic motivations may prove healthy within certain collectivistic religious groups that value group loyalty and obligation (A. B. Cohen, Hall, Koenig, & Meador, 2005). Clinically, this suggests it can be beneficial to try to understand the basis of clients' spiritual and religious motivations and commitments while viewing them in the context of their cultures and traditions.

Practices That Enhance Self-Regulation

Healthy forms of spiritual dwelling are also characterized by embodied rituals or practices that can facilitate emotional and spiritual regulation. For example, meditation, prayer, and other spiritual practices potentially provide a sense of centering and self-regulation for anxiety and other emotions. Eliade (1959) suggested that humans inhabit the body in ways that parallel inhabiting a house or other dwelling place, and this connection between spirituality and embodiment invites consideration of how differing forms of spiritual dwelling may be psychologically and spiritually helpful or harmful (Griffith, 2011). Most spiritual and religious traditions recognize the importance of embodiment and have developed practices that constructively engage the body—including meditating, dancing, holding poses, eating, fasting, making physical gestures, prostrating oneself, drumming, smelling incense, sweating, anointing with oil, and many others. Spiritual and religious traditions may also identify spiritual meanings in physical functions such as breathing, eating, drinking, sleeping, and sexuality. However, some streams within certain traditions hold sharply dualistic worldviews that try to segregate the spiritual dimension from the physical/human dimension of life (the sacred from the profane), which can lead to views of the body as more of a "prison than temple" (see Jacobson, Hall, Anderson, & Willingham, 2016). These "body-negative" forms of relational spirituality may be associated with practices that are more dissociative or disruptive than growth-producing, and some individuals may be very earnest in their spiritual practices but find it does not seem to help with emotional regulation or relational development.

This highlights several potential clinical assessment questions we might ask spiritually- or religiously committed clients related to dwelling dimensions:

- Do they have spiritual or religious practices that are important to them? If so, how do those practices impact how they feel about themselves (relational selfhood) and their bodies? What do those practices mean to them?

- Are they finding those practices helpful at this time?

- Can they see ways those practices could be integrated into what they are working on in therapy?

- Is there a particular goal for those practices within their traditions (if relevant)?

- Are there new spiritual practices they have been considering?

- Are there practices that haven't been helpful?

- Note that it is important to also be sensitive and attuned to struggles or inconsistency clients may have with spiritual practices, and the guilt or shame some may feel when asked about practices. This would be an important part of understanding the relational spirituality dynamics of that client, and we discuss these issues further below.

Safe Haven for Emotion Regulation

Based on attachment theory (which is the focus of Chapter 5), spiritual dwelling is also consistent with the safe haven function of attachment that provides emotional and physical security and the regulation of fear, sadness, shame, anger, and other emotions (see Table 3.1). Safe haven themes are found within many spiritual traditions, and attachment security has been empirically associated with a wide range of indicators of spiritual, psychological, and relational well-being (Granqvist & Kirkpatrick, 2016). As one example, Bonab, Miner, and Proctor (2013) integrated attachment theory and Islamic spirituality, noting Allah's divine attribute of *Al-Mu'min*—the preserver and bestower of security, as evident in this dwelling-oriented prayer: "You are the faithful who rests in security, and I am God the Faithful who bestows security. . . . There shall be no fear for you, nor shall you be sad. . . . You are in My abode" (Ibn Arabi, 2004).

From a relational spirituality perspective, spiritual well-being generally involves positive or securely attached forms of connection with the sacred which contribute to a sense of meaning, purpose in life, and overall well-being (see E. B. Davis, Granqvist, & Sharp, 2018; Jankowski & Sandage, 2011; Unterrainer, Ladenhauf, Wallner-Liebmann, & Fink, 2011; Worthington & Sandage, 2016). However, some individuals are committed to their spirituality or religion, but their insecurely attached style of relational spirituality does not facilitate a spiritual safe haven, and they may not have developed spiritual practices that foster spiritual and emotional regulation to help achieve well-being. For example, a theistic person whose shame-prone relational spirituality template is organized around a schema of God's disappointment in them might engage in verbal prayers for divine assistance, but their internal conflicts and projected image of God makes these experiences of prayer stressful (Paine & Sandage, 2015). Trauma can also overwhelm internal working models of relational spirituality in ways that create insecurity; thus, spiritual dwelling may feel unsafe or even dysregulating. This was the case for Sofia in Chapter 1, as she perceived her suffering as an ambiguous spiritual punishment. When clients have highly insecure internal working models leading to patterns of relating with the sacred characterized by extreme mistrust, shame, fear of persecution or abandonment, or anger, certain highly cognitive or verbal spiritual practices may be discouraging or ineffective until corrective relational experiences can begin to revise limbic-based relational spirituality templates. Some forms of mindfulness, meditative prayer, and other embodied spiritual practices may prove helpful in these cases, but the relational dynamics of the client's spirituality will need to be carefully considered.

Relational sensitivity to the effects of trauma is essential if therapists are to cultivate a working relationship with clients that can become a dwelling place of safety and meaning reconstruction. Stolorow (2016) took an existential stance that severe emotional pain becomes traumatic when it must be experienced alone and without a "relational home" provided by a therapy relationship where unbearable feelings can be "shared and held" (p. 72). He advocated a therapeutic stance of "emotional dwelling" (p. 72) in which therapists move beyond empathy toward actively entering and participating with clients in their emotional pain. Stolorow explained his view of therapeutic dwelling using the language of the sacred to describe a core dynamic that we associate with relational spirituality:

> If we are to be an understanding relational home for a traumatized person, we must tolerate, even draw upon, our own existential vulnerabilities so that we can dwell unflinchingly with his or her unbearable and recurring emotional pain. When we dwell with others' unendurable pain, their shattered emotional worlds are enabled to shine with a kind of sacredness that calls forth an understanding and caring engagement within which traumatized states can be gradually transformed into bearable painful feelings. Emotional pain and existential vulnerability that find a hospitable relational home can be seamlessly and constitutively integrated into whom one experiences oneself as being. (p. 73)

We are not suggesting therapy can replace other sources of community for clients, including spiritual and religious communities. But we do agree with Stolorow (2016) that clients benefit from safe places of emotional connection with therapists who have the courage to personally journey with them into spaces of existential vulnerability, and we also consider this a sacred process.

Community as Support or Source of Conflict

While therapy can sometimes provide a sense of relational home as Stolorow (2016) described, the community dimension of spiritual dwelling is much broader and includes relational connections involving the sacred in a client's life. As suggested earlier, such connections to formal or informal sources of spiritual or religious community can be tremendous sources of support and provide opportunities for developmental growth and prosocial service to others. But lest we be idealistic, we must also recognize spiritual and religious communities can also at times be sources of conflict, and dysfunctional dynamics within sacred communities can be particularly painful sources of spiritual disappointment. Some spiritual or religious communities are relatively closed systems (e.g., fundamentalist groups of various types) that may serve sociobiological functions for peer affiliation and kin recognition but become too relationally enmeshed and restrictive to facilitate the spiritual and psychological development of certain members or openness to constructive relationships with outgroup members and resources (Griffith, 2011; Van Tongeren, Hakim, et al., 2016). Thus, certain forms of spiritual dwelling may involve high levels of anxiety and low levels of differentiation and intersubjectivity, particularly when individuals engage in spiritual seeking by asking existential questions or exploring ideas or behaviors that differ from community norms.

Several questions can be helpful in assessing a client's dwelling-oriented spiritual and religious dynamics of community:

- Do they have access to and are they involved in spiritual or religious communities that fit their particular spiritual or religious orientation?
- How are they experiencing those communities?
- Are there important sources of healing or support within those communities that we/I need to understand?
- Do dynamics within their communities work against access to mental health resources or stigmatize or even increase clients' struggles?

Awareness of, or Intimacy With, the Divine

Another dimension of spiritual dwelling in the RSM is spiritual awareness, which references a variety of ways differing spiritual traditions encourage mindful awareness of sacred presence or sacred realities. Clearly, traditions differ in their understandings of the nature of spiritual awareness and the related practices, but we want to highlight a common dwelling-oriented theme of valuing spiritual awareness beyond normal cognitive processing (de Castro, 2017). In some traditions, this will take the form of dwelling in intimacy with the divine, whereas in many mindfulness traditions the dwelling focus is on more general, nonjudgmental, and purposeful awareness of the present moment. The neuroimaging research of Azari, Missimer, and Seitz (2005, p. 275) suggests that among both Christians and Buddhists, dwelling-oriented spiritual experiences of a "perceived relationship" with the sacred are mediated through prefrontal structures involving social–relational cognitive processes. This raises questions about individual differences in personality and neurobiological function that might impact a person's ability to engage in calming or intimate forms of spiritual dwelling.

Clinically, it is also important to understand that some individuals may report high levels of spiritual awareness that is not well-integrated with healthy psychosocial functioning. For example, research on spiritual grandiosity shows that self-reports of high levels of spiritual awareness combined with interpersonal superiority and entitlement are associated with difficulties with forgiveness, humility, and relating well across cultural differences (Sandage & Crabtree, 2012; Sandage & Harden, 2011; Sandage, Jankowski,

Bissonette, & Paine, 2017). It seems that over the life span, the integration of spiritual dwelling with authentic relational virtues and spiritual maturity will typically require periods of spiritual seeking in order to grow in more complex understandings of self and others.

DYNAMICS OF SPIRITUAL SEEKING

Spiritual seeking in the RSM references processes of exploring the sacred, movement into existential questioning, and potential transformation into new and more complex forms of relational spirituality (Sandage & Moe, 2013). In contrast to the themes of spiritual dwelling, home, and abode, Eliade (1959) described the theme of spiritual seeking as *passage* and noted "human existence gains completion through a series of 'passage rites'" (p. 181); that is, passing from one mode of being to another. In many religious and cultural narratives, this process of spiritual passage may be symbolized by crossing a bridge, entering a narrow gate, or going on a sacred journey or quest. Each requires the courage to leave one's familiar dwelling places to venture into unknown territory even if that exploration involves wrestling with a deeper understanding of one's own spiritual or religious tradition.

In contrast to conserving forms of spiritual and religious coping, Pargament (2007) described the transforming types of spiritual and religious coping as involving seeking changes in the place or the character of the sacred in a person's life, or pathways employed in pursuit of the sacred (see also Sperry, 2012). A large body of literature in the empirical psychology of religion has compared and contrasted intrinsic and quest orientations toward spirituality and religion, with intrinsic being oriented toward internalized commitments of dwelling and quest toward the exploration and tentativeness of seeking (Beck, 2006; Edwards, Hall, Slater, & Hill, 2011; Hood, Hill, & Spilka, 2018; Sandage, Hill, & Vaubel, 2011; Van Tongeren, Davis, Hook, & Johnson, 2016). Like spiritual dwelling, spiritual seeking is complex to define but we view it as a multidimensional construct including spiritual exploration, tolerating spiritual ambiguity, spiritual openness, and spiritual complexity (see Table 3.1).

Willingness to Explore

Spiritual seeking involves a willingness to search and engage in exploration of spiritual and existential questions and new ways of relating to the sacred, and this involves certain neurobiological processes. Panksepp and Biven (2012) described the neurobiology of what they call the *seeking system* in humans and animals, an emotional system involved in approach motivations and appetitive behaviors of exploration and foraging for needed resources. When the seeking system is aroused in humans via brain chemicals (e.g., dopamine, glutamate), there is an increased sense of curiosity about novelty in our environment and agency about searching for things we want or ways to escape potential problems. The subcortical seeking system in the ventral tegmental area informs medial frontal neocortical regions in humans to activate intellectual curiosity in making sense of how the world is organized. Overactivity of the seeking system might generate either narcissistic or manic overconfidence about impacting the world or repetitive and addictive pursuit of desired resources (e.g., substances). Underactivity of the seeking system can lead to depression and a lack of agency about finding what one desires, and this may result in part from habituation effects and a lack of novelty in our experiences of stimulation and reinforcement. In colloquial language, we say, "same old, same old."

Panksepp and Biven (2012) suggested "the seeking system might explain a great deal about the roots of religious belief" (p. 116) because it can promote ritualistic behaviors (e.g., prayer) that involve a sense of agency in impacting the world. This emotional system is crucial to the health and well-being of humans because we do periodically need to be activated in hopeful expectancy that we can find the resources we need through active seeking. In the New Testament, Jesus is quoted as saying "seek and you will find" (Luke 11:9). Panksepp and Biven described neurobiologically a part of what we mean by spiritual seeking, particularly the spiritual exploration dimension, or what we like to call "spiritual foraging."

Spiritual seeking maps onto the secure base function of attachment, which can ultimately lead to personal and relational growth (see Table 3.1). Attachment theory suggests humans need to internalize securely attached connections to caregivers and other attachment figures in order to feel confident in venturing out to explore their environment and unfamiliar territory. This is obviously very concrete for infants and young children; for example, in engaging with a new toy or crawling out of the lap of a caregiver into the grass to explore a field. But this kind of process continues throughout development, such as when an adult enters transitions of a new workplace, moves to a new town or dwelling place, or enters a different life-cycle phase. Attachment dynamics help us understand how a person's seeking system interacts with the anxiety and arousal often inherent in exploring the unfamiliar, as well as the variety of individual differences in relational dynamics related to seeking. We return to these issues below and also in Chapter 5 on attachment. The main point here is that, for some persons, spiritual seeking may become either highly anxious, compulsive, emotionally conflictual, or disorganized, and for other persons anxiety may shut down the seeking system altogether. For the seeking system to operate in optimal ways under stress and transition, relational experiences of secure attachment will be necessary to form differentiated and intersubjective capacities for secure base behavior.

Tolerating Ambiguity

Spiritual seeking also involves capacities to tolerate spiritual ambiguity, which are necessary to mentalize and explore new meanings or ways of relating with the sacred. Mentalization involves feeling secure enough to tolerate ambiguity and to be curious and explore personal meaning and the perspectives of others, and this fosters the developmental ability to construct coherent narratives of personal experience. Deficits in mentalization have been found in personality disorders and autism spectrum disorder, which involve difficulties in self–other awareness and perspective taking.

Mentalization-based therapy (MBT) is an approach to psychotherapy that integrates the dynamics we are calling dwelling and seeking. MBT is based on attachment theory and theory of mind research and uses relational regulation dynamics, intersubjective attunement, and an emphasis on curiosity to help clients develop a capacity to mentalize or effectively attend to the mental states of both self and others (Allen, Fonagy, & Bateman, 2008). Forms of relational spirituality that are low in mentalization can involve ways of relating to the sacred that are characterized by mental rigidity and dichotomous thinking, narcissism or egocentrism, and a lack of empathy or compassion. Mentalization has been described as a common factor in numerous approaches to psychotherapy; however, some therapies tend to emphasize individual self-awareness rather than the more complex self and other or intersubjective awareness involved in mentalization and mature forms of relational spirituality (Allen et al., 2008; Worthington & Sandage, 2016).

Growth in capacities to tolerate ambiguity is central to many forms of psychotherapy because progress is not always immediate, and change can often follow a nonlinear trajectory of feeling worse before clients feel better. Developmentally, this is because a certain way of organizing our understanding of ourselves and the world around us may be deconstructed before a new developmental form takes shape. The time between this deconstruction and formation of the new can be described as a liminal phase. Symbolic anthropologist Victor Turner (1969) described the liminal phase of ritual process in African tribal initiations as a kind of deconstructed "between-state." In liminality, the person is not the same as before, but they have not yet crossed the threshold into transformed identity and meaning. Spiritual and religious traditions often use narratives and metaphors of a descent into a dark passageway or a dark container to depict this liminal phase of the spiritual transformation process (Frankel, 2003; Shults & Sandage, 2006). There is the loss of familiar ways of relating to the sacred, which 16th-century Spanish mystic and Carmelite friar Saint John of the Cross (ca. 1578/1990) depicted in *Dark Night of the Soul*. The Jonah story in the Hebrew Bible offers what some see as an archetypal version of this liminal process, with Jonah running from God and avoiding certain spiritual dilemmas until he ends up going underwater to be swallowed by a sea beast, with the "belly of the whale" becoming the container of his spiritual transformation.

Parallel to the concept of liminality in ritual process, Hager (1992) used the metaphor of "gestation states" (p. 379) in psychotherapy to describe disruptive or chaotic states in clients who may be struggling with ambiguity early in the process of developmental reorganization. He explained:

[these particular] Client chaotic states are not due to resistance, regression, psychosis or borderline states, mystifying therapist communications, or organic conditions (e.g., fatigue, intoxication), they represent developmental bridges between former constructions of reality and modified versions that have not yet crystallized. In growth, the individual's organization of experience (Atwood & Stolorow, 1984) becomes temporarily relaxed as the person works preconsciously to pull together a new order. Thus these chaotic states are referred to here as gestation states, for they stand as periods of incubation out of which emerge new syntheses and directions for living. (p. 379)

We say more in Chapter 6 about how therapists can respond to client seeking and gestation based on our model, but Hager (1992) made the valuable point that therapists might seek to recognize gestation states when clients go silent while seeming to contemplate or mentally scan for something just out of reach, express confusion in trying to articulate a new goal or insight, or use transition metaphors (e.g., bridges, feeling lost, searching through a tunnel, ice breaking up) to depict a reorganization process underway. Hager explained that "in gestational states, the client is working, preconsciously, to resolve conflicts and integrate previously warded off elements" (p. 380). Client transferences may intensify at this point, and we suggest this is due to limbic-based attachment dynamics that are necessary for the secure base of spiritual seeking. The therapist will need to tolerate ambiguity at this point and resist the urge to rescue or organize things for the client. Wise clinical strategies can include asking exploratory questions to help the client work "from the inside out" (p. 381) and offering brief comments that could help frame the process with the client (rather than long interpretations). We agree with Hager that the therapist will need faith "that the client will eventually find light at the end of the tunnel" (p. 382), but this is best communicated nonverbally. This form of "faith" is a core capacity of relational spirituality we must develop and periodically rediscover as therapists and emerges from our own respect for the value and potential benefit of spiritual seeking.

Certain psychological and spiritual traditions agree that developmental growth can emerge out of losing familiar and cherished understandings of self and the sacred. Jones (2002) insightfully integrated apophatic, or deidealizing forms of relating to the sacred through the ambiguous negation of unknowing (the "via negativa," p. 108), with psychoanalytic insights about the need to face and process losses of our earlier idealizations. Many spiritual and psychological writers agree on the developmental need to enter dark empty spaces through spiritual seeking and to surrender to the limits of our human understanding in order to grow into relational maturity (Sperry, 2012). This does not necessarily mean permanently losing all relation to the sacred, as Freud seemed to suggest, but an unknowing and losing that transforms spiritual grandiosity and can lead to a more differentiated form of relational spirituality (Paine, Jankowski, & Sandage, 2016; Shults & Sandage, 2006). A longitudinal study of Christian seminary students found increases in measures of both dwelling and seeking over the course of their training, suggesting many students were working to balance these dialectical aspects of spiritual development (Williamson & Sandage, 2009).

Experiences of trauma and suffering involve ambiguities of meaning and may activate the liminal, gestation processes we associate with spiritual seeking. There is empirical evidence that exposure to tragedy is associated with higher levels of quest religiosity or a tendency to engage existential and religious questions (Krauss & Flaherty, 2001). However, it is obvious that trauma and suffering do not automatically increase spiritual seeking or conscious exploration of existential questions. In fact, traumatic experiences can produce pulls toward emotional numbing but also levels of anxiety that prevent conscious spiritual seeking with considerable energy focused on trying to regain a sense of security. A person needs to be able to tolerate ambiguities of meaning and certain levels of cognitive and emotional dissonance to engage in seeking, and preoccupation with emotional or physical survival may overwhelm capacities for spiritual seeking. There may be powerful emotional and relational pulls to close down questioning or seeking and to either avoid the questions or simply try to return to former understandings. Those with personalities involving a strong need for epistemological closure may also have difficulty engaging in spiritual seeking.

Openness to New Meanings

Therefore, spiritual seeking necessitates a level of psychological and spiritual openness and further cultivates openness to new meaning and new ways of relating to the sacred. In systemic terms, this is an open-system (as opposed to closed-system) approach to spirituality with a willingness to receive new inputs of information and new perspectives that challenge one's prior system of self-organization. Psychological flexibility has been associated with both health and the resilience to cope with adversity (Kashdan & Rottenberg, 2010), and we believe flexibility and openness are important aspects of spiritual resilience. As suggested earlier, individuals from highly enmeshed families or religious systems may have considerable anxiety about the relational implications of spiritual seeking that could result in conflicts with one's family or spiritual community. A study with undergraduates found students' level of triangulation in their families was related to less existential and religious questing, supporting this idea that relational anxieties and conflict might limit a young adult's emotional freedom to differentiate by spiritual seeking (Heiden-Rootes, Jankowski, & Sandage, 2010).

Spiritual seeking can also foster openness to diversity and relating effectively across social and religious differences (i.e., with outgroup members). Those high in spiritual seeking tend to view the human community in broader terms, recognizing differences but feeling less need for homogeneity in their relationships than those low in spiritual seeking. Kimball and colleagues found longitudinal evidence that ongoing spiritual seeking actually predicted the development of a communal orientation to spirituality among recent graduates of a Christian college, whereas students lower in seeking tended to develop a more personally focused spirituality (Kimball, Cook, Boyatzis, & Leonard, 2016). Measures of spiritual seeking or questing have also been positively associated with intercultural competence (Sandage & Harden, 2011) and fair and positive attitudes toward religious outgroup members (Beck, 2006; Van Tongeren, Hakim, et al., 2016). These findings are consistent with our RSM that secure-base forms of spiritual seeking can be part of developmental growth in relational complexity and maturity.

Growth in Complexity and Maturity

Ultimately, spiritual seeking may lead to growth in spiritual complexity and maturity. Complexity can be understood in various ways, but we have in mind the ways open systems can develop and flexibly adapt to new challenges through spiritual emergence—new and more differentiated forms of systemic reorganization of a person's relational spirituality (Albright, 2006). Complexity theory and developmental systems theory (Gelo & Salvatore, 2016) both suggest that transformations into greater dynamic complexification of a system unfold through nonlinear processes and happen when neither order nor chaos dominate; in other words, the liminal conditions Turner described. Thus, spiritual seeking is likely related to ways most spiritual and religious traditions offer a vision of spiritual maturity that is more complex than found among spiritual novices or beginners. Traditions will define this complexity or maturity in differing ways, and in the chapters that follow we unpack to our own view of relational spirituality maturity centered around the developmental capacities for secure attachment, differentiation of self, and intersubjectivity we described in Chapter 2. But a key issue is that spiritual complexity and maturity will involve integrating the dialectical processes of spiritual dwelling and seeking.

In the clinical contexts of working with extremes of suffering and trauma, this will include several complex dynamics that can be related to *wisdom* (Baltes & Smith, 2008; Shults & Sandage, 2006): (a) facing the ambiguity of existential questions and eventually coming to some internalized commitments (which may change over time); (b) accepting with humility certain human limitations (finitude), such as limitations in our capacities to know and to care for ourselves without help from others; and (c) understanding and valuing the realities of human differences and differing social contexts that will lead others to alternative forms of relational spirituality. Healthy and adaptive forms of complexity should also help people take necessary action to cope with suffering or to make life decisions. There will be a reflective ability to hold paradoxes and to "cast one's bread upon the water," a metaphor used by Qohelet (pseudonym for the author) in the Jewish wisdom book of Ecclesiastes to describe taking risks in living life despite the existential realities of death and loss.

An important tenet of the RSM is that spiritual well-being and spiritual maturity are different goals that form a complex relationship (Shults &

Sandage, 2006; Worthington & Sandage, 2016). This is similar to the ways that psychological well-being and psychological maturity can be differentiated (McAdams, 2006). Psychological and spiritual well-being can, in some cases, indicate use of primitive defense mechanisms or positive illusions about oneself and the world that lack depth and complexity. A person might feel happy or satisfied with their spirituality or sense of self while remaining relatively unaware of their personal impact on those around them or wider realities of suffering in the world. Based on our RSM, we suggest that both psychological and spiritual maturity involve well-developed capacities for relational attunement and self-awareness along with skills in emotional regulation, empathy, and diversity competence. These mature psychological and spiritual capacities are conducive to cultivating and regaining a sense of authentic well-being while also facing pain (Bailey et al., 2016) and tolerating suffering needed for growth, which Schnarch (2009) called "meaningful endurance" (p. 72). We recognize that experiences of suffering do not automatically lead to complexity or spiritual maturity, but spiritual maturity cannot be developed without some level of suffering, struggle, and spiritual seeking that facilitates wisdom, humility, and compassion for the suffering of others.

Although we are pointing to the benefits of spiritual complexity, we also affirm there can be a healthy simplicity to well-developed spirituality. Ricoeur (1967) referred to a "second naivete" (p. 358) in which persons return to a form dwelling with symbols and narratives from their tradition after a period of critical reflection and gaining some distance from earlier, precritical understandings. Fowler (1995) related this second naivete to a mature, conjunctive stage of faith development in which adults may regain "appreciation for the primitive stories . . . and beautiful truths" they lost during times of critical reflection and questioning (McAdams, 1993, pp. 183–184). McAdams (1993) noted that the spiritual simplicity of a second naivete can be held in an ironic way within a broader awareness of the complexity and paradoxes in life and the ability to navigate dialectical tensions within spirituality (e.g., faith and doubt, law and grace, justice and compassion). This second naivete is consistent with the aspects of wisdom we described above and the cognitive capacity to appreciate symbolic aspects of spirituality.

SPIRITUAL STRUGGLES

Spiritual struggles are another key dimension of the RSM and refer to relational spirituality dynamics that generate distress or conflict. Hathaway and colleagues noted that mental health problems can, in some cases, lead to clinically significant religious/spiritual impairment, defined as "a reduced ability to perform religious/spiritual activities, achieve religious/spiritual goals, or experience religious/spiritual states because of a psychological disorder" (Hathaway, Scott, & Garver, 2004, p. 97). For example, individuals who suffer from attention-deficit/hyperactivity disorder may struggle with "spiritual focus, socialization into religious traditions, internalization of faith" (p. 98) or other forms of clinically significant religious/spiritual impairment. This suggests clinicians should go beyond the assessment of the impact of mental health symptoms on social and occupational functioning to also consider religious/spiritual impairment, which could hinder important dimensions of life for clients who value spirituality and religion.

While Hathaway has considered the impact of mental disorders on religious/spiritual functioning, Exline, Pargament, Grubbs, and Yali (2014) considered the opposite sequence—religious and spiritual struggles impacting mental health functioning (see also Peteet, 2010, on spiritual struggles and depression). Their program of research has investigated ways religious and spiritual struggles can "become a focus of negative thoughts or emotions, concern or conflict" (p. 208). Studies have shown religious and spiritual struggles are common (Bryant & Astin, 2008; Nielsen, 1998). Exline's research has identified a set of six different religious and spiritual struggles with an associated measure (note that we use the shorter term *spiritual struggle* to reference struggles in relational spirituality). *Divine Struggles* involve negative relational dynamics with a deity; for example, feeling angry at God. *Demonic struggles* involve feeling attacked or persecuted by the devil or evil spirits as the cause of illness, trauma, or other negative events. *Morality struggles* involve feelings of shame or guilt related to a failure to follow certain spiritual or religious values and principles. *Doubt-related struggles* involve distress related to doubts about one's spiritual or religious beliefs. *Ultimate meaning struggles* involve existential struggles or conflicts related to a loss or absence of ultimate meaning in life. *Interpersonal struggles* in this context refer to conflicts or difficulties related to spiritual or religious issues in important personal relationships or relationships with larger systems (e.g., a religious congregation). This model of religious and spiritual struggles does not have a specific category for being the victim of religious bigotry, discrimination, or microaggressions, but such experiences of religious oppression could lead to any of the struggles above or a combination thereof (Sandage, Bell, Moon, & Ruffing, 2019).

Spiritual struggles may generate differing levels of distress, but they sometimes contribute to clinical levels of psychosocial and spiritual impairment. Measures of spiritual struggle have been associated empirically with a wide range of emotional and mental health problems, including depression, anxiety, anger, body image concerns, compensatory behaviors related to eating (e.g., purging), loneliness, moral injury, suicidal ideation, reduced immune functioning, reduced life satisfaction and well-being, and elevated mortality rates (Evans et al., 2018; Exline, Homolka, & Harriott, 2016; Exline et al., 2014; Pargament, Koenig, Tarakeshwar, & Hahn, 2001; Rosmarin, Bigda-Peyton, Öngur, Pargament, & Björgvinsson, 2013; Weber & Pargament, 2014; Wilt, Grubbs, Exline, & Pargament, 2016). Spiritual struggles have also been linked to posttraumatic stress disorder (PTSD) symptoms in several trauma-exposed samples (see Feder et al., 2013; Wortmann, Park, & Edmondson, 2011), and trauma survivors reporting spiritual struggles have demonstrated greater PTSD symptom severity than survivors not reporting spiritual struggles (Harris et al., 2012). Spiritual struggles have also mediated (partially or fully) the impact of trauma on moral injury and PTSD symptoms (Evans et al., 2018; Wortmann et al., 2011), suggesting that spiritual struggles are an indicator of distress in the process of making meaning of suffering and coping in response to traumatic events (Park et al., 2017).

The *Diagnostic and Statistical Manual of Mental Disorders* (5th ed.; *DSM–5*; American Psychiatric Association, 2013) does include a diagnostic code for *Religious or spiritual problems* (Z65.8) for use when it is determined that a focus of clinical treatment will be struggles related to the religion or spirituality of a client. Examples from the *DSM–5* include problems related to questioning or loss of faith, conversion to new religious/spiritual beliefs, and questioning values not necessarily part of organized religion. However, as suggested above, these kinds of spiritual and religious questioning or change processes can often represent cycles of spiritual seeking that are common experiences within psychological and spiritual development. Clinicians need to assess and understand the larger developmental context of a client's spiritual struggles, which might potentiate spiritual transformation with support and assistance in making sense of questioning and adjusting to changes that are unfolding (Pargament, Murray-Swank, Magyar, & Ano, 2005; Wilt et al., 2016; Worthington & Sandage, 2016). At the same time, even if a client's spiritual struggles are combined with seeking and developmental changes, we should not underestimate the potential for emotional distress and should assess the impact on the client's overall psychosocial functioning. Spiritual struggles also typically unfold in a relational context, and it is important to understand the relational and social impact of these struggles for a client.

Authentically expressing spiritual struggles is more normative in some traditions than in others. For example, A. B. Cohen and Johnson (2017; see also L. Miller, 2016; Silverman, Johnson, & Cohen, 2016) noted that lament (authentic spiritual complaint) is a valued part of Jewish spirituality. Whereas Exline and Pargament largely framed their understanding of spiritual struggles through a stress and coping perspective, our relational orientation leads us to assess the implicit relational dynamics of spiritual struggles and the impact of those struggles on relational spirituality (which we illustrate further in later chapters). In particular, we are concerned about ways in which spiritual struggles may represent (a) spiritually complicated losses, (b) dynamics of chronic spiritual or existential dysregulation, (c) spiritual internalization of negative relational introjects (e.g., contempt), or (d) barriers to ongoing development in relational spirituality due to underlying and long-term dynamics of fear, shame, mistrust, or hostility in relation to the sacred. In these relational forms, spiritual struggles may become chronic, circular patterns of negative relational spirituality which perpetuate further difficulties with coping and development (Park et al., 2017).

INITIAL CLINICAL RESEARCH FINDINGS

We investigated whether the relational spirituality constructs discussed previously in this chapter would show incremental validity in predicting psychosocial functioning among clients at our clinic over and above the effects of mental health symptoms. This is an important question because the medical model correlates mental health symptoms rather tightly with problems in psychosocial functioning without attention to spiritual or existential dynamics, and this forms the basis of mental health diagnoses and the determination of insurance-reimbursable mental health services in the United States. These connections between unidimensional interpretations of symptoms, the power–knowledge dynamics of diagnosis, and economic forces of health care access represent one fulfillment of Foucault's (1963/1994) sociopolitical concern about reductionism in modern medicine (described in Chapter 1; see also Ghaemi, 2010). This creates a need to demonstrate empirical evidence that relational spirituality is clinically relevant to actual client functioning.

Adult clients ($N = 107$) at our clinic who indicated spirituality or religion held some level of importance to them completed measures of spiritual well-being, spiritual struggles, spiritual seeking, psychological well-being, mental health symptoms, and psychosocial functioning (Sandage, Paine, Ruffing, et al., 2017). Spiritual well-being was chosen as an index of healthy spiritual dwelling in this study and operationalized using an inclusive, multidimensional measure that included personal, communal, environmental, and transcendental domains of well-being (Gomez & Fisher, 2003), and spiritual struggles was operationalized using the scale from Exline et al. (2014) mentioned above. Spiritual well-being and spiritual seeking were moderately positively correlated in this clinical sample, suggesting many clients were attempting to integrate or balance spiritual dwelling and seeking. Spiritual struggles showed a modest positive correlation with spiritual seeking and a modest negative correlation with spiritual well-being, which fits our understanding that spiritual struggles might be associated with increased spiritual seeking and reductions in spiritual well-being among some, but not all, persons. There can be complex patterns of association among these factors, necessitating careful clinical assessment.

On the key incremental validity questions, we found client ratings of their spiritual well-being (positively) and spiritual struggles (negatively) predicted psychosocial functioning over and above the statistical effects of mental health symptoms (see Figures 3.1 and 3.2). Spiritual well-being and psychological well-being both predicted unique variance in psychosocial functioning in the same statistical model, which means both dimensions of well-being were important to client functioning. Spiritual well-being cannot be reduced to the same thing as psychological well-being and vice versa. Overall, these results suggest relational spirituality influences on clients' psychosocial functioning would not be accounted for if we only considered their mental health symptoms and psychological well-being. If we neglect clinical assessment of relational spirituality, we would miss influential factors related to client

FIGURE 3.1. Spiritual and Psychological Well-Being Predict Psychosocial Functioning Over and Above Symptoms

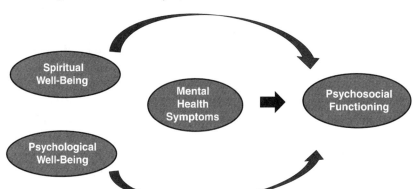

functioning, which is typically considered the bottom line in mental health treatment.

These are only preliminary cross-sectional findings in need of further replication over time, but these results with psychotherapy clients are consistent with other emerging research on the roles of spirituality and religion in mental health in community samples. For example, there is some evidence that measures of spiritual well-being and spiritual struggles can predict unique variance in psychological distress, well-being, and psychosocial outcomes among U.S. adults, in some cases over and above religiousness, personality (e.g., neuroticism), and other risk factors (Abu-Raiya, Pargament, Krause, & Ironson, 2015; Douglas, Jimenez, Lin, & Frisman, 2008; Hammermeister, Flint, Havens, & Peterson, 2001; Wilt et al., 2016).

DIALECTICS OF DWELLING AND SEEKING

To summarize, our RSM suggests that spiritual dwelling and seeking form a dialectical relationship that can shift at various points across the developmental life span depending on certain changes in stressors or contexts. It is challenging

FIGURE 3.2. Spiritual Struggles Predict Psychosocial Functioning Over and Above Symptoms

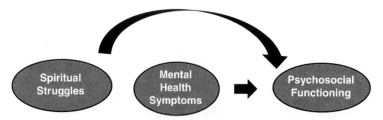

to balance spiritual dwelling and seeking since systems have homeostatic processes that pull for stability (dwelling) and make change (seeking) anxiety-provoking. Spiritually transformative changes can involve shifts in the balancing of dwelling and seeking, and we found some empirical support for this in graduate student samples (Sandage, Hill, & Vaubel, 2011; Sandage, Jankowski, & Link, 2010). Over time, it is possible for individuals and larger systems to integrate capacities for spiritual dwelling and seeking (Bailey et al., 2016; Cook, Kimball, Leonard, & Boyatzis, 2014; Kimball et al., 2016), as depicted in this meditation from Howard Thurman in *Deep River*: "This is the greatest disclosure: there is at the heart of life a Heart . . . do not shrink from moving confidently out into choppy seas. Wade into the water, because God is troubling the water" (Thurman & Smith, 2006, p. 41). In attachment terms, we read this as a powerful relational spirituality invitation to trust in the sacred as both a safe haven ("a Heart") and a secure base for growth ("Wade into the water because God is troubling the water"). Using the language we develop further later, Thurman is describing the water as a spiritual crucible that is being stirred up or "troubled" by the benevolent power of God. He is obviously using language that fits African American Christian traditions, but many spiritual traditions speak to this dialectic of spiritual dwelling and seeking that is both *limbic* and *liminal*, holding and provoking of growth. Some therapists may tend to think spiritual and religious resources are useful to the extent they are comforting for clients, but it is important to remember that many traditions also depict this challenging, provoking, and transformative side of spirituality (Pargament, 2007).

We have been struck that many other theorists have articulated related dialectical themes that have informed our thinking about dwelling and seeking (see Table 3.2). We are not saying these other dialectical perspectives are synonymous with dwelling and seeking, which would be unfair to those theorists. But we do want to communicate our appreciation and briefly draw attention here to some of the dialectical wisdom from authors referenced in various parts of this book, and encourage readers to become familiar with these works. We already discussed Tuan's (1977) dialectic of place and space.

TABLE 3.2. Other Dialectics Related to Themes of Dwelling and Seeking

Dialectical theme	Reference
Place and space	Tuan (1977)
Cosmos and chaos	Eliade (1959)
Conserving and transforming functions of religion	Pargament (2007)
Safety and adventure	Mitchell (2002)
Pacing and leading	Maddock & Larson (2004)
Stability and growth cycles in couples	Schnarch (1997)
Acceptance and change	Linehan (1993)
Communion and agency	Bakan (1966)
Union and separation	Rank (1978)
Integration and differentiation	Kegan (1994)

Eliade (1959) held up the archetypal spiritual themes of cosmos and chaos. Cosmos is the world we inhabit (dwelling) which is sanctified by sacred traditions, and everything outside that sanctified environment is chaotic space which is anxiety-provoking and both potentially dangerous and spiritually transformative (if one survives the chaos through seeking).

Bakan's (1966) classic work *The Duality of Human Existence* put forward the dialectic of communion and agency as two fundamental human modalities or motivations, and Bakan's work went on to influence a large body of psychological research. The pull toward communion is to connect or dwell with others in a larger whole of cooperative relations, whereas agency involves the pull toward self-assertion, individuation, and self-efficacy. Rank (1978) similarly described a developmental dialectic of the human desires for, and fears of, both union and separation. The pull toward union or merger activates existential fears of death and the pull toward individuality and separation involves the fear of living. Mitchell's (2002) psychoanalytic work on romantic love described the human desires for both safety and adventure, a sense of home and the freedom of escape. He noted the "archetypal dark side to the sense of home . . . homes turn into prisons; enclosures become confinements" (p. 37). He theorized the following:

> [Safety and adventure are] two fundamental, conflictual human needs: on the one hand, a need for grounding that feels completely known and predictable, a reliable anchoring, a framework, as Erich Fromm put it, for "orientation and devotion"; on the other hand, a longing to break out of established and familiar patterns, to step over boundaries, to encounter something unpredictable, awesome, or uncanny. Romantic passion emerges from the convergence of these two currents. (p. 39)

We would draw the parallel that healthy relational spirituality often emerges from the convergence of these two currents—safety and adventure, dwelling and seeking. Several clinical theorists have described dialectics related to stability and change. Maddock and Larson (2004; Worthington & Sandage, 2016) applied the dialectic of pacing and leading from Eriksonian hypnosis to more general relational processes in psychotherapy. Pacing involves dwelling with or embodied attunement to a client's behavior and concerns through empathy, reflection, validation, using the client's language and terminology, and even mirroring physical posture and emotional intensity. Leading involves offering new inputs into a client system to prompt seeking, such as suggesting a reframe, changing the focus of discussion or challenging a client's perspective, or altering one's physical position and intensity in the room. Lead moves prior to careful pacing tend to be ineffective; thus we would say that dwelling needs to precede seeking. Some clients need considerable pacing or dwelling with a well-attuned therapist over a long period of time before they will be open to seeking.

Linehan (2015) drew on Zen philosophy to describe the therapeutic value of the acceptance and change dialectic; that is, the need to accept oneself and the given realities of one's life and the value of working toward changing oneself and one's life. Linehan considered this "the most fundamental tension in any psychotherapy" (p. 5). Schnarch (1997, 2009) has described stability and growth cycles in couples' relationships, which involves movement between dwelling within stable systemic patterns of relating and the periodic needs for anxiety-provoking growth cycles through seeking change (described further below). Kegan's (1980, 1982, 1994; Kegan & Lahey, 2009) unique and complex developmental theory combined dialectical emphases on inclusion and independence (or integration and differentiation) with an existential perspective on the ongoing need for stability and growth as part of "meaning-constitutive evolutionary activity" (1980, p. 407). Like these other theorists, Kegan highlighted the relation between integration with others in specific ways of relating to the world and the periodic need for developmental change.

CRUCIBLE PROCESSES OF TRANSFORMATION

The crucible is a metaphor of intensification and containment that we use in the RSM to reference the process of transformative changes in dwelling and seeking in psychotherapy. Earlier versions of this model have been described in other publications (Sandage, Bell, Moon, & Ruffing, 2019; Sandage, Jensen, & Jass, 2008; Sandage & Shults, 2007; Shults & Sandage, 2006; Worthington & Sandage, 2016). By transformative change, we mean what systems theorists call *second-order change*, or changing the ways an individual or relational system operates in terms of goals, values, and ways of relating. Numerous clinical and spiritual writers have invoked images of crucibles, furnaces, or melting pots to depict a container as a kind of symbolic dwelling place that holds a heat-filled intensification process that transforms base metals into precious ones as an analogy to the stressful seeking process of human transformation. Saint John of the Cross (ca. 1578/1990) portrayed the *dark night of the soul—* a stressful developmental process of spiritual dryness and darkness leading to transformation—as a purifying "furnace, like gold in a crucible" (p. 107). Jewish Hasidic Rabbi Levi Yitzchok (1740–1809) described "the divine crucible of *ayin*," with *ayin* representing the liminal dynamic of divine nothingness out of which the world is continually repaired and re-recreated (Frankel, 2003, p. 60). The *Jap Ji* is a collection of Sikh holy scriptures attributed to Guru Nãnak, (1469–1539) that also includes the crucible as a metaphor of liminality and spiritual transformation within the fires of the blacksmith's workshop ("smithy" and "forge"; Sundararajan & Mukerji, 1997, p. 558; also Singh, 2005):

> Let smithy be the continence, patience the goldsmith.
> Let anvil be wisdom; knowledge the hammer.
> Let bellows be divine fear and fire be inner control and heat;
> On the crucible of divine love, let the ambrosial gold flow;
> In this True mint forge the transcendent word.
> Such fulfillment comes to those blessed with the Gaze;
> Says Nãnak, happy are those who are gazed upon by the Divine. (Sundararajan
> & Mukerji, 1997, p. 558)

Carl Jung (1944/1953) may have been the first psychotherapist to use the crucible metaphor in his work drawing parallels between the ancient practice of alchemy and the individuating processes of psychospiritual change, noting that alchemy "blended empirical science and mystical philosophy" (p. 228). Jung's text is surrounded by ancient drawings and artwork showing crucible-like images—round or egg-shaped sealed vessels, melting furnaces, or a sacred *vas*—as symbolic containers of dark space to receive psychological and spiritual projections of the unconscious and to hold intense chemical transformations. This crucible metaphor for the change process points to the crucial resiliency and nonreactivity of the container (or crucible). Crucibles or containers with melting points lower than the chemical reaction inside will crack under pressure and spill out the potential transformative process (Schnarch, 1991), which is why the anxiety tolerance or characterological formation of a psychotherapist or spiritual healer is so critical to their capacity to help relationally contain the process of transformation (Moore, 2001). We resonate with Jung's effort to integrate symbolism, science, and spirituality around crucible themes.

Crucible as Therapeutic Process

Napier and Whitaker's (1978) classic work *The Family Crucible* portrayed family therapy as a crucible-like process, "a boiling cauldron of feeling" contained in the relational matrix of the family (p. 10). They described the family's need to be able to trust that the therapist can handle the stressful process of change and is strong enough to give a "shape, a form, a discipline of sorts" (p. 11) to the process, with families even unconsciously presenting the therapist with certain tests of this in the early phases of therapy. Napier and Whitaker's application of the crucible metaphor to family therapy registered the view that therapists need more than great insight and technical skill, but also the personal formation (or self of the therapist) capacity to relate wisely and flexibly with client systems amidst the anxious push and pull of the crucible tensions in therapy.

Several recent clinical theorists have also explicitly invoked the crucible metaphor to convey the roles of relational tension and conflict in generating opportunities for developmental growth in psychotherapy (David Schnarch, Jeremey Safran, David Wallin, and Steven Cooper). These theorists have articulated some overlapping and some unique understandings of crucible processes in psychotherapy, and we will draw key relational spirituality themes from each theorist for an integrative RSM approach to crucible processes (see Table 3.3).

Schnarch (1991; also see 1997, 2009) used an understanding similar to Jung's in defining a crucible as a "resilient vessel in which metamorphic processes occur" (p. xv) and applying this image to his differentiation-based crucible model of couple and sex therapy. Schnarch focuses on the ways that intimate relationships involve a systemic balancing of cycles of stability and growth. Relational stability involves familiar forms of relating, which can

TABLE 3.3. Key Clinical Theorists Describing Crucible Processes in Psychotherapy

Theorist	Crucible emphases	Relational spirituality dynamics
Schnarch	Self-confrontation	Integrity and justice
	Courage to grow	
Safran	Rupture and repair	Grace and compassion
	Optimal disillusionment	
Wallin	Deconstruction and new construction of attachment	Awareness of awareness
	Double helix: mindfulness and mentalization	
Cooper	Benevolent disruption	Hope
	Containment and spontaneity	

generate feelings of safety and security. However, Schnarch believes that stability will inevitably become dull, dissatisfying, or problematic at some point for one or both partners when growth becomes necessary, which offers striking parallels to St. John's dark night of the soul process. For couples, Schnarch (1997) described how this state of relational gridlock may eventually lead to a systemic destabilization and integrity crisis he calls "critical mass" (p. 338; see also Napier & Whitaker, 1978) in which one or both partners tolerate the anxiety that intensifies as crucibles of change take form in a transforming growth cycle. Schnarch's crucible emphasis was on the need for personal self-confrontation about one's own integrity and the courage to overcome internal resistance to growth. He invoked Jung's (Jung & Foote, 1976) statement "To become acquainted with oneself is a terrible shock" (p. 206) and highlighted the need for solid differentiation of self and personal agency to both stretch into growth and self-soothe the accompanying anxiety of change. Schnarch's tone in describing relational crucibles could be likened to religious prophetic traditions as he explains, "There is a place within each of us that recognizes the truth when we are confronted with it. That moment of recognition comes from the part that knows right from wrong and values justice" (Schnarch, 1997, p. 340).

In contrast to Schnarch's emphasis on the prophetic crucible themes of self-confrontation, personal agency, integrity, and justice, Safran focused on the therapist–client relationship as a crucible of developing capacities for repairing interpersonal ruptures or conflict and engaging in collaborative exploration, with the latter similar to our notion of seeking (Safran & Muran, 2000). In a subsequent article on agency, surrender, and grace, Safran (2016) advocated for the potential therapeutic value of surrendering to the *other-power* of grace and compassion as a dialectical counterpart to the common Western psychotherapy emphasis on *self-power* or agency. He described the ways many spiritual and religious traditions diagnose the human problem of feeling something is missing and what Balint (1979) called "a basic fault—

a fundamental sense of emptiness or basic lack of being" (p. 59). Safran noted that for some clients, the core challenge of the crucible of psychotherapy may be less about personal agency, self-validation, and justice and more oriented toward internal resistance to surrendering to dependence on another person and actually taking in relational experiences of grace and compassion. This is worked out, in part, by the therapist's dwelling-oriented attunement to ruptures in the relationship with the client combined with humble and empathic efforts at repair, which can help clients achieve a kind of "optimal disillusionment" with their therapist and an implicit encounter with interpersonal forgiveness (Safran & Muran, 2000, p. 99). This notion of certain crucibles of surrender in contrast to self-assertion requires awareness of gender, cultural, and other diversity factors that might impact whether a person has been socialized toward dependence or independence and the systemic influences on what has been "allowable."

Like Safran, Wallin (2007) focused on "the therapeutic relationship as a developmental crucible" (p. xii), one that can transform the client's "experience of internal and external reality" (p. 3). Wallin employed attachment theory to suggest the therapist's role is to help the client "deconstruct the attachment patterns of the past and to construct new ones in the present" (p. 3). Drawing on Buddhism, Wallin described psychotherapy as a crucible for healing emotional injuries to the self and the spiritual cultivation of mindfulness through relational help from another person's mind. He is among the few clinical writers to deeply integrate mindfulness and mentalization as partially overlapping and complementary ways of knowing and responding to experience with open presence, calling them "the double helix of psychological liberation" (p. 307). Wallin's double-helix metaphor is interesting to us in light of our RSM association of mindfulness primarily with spiritual dwelling and mentalization with spiritual seeking (though both constructs can involve aspects of dwelling and seeking). Wallin (2014) has disclosed his own psychospiritual autobiography as including both the intergenerational trauma of the Holocaust within his Jewish heritage and his spiritual encounter with "awareness of awareness itself" (p. 64) through mindfulness. For Wallin, the crucible of psychotherapy can potentially generate interpretive understanding (mentalization) and acceptance and awareness (mindfulness) through relational development.

S. H. Cooper (2000) also focused his use of the crucible metaphor on the relational dynamics between client and therapist, specifically the "crucible of transference and countertransference" (p. 138). His unique contribution to this discussion on psychotherapy crucibles is the theme of transference as hope and therapists as objects of hope who can instigate a "benevolent disruption" (p. 95) of old relational patterns and experiences. As an object of hope, the therapist may stir tension and longing in the client—the unconscious hope of a new and healthier relational experience. But, like many relational psychoanalysts, Cooper advised us to understand that hope is a challenging crucible because most of us have ambivalence about grieving over old objects and taking the risk of actually imagining and encountering hoped-for objects. Dwelling within old relational experiences may be painful or disappointing, but it may also offer the safety of familiarity whereas hopeful seeking of a new relational experience can feel quite dangerous.

S. H. Cooper (2000) also highlighted the dialectical contrast between containment functions of the therapist for the metabolization of affect, which we relate to the theme of dwelling, and expressive, spontaneous, and playful modes of relational improvisation by the therapist that prompt seeking (if not too overwhelming to the client). His model invites questions about how we as therapists hold the projected hopes of our clients in the crucible process, and also how we manage the rising and falling levels of our own hopefulness we experience internally about a given case or clinical practice, in general, as part of our own relational spirituality. Cooper's approach fits our RSM emphasis on the need to develop complex and mature forms of hope which can sustain hopefulness about the potential for change and growth along with realism about the existential processes of suffering and loss that are often a part of growth (Worthington & Sandage, 2016; see also Grace, 1994; West, 2004).

Crucible Dangers

We think this integrative, multidimensional approach to crucible processes in psychotherapy can assist in nuanced treatment planning by highlighting multiple therapeutic dynamics needed across differing client cases or differing points in a treatment process with the same client(s). However, we also want to be mindful of certain clinical dangers of uncritical therapist–client engagement in the relational intensity of crucible-like processes. For example, Schnarchian emphasis on inviting clients to self-confrontation may be too confrontive for some clients with unaddressed trauma histories or fragile psychological functioning. With respect to development, we could also question the therapeutic efficacy of inviting clients to self-confront if they do not have much sense of self-development. Similarly, repairing ruptures is an important therapeutic process, but some clients may benefit more from exerting agency and the space of difference from their therapists than engaging in repair. We need to balance support and challenge, connection and autonomy, in psychotherapy, and this kind of balanced case-by-case positioning will necessitate that clinicians have relationships with wise colleagues in the context of regular consultation to dialogue about positioning and diversity sensitivity in cases (see Chapter 11). The therapeutic balancing of challenge and support needs to be informed by awareness of various diversity and power dynamics in client–therapist relationships and the meanings those dynamics hold for negotiating and renegotiating a constructive therapeutic alliance.

Crucible processes can also be very taxing to clinicians, and so relational resources of dwelling for support, personal growth, and self-care are crucial to prevent vicarious trauma effects and burnout. We also believe ongoing healing and formative experiences through one's own crucibles of personal psychotherapy are crucial for becoming an effective steward of crucible processes as a therapist.

BALANCING SPIRITUAL DWELLING AND SEEKING

We will now attempt to provide an integrative understanding of the dynamics of spiritual dwelling and seeking within crucible processes of change. Worthington and Sandage (2016; see also Sandage, Jensen, & Jass, 2008; Sandage & Shults, 2007; Shults & Sandage, 2006) offered a symbolic depiction of the crucible process of spiritual transformation which serves to systemically and dialectically balance spiritual dwelling and seeking. Clearly, the psychological and spiritual processes of second-order change are too complex to visually depict as a figure in a book, and it is impossible to arrive at universal language that can apply across all traditions (W. R. Miller & C'de Baca, 2001). Nevertheless, we do find this figure to be a useful heuristic for our RSM, and we encourage readers to consider it in a symbolic rather than literal fashion.

The inner ring on the left side of Figure 3.3 represents the cycle of spiritual dwelling, which involves relating to the sacred in usual or familiar ways. Familiar does not necessarily mean healthy or securely attached, and could include distance, inconsistency, or avoidance or some form of spiritual bypass. Due to habituation effects or developmental and context life changes, it is inevitable that spiritual disappointment or complacency will set in over time for individuals. This might take the form of a reduced sense of spiritual well-being and vitality, or certain stressors or trauma may require individuals to seek new ways of relating to the sacred. The former ways of spiritual dwelling no longer work.

In this model, transformation starts with contemplation of change (Prochaska, Norcross, & DiClemente, 2007) and movement into the awakening pathway (depicted on the left side of Figure 3.3), which leads the person into the intensification of anxiety that comes with the cycle of spiritual seeking (outer ring). Spiritual traditions describe spiritual awakenings and transformations in many different ways (de Castro, 2017; Sandage & Moe, 2013; Starr, 2008), and the spiritual seeking that follows is often stressful and destabilizing of homeostasis while focusing attention on certain personal struggles and existential dilemmas. For example, a person might begin to wrestle with questions of meaning and the place of the sacred in their present suffering or prior traumatic experiences. As described previously, this could start as an existential or spiritual struggle that prompts seeking.

The cycle of spiritual seeking can be both enlivening and frightening. If a person's need for stability and safety exceeds their motivation to tolerate anxiety and ambiguity of seeking, they might resume familiar forms of spiritual dwelling to de-escalate the anxiety. In contrast, if the person continues in the spiritual seeking cycle they will enter liminality and what some contemplative

FIGURE 3.3. Spiritual Transformation: Balancing Spiritual Dwelling and Seeking

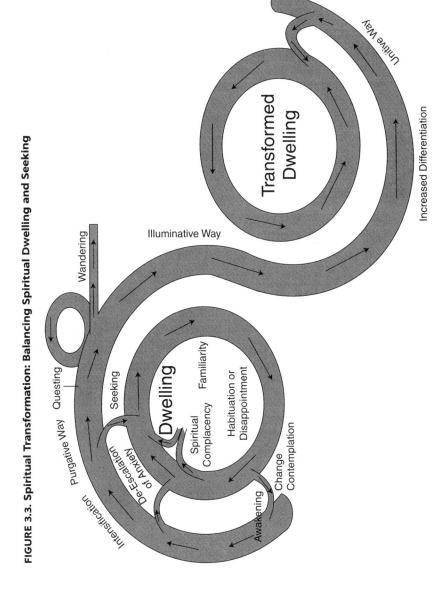

traditions have named the *purgative way*, which refers to an intensified existential and spiritual confrontation and focusing of attention on necessary changes that include a willingness to face painful realities and internal conflicts and a redirecting of values and priorities. Integrating Jewish mysticism and psychoanalysis, Starr (2008) described this kind of pull toward transformation as "a willingness, for the sake of discovering one's authentic being . . . to face the truth in all of its aspects" (p. 208).

The questing of the purgative way can potentiate an illumination of new and more differentiated understandings of self in relation to the sacred, often in response to the conflicts or existential dilemmas that activated the seeking. Some contemplative traditions have described this as the "illuminative way." For example, a person may shift from trying to prove their self-worth through various behaviors to a deeper sense of self-acceptance and spiritual security and compassion toward others. Illumination in response to episodes of significant suffering or trauma might take various forms, such as forgiveness of self or others or reduced despair, and increases in hopeful self-agency.

Spiritual seeking may immediately lead to illumination and spiritual transformation but could result in a period of spiritual wandering and arrested spiritual development. We illustrate this in Figure 3.3 in the top center portion. The term *spiritual wandering* could sound pejorative, but we mean it descriptively to reference a kind of spiritual moratorium period or avoidance of actively engaging spiritual and existential struggles through spiritual seeking. Suffering and trauma might overwhelm capacities to engage in spiritual seeking for some, and in such cases the term *wandering* is not meant to imply a casual approach to relational spirituality. Some will have had very negative or even oppressive experiences in spiritual and religious communities or other relational holding environments (e.g., psychotherapy) and may prefer an autonomous path focused on other pursuits or coping strategies. One subgroup here could also be highly narcissistic seekers with a limited capacity to attach or receive feedback and input from others, and this kind of avoidantly attached narcissism might also be a result of developmental trauma (see Chapter 4). Spiritual and religious minorities may have trouble finding helping professionals in their contexts whom they trust to understand their relational spirituality traditions and perspectives, so their "wandering" may be due to limited relational resources or systemic marginalization. Clinicians who work with clients returning from the "exile" of wandering may need high levels of differentiation, relational sensitivity, and patience to tolerate their ambivalence, guardedness, and mistrust.

The *unitive way*, or spiritual union, described by contemplative traditions is depicted in the lower right area of Figure 3.3 and results from the developmental growth in relational spirituality of the illuminative way. Spiritual traditions use differing language for the ultimate goals of transformation, such as enlightenment, and may sometimes orient toward different outcomes than is the typical focus of psychotherapy (Jennings, 2010). Psychotherapists might describe the unitive way psychologically as representing constructive changes in selfhood toward greater differentiation and accurate self-knowledge that can increase capacities for relational connection and intimacy (Starr, 2008). The winding path in Figure 3.3 is intended to depict the nonlinear movement of seeking cycles toward transformed spiritual dwelling characterized by greater spiritual maturity and enhanced capacities to cope with pain and anxiety; reflect upon suffering, meaning in life, and personal values and commitments; and relate effectively across cultural, spiritual, and other social differences. Mystical traditions are diverse but often associate transformative growth in spiritual union with love or an intimate connection or bond with all of reality (Dupré, 1989; Frankel, 2003).

When the transformation of self-organization occurs in the context of psychotherapy, we view the relational dynamics as key sources of gain that shape the container or holding environments for crucible processes. This requires therapists and other helping professionals who have the relational flexibility to cultivate and repair a constructive therapeutic alliance and who can resist the urges to "rescue or run away" when crucible dynamics heat up. We will further explore dynamics in the client-therapist alliance and the wider relational ecology of treatment that facilitates this approach to psychotherapy in Chapters 8, 9, 10, and 11.

CONCLUSION

We have drawn on various disciplines to elucidate some of the key constructs and dialectics of the RSM, including spiritual dwelling, spiritual seeking, spiritual struggles, and crucibles of transformation as they emerge in individual differences and the process of psychotherapy. Each of these constructs are multidimensional and can be clinically applied within a highly personalized case formulation that differs across clients. In Chapter 4, we describe our RSM understanding of the interrelated dynamics of anxiety, relational trauma, and suffering as they can factor into clinical practice.

4

Anxiety, Relational Trauma, and Suffering

Psychotherapy cannot remove ontological anxiety, because it cannot change the structure of finitude.

—P. TILLICH, *SYSTEMATIC THEOLOGY* (1973, P. 191)

Anxiety is one of the core topics in our relational spirituality model (RSM) of psychotherapy, but when combined with Tillich's existential statement above about the anxiety-removing limits of psychotherapy this may not seem like a strong selling point. Problems with anxiety are the most common reason people seek mental health treatment, and many therapeutic approaches have been shown to be empirically effective in reducing symptoms of anxiety. However, we locate the RSM within streams of psychodynamic, existential, and systemic psychotherapy traditions and the many spiritual, religious, and philosophical traditions that invite us to consider the depth functions of ontological anxiety in human experience even as we seek to alleviate suffering. It is good that we can reduce symptoms of anxiety, yet we believe diversity-sensitive treatment aimed at healing and growth requires that we also understand deeper dimensions of anxiety that can ultimately catalyze the relational spirituality meaning-reconstruction process for those who are suffering. In this chapter, we start by considering differing dynamics of anxiety and trauma and then move on to consider diverse existential themes and views of suffering than can inform RSM-based treatment.

http://dx.doi.org/10.1037/0000174-005
Relational Spirituality in Psychotherapy: Healing Suffering and Promoting Growth,
by S. J. Sandage, D. Rupert, G. S. Stavros, and N. G. Devor

DEPTH AND SURFACE VIEWS OF ANXIETY

The *Diagnostic and Statistical Manual of Mental Disorders* (5th ed.; *DSM–5*; American Psychiatric Association, 2013) defines anxiety as "the apprehensive anticipation of future danger or misfortune accompanied by a feeling of worry, distress, and/or somatic symptoms of tension. The focus of anticipated danger may be internal or external" (p. 818). This definition closely connects anxiety to worry, distress, and symptomatology and shapes the dominant view in Western mental health systems that anxiety is pathological. The existential philosopher Soren Kierkegaard (1844/1980a) viewed anxiety much more broadly and deeply as ontologically rooted in human finitude and related anxiety to the German concept of *angst*, which implies dread of human vulnerability to existential realities such as loss, failure, and death. We would call this existential perspective a *depth view* of anxiety, and this view suggests that anxiety can be problematic but can also serve an important activating function in the discovery and construction of meaning related to ultimate concerns about life and death (Weems, Costa, Dehon, & Berman, 2004). Similarly, existential theologian Paul Tillich (1952) defined anxiety as awareness of finitude and suggested that the deepest ontological anxiety is about death, disintegration, or losing one's ontological structures in a fall into the nothingness of nonbeing. The quote by Tillich we use to open the chapter reflects the existential perspective that ontological anxiety about human finitude needs to be faced rather than denied in order to cultivate an integrated sense of meaning in the face of suffering and loss. Thus, psychotherapy cannot (and should not) alleviate all anxiety but can effectively reduce what Tillich called "neurotic" (p. 68) forms of anxiety that distract from awareness of deeper questions about the meaning of one's life.

Psychiatrist Irvin Yalom (1980) built on this existential tradition by suggesting that the symptoms of anxiety are related to ultimate existential concerns such as death, freedom, isolation, and meaninglessness; and he argued that psychotherapy can offer relationships to support individuals as they courageously grapple with these kinds of deep concerns and construct meaning in the midst of existential anxiety. From an existential perspective, human capacities for symbolic consciousness and awareness of biological finitude contribute to the psychological challenges and possibilities of reflecting on one's mortality and other sources of negation, which shapes the periodic collisions between existential issues and our culturally and religiously derived meaning frameworks (Sullivan, 2016). Depth perspectives on anxiety suggest trying to get "underneath" surface-level anxiety to understand existential concerns that are a natural part of human finitude.

Behaviorists in the field of psychology conflated anxiety with fear and suggested both have an identifiable cue (for a historical overview, see Barlow, 2002), which served to highlight the ways specific patterns of anxiety are learned through experiences of conditioning and reinforcement. This behavioral, and later cognitive behavioral, psychology tradition generally divorced symptoms of anxiety from any spiritual or existential meaning tied to human finitude and led to the scientific development and testing of specific interventions to reduce symptoms of anxiety. We call this a *surface view* of anxiety because the sole focus is the surface manifestation of embodied symptoms that perpetuate self-defeating patterns of behavior rather than any deeper existential or symbolic significance to anxiety. This approach has led to the development of multiple effective therapeutic interventions that have helped many people suffering from symptoms of anxiety. In fact, mindful awareness of embodied symptoms of anxiety is a key part of growth in capacities for self-regulating anxiety and other emotions (Barlow & Farchione, 2018; Boettscher, Sandage, Latin, & Barlow, 2019).

However, the personal meaning of a client's suffering and overall developmental trajectory is typically left unaddressed in surface approaches to anxiety. This is acceptable to some clients, but it does invite questions in cases like that of Sofia (see Chapter 1, this volume), with clients who are struggling with the meaning of their lives and contending with existential threats of nihilism. It may also help explain why symptom reduction may be temporary for some clients when a more holistic sense of a meaningful life is not developed and existential concerns reemerge. Tillich and the existentialists would say that once neurotic anxieties lessen, ontological anxieties about the fragile structures of finitude (i.e., losses, disappointments, failures, etc.) will eventually intensify and pull for the construction of a meaning system that can sustain self-esteem and motivate the person even in the face of those deeper threats to the human ego (i.e., their "symbolic structures of meaning and value"; see Sullivan, 2016, p. 47). Thus, we see a benefit in integrating clinical attention to both surface and depth perspectives on anxiety.

EXISTENTIAL FEELINGS

Ratcliffe (2008) offered a helpful distinction between emotional feelings and existential feelings in supporting the relevance of a depth perspective. The former relate to specific episodes and cues, as the behaviorists indicated, whereas existential feelings do not relate to anything specific but represent a background orientation or "how we find ourselves in the world" (p. 36). Ratcliffe explained:

> The world as a whole can sometimes appear unfamiliar, unreal, distant or close. It can be something that one feels apart from or at one with. One can feel in control of one's overall situation or overwhelmed by it. One can feel like a participant in the world or like a detached, estranged observer staring at objects that do not feel quite "there." Such relationships structure all experience. (p. 37)

Stephan (2012) built on this framework to suggest existential feelings can relate to self, the social environment, and the world at large. For example, one might generally feel dead inside or quite vibrant and alive (self), welcomed or rejected (social environment), at home or as a stranger (larger world).

It would be common for psychotherapists to view these dynamics as purely emotional or aspects of personality functioning; however, they connect to powerful existential themes and ultimate concerns related to our sense of dwelling and the security to engage in seeking (see Chapter 3). We return to these and other existential themes or *predicaments* below.

Existentialists have also used the term *angst* to reference these negative existential orientations that go beyond discrete feelings and specific anxieties and move into states of generalized insecurity or meaninglessness (Peteet, 2010; Sullivan, 2016). Angst could involve depressive feelings that one's life goals are empty or one's basic worldview system is faulty, and could also be located in the embodied self as basically defective, unworthy, shameful, or alone. From an existential perspective, feelings of angst may shape or mutually constitute perceptions of reality but can also arise from an awareness of actual sources of human negation, including natural processes of finitude and death but also social and systemic pathologies such as discrimination, bigotry, and exclusion. The dominant rationalistic framework in Western psychology tends to pathologize symptoms of angst as cognitive distortions, whereas our RSM starts with respecting the existential functions of anxiety, and we tend to assume angst is typically a reflection of genuine existential threat. This makes further sense when we also consider the relational functions of anxiety.

RELATIONAL FUNCTIONS OF ANXIETY

In addition to existential functions, anxiety can also serve relational functions. Systems theorists (e.g., Kerr & Bowen, 1988) and attachment theorists (e.g., Wallin, 2007) have argued that a key function of anxiety is to regulate the balancing of closeness and distance in relationships. Individual differences in personality influence how this plays out. When anxious, some people distance from others through emotional cutoff by ignoring and/or not thinking or caring about others. In contrast, some people cling to others through emotional fusion or enmeshment by trying to maintain constant closeness or sameness. Others oscillate between these relational strategies.

As interpersonal boundaries become porous or diffuse, anxiety can also become contagious or "an increasingly infectious agent" (Kerr & Bowen, 1988, p. 77) in relational systems. Tillich (1952) noted this relational dynamic, observing that "outbreaks of anxiety are always contagious" (p. 92). Some families, religious communities, or social organizations suffer from chronic anxiety—an ongoing anticipatory fear of what might happen next. While situational anxiety can be adaptive for dealing with certain stressors or threats and facing important issues, chronic anxiety is nonadaptive and typically involves a lack of flexibility in how a system copes with challenges. The anxiety-driven "immunity to change" in some systems (Kegan & Lahey, 2009, p. 37) results in a resistance to new information from outside the system that might interrupt maladaptive patterns of response and foster positive growth. Chronic anxiety in relational systems can also generate circular homeostatic loops that maintain stances of vigilance against perceived threats while interpreting feedback in ways that reinforce or even intensify anxiety.

Thus, in the RSM, we view anxiety as a dialectical phenomenon that is both stressful and potentially constructive. Much anxiety is unconscious and occurs at the cellular level to mobilize valuable immune functioning to protect against threats and maintain the stability of an organism or system (Kegan & Lahey, 2009; Kerr & Bowen, 1988). Overwhelming anxiety can lead to trauma (discussed below) and prove damaging to human well-being, whereas an optimal level of anxiety may be activating and contribute energy for facing important issues, conflicts, or facets of nonintegration and non-being (Tillich, 1952). If handled with a healthy balance of self-confrontation and emotional regulation in a supportive relational context, certain levels of anxiety can arouse or catalyze growth, creativity, and spiritual transformation (Sandage, Jensen, & Jass, 2008).

Given the possible constructive role of anxiety for relational spirituality and meaning-making, it will be helpful to examine the influence of anxiety on individual differences in relational dynamics during stress and transitions. When thinking about the dynamics of relational spirituality within a relational system (e.g., a couple, family, religious congregation, mental health clinic), it is useful to attend to the overall level of anxiety in the system and whether the system has been able to navigate successfully other recent change involving new perspectives. Some systems with high levels of anxiety will have rigid boundaries and be impermeable to new inputs, while other systems might be overly porous to a cacophony of new inputs and show limited capacities for integrative coherence.

As we have suggested at multiple points in this book, various forms of relational spirituality can serve to help defend against, buffer, or metabolize anxiety and suffering, but certain forms of relational spirituality can also become sources of anxiety and suffering. Our RSM posits that humans have needs for both dwelling and seeking, and that because these needs are complex, they must be integrated over time. When individuals struggle to develop healthy forms of dwelling and seeking, there are risks for disorientation (dwelling problem) and despair (seeking problem). Nietzsche (1887/1964; see also Reginster, 2009; Sullivan, 2016) said that nihilism or the severe absence of meaningful goal pursuit can result from the loss of either orienting values (disorientation) or of the belief in our own capacities to achieve those goals (despair). Mild levels of disorientation anxiety through the negation of our orienting beliefs, values, and worldview is a challenge to spiritual dwelling and may prompt attempts to recover our beliefs and/or connect with sources of orienting community. Moderate to severe disorientation anxiety may prompt either seeking behaviors, which may potentiate a spiritual transformation (Chapter 3), or some form of marginality, helplessness, or acting out that reflects existential feelings of nihilism and meaninglessness.

Despair anxiety is related to a loss of confidence in the self or the capacity to achieve one's goals. Rather than trying to return to sources of orienting community outside the self, despair anxiety can often promote the self-reflexivity and interiority of seeking in an attempt to understand these struggles and/or despondency toward larger social forces that do not seem to validate and support the person's goal quest (Sullivan, 2016). At manageable levels, despair anxiety may activate further spiritual–existential–religious–theological (SERT) exploration and efforts to transform societal structures, religious communities, and the like. But at extreme levels, despair anxiety generates feelings of meaninglessness and hopelessness, which could lead to self-harm or suicidality.

ASSESSMENT AND CLINICAL ENGAGEMENT OF ANXIETY

For the theoretical reasons outlined here, we view anxiety as a core human dynamic related to finitude and suffering that we want to assess and clinically engage in all cases. This starts by introducing the language of "anxiety" to clients and taking the dialectical stance of both normalizing realities of anxiety while remaining empathic to the distress anxiety can generate. We want to help clients become self-aware of how anxiety manifests for them as somatic, psychosocial, and ultimately existential and relational spirituality processes. Somatically, anxiety can be related to numerous physical symptoms, such as

- accelerated heart rate,
- accelerated breathing or shortness of breath,
- muscle tension in certain parts of the body,
- abdominal or digestive distress,
- physical shaking,
- numbness or sleepiness,
- choking sensations or difficulty swallowing,
- feeling dizzy or light-headed, and
- sweating.

It is important to help clients mindfully inhabit (or *dwell*) within their bodies to understand and begin to regulate their own anxiety. We also want to help clients identify psychosocial or relational stressors that tend to trigger their anxiety and help them begin to track patterns of how they respond and attempt to cope with these anxieties. We give particular attention to relational stances, beliefs, and practices in their coping processes. In relational modalities of treatment (couple, family, or group therapies), it can be particularly useful to draw out (i.e., differentiate) points of similarity and difference in anxiety processes (i.e., how anxieties manifest, how each individual attempts to cope, and what anxiety means). For example, a married couple shows a chronic pattern within which one spouse becomes anxious when feeling controlled or crowded by their partner's desire for closeness and responds by creating emotional and physical distance through work preoccupation. In complementary fashion, the other spouse becomes anxious in the face of her partner's emotional and physical distancing (perceived as abandonment) and responds with intensifying demands for more closeness, further escalating the anxiety and reactivity in the couple system.

This assessment of anxiety and related patterns can often present an opportunity to explore where clients may have learned these coping strategies, which probably proved adaptive in family of origin and other past situations but may not fit their current life contexts. Again, we want to take the dialectic stance of communicating respect for survival strategies clients have learned to make it through prior episodes of suffering while also inviting flexibility and openness to considering new relational strategies.

Embodied and relational themes of anxiety can often lead to understanding a client's implicit existential and relational spirituality dynamics. We discuss many clinically powerful existential and relational spirituality themes below, but a key point here is to recognize that many clients have not previously been able to consistently mentalize or reflect on their anxieties in their prior relationships. Thus, key relationships that might provide the safety and strength to hold clients during crucible processes related to existential and spiritual dilemmas (see Chapter 3) have not been able to do so. This often has the effect of freezing the processes of meaning-making and relational spiritual development. And, this is also why our RSM suggests it is particularly important to assess how clients have handled or avoided transitions in life where processes of meaning-making and relational growth can be particularly stressful (e.g., birth or adoption of a child, leaving home, moving to a new place, marriage, divorce, death of a family member, loss of a job, retirement), since existential difficulties like this can become highly influential on internal working models of relationships, including relational spirituality.

DYNAMICS OF TRAUMA

When individuals and relational systems experience overwhelming levels of anxiety, it is traumatic. The *DSM–5* orientation toward trauma focuses on traumatic stressors or events, and a traumatic stressor is defined as "any event (or events) that may cause or threaten death, serious injury, or sexual violence to an individual, a close family member, or a close friend" (American Psychiatric Association, 2013, p. 830). The anxiety related to traumatic experiences can overpower a person's capacity to cope and to integrate such experiences into a coherent set of memories and narratives (Levine, 2008). Trauma expert Bessel van der Kolk (2014) put it succinctly: "Trauma, by definition, is unbearable and intolerable" (p. 1). Trauma has also been described symbolically and existentially as a timeless "black hole" (Pitman & Orr, 1990, p. 469) that has a psychic gravitational pull "within which the light of awareness, of peace, and of wholeness is absorbed" (Bloom, 2010, p. 210; see also van der Kolk & McFarlane, 2007).

The effects of trauma can include a range of conflicting symptoms, such as

- intrusive thoughts and memories,
- numbing or dissociation,
- constriction of affect and experience,
- inability to regulate affect and arousal,
- hypervigilance,
- problems with concentration,
- self-destructive behavior,
- feelings of detachment or estrangement from others,
- nightmares and sleep disturbance,
- chronic anger,
- feelings of helplessness,
- chronic pain,
- avoidance of symbolic reminders of trauma, and
- compulsion to reexperience aspects of the traumatic event.

Herman (2015) noted "the dialectic of trauma" (p. 2), which is represented in the various contrasting themes and symptoms related to intrusion and constriction, and hypervigilance and dissociation, as a person unconsciously tries to balance these opposing psychic forces in the absence of the integrative dynamics involved in healing. Trauma often instills a deep sense of shame or humiliation over the extreme helplessness and self-disappointment a traumatized person can experience during (or after) dis-integrating and overwhelming experiences that transcend their coping resources.

The language of "trauma" has become ubiquitous and expansive in both public and clinical discourse to a point that the crushing nature of traumatic experience can sometimes be trivialized. One of our clients, a survivor of a gang rape, was deeply offended by the title of Mark Epstein's (2013) book, *The Trauma of Everyday Life*, saying of the author, "He must not understand *real* trauma!" Traumatic symptoms that become clinically impairing of functioning for more than one month may represent posttraumatic stress disorder (PTSD; American Psychiatric Association, 2013). Actual experiences of clinical-level trauma may be more prevalent than is often recognized by laypersons, yet it is also important for clinicians to exercise clinical discipline in use of the language of trauma. It is worth noting that experiences of trauma for some individuals, families, and groups can become chronic, particularly in the context of systemic oppression (Tummala-Narra, 2016), so the symptoms of trauma may become less tied to events and more a part of daily life. For all these reasons, it can be challenging to find the most meaningful and accurate ways to use the language of trauma and to differentiate types and levels of intensity or chronicity.

Herman (2015) proposed a more severe diagnostic category of complex PTSD (C-PTSD), which can result from chronic or repeated traumatic experiences of abuse, neglect, exploitation, violence, entrapment, and other forms of repeated victimization. It is noteworthy that Herman's definition of C-PTSD has a decidedly relational orientation in that trauma is understood as most frequently experienced through relationships. C-PTSD is not yet an official diagnostic category in the *DSM* system. However, the World Health Organization Working Group on the Classification of Stress-Related Disorders has proposed including C-PTSD as a diagnostic category distinct from PTSD (Maercker & Perkonigg, 2013), and empirical evidence is accumulating to support that distinction (Cloitre, Garvert, Weiss, Carlson, & Bryant, 2014). C-PTSD is characterized by symptoms of PTSD but also more severe self-identity disturbance, relational impairment, and "loss of sustaining faith" or a "sense of hopelessness and despair" (Herman, 2015, p. 121), which speaks to our interests in the existential and spiritual dynamics of trauma. Research comparing C-PTSD and PTSD client profiles has found a longer duration of trauma exposure and higher levels of consistently negative self-identity (i.e., high levels of worthlessness and guilt), relational avoidance, reactive anger, feelings of emptiness, and overall impairment in the former.

Van der Kolk (2005, 2014) proposed the diagnostic category of *Developmental Trauma Disorder* to relate the idea of C-PTSD to the developmental impact of trauma on children, which impairs key aspects of healthy development such as affect regulation, interpersonal trust and collaboration, forming and executing plans and goals, and delaying gratification. He also briefly referenced the existential impact and notes these children "develop a view of the world that incorporates their betrayal and hurt. They expect the trauma to recur" (van der Kolk, 2005, pp. 406–407). He suggested they often have frozen reactions to the process of meaning-making and, in addition to help with affect regulation, these individuals need help "to re-awaken their curiosity and to explore their surroundings" (p. 408). In the language of the RSM, van der Kolk described the impact of developmental trauma on impaired dwelling *and* seeking.

Trauma Matrix

The perspectives above lead us to two key summary points in our RSM approach to psychotherapy. First, trauma is always existential. In addition to the physical and psychosocial aspects, trauma is always an existential process of responding to the ontological anxieties inherent in threats to existence, selfhood, and relational and spiritual security within the "trauma matrix" (Yansen, 2016, p. 70), a concept that refers to worldview assumptions used to filter experiences of trauma and existential threat (Sullivan, 2016). Janoff-Bulman (2002) suggested the core of human assumptive worlds include beliefs about self, the external world, and the relations between the two, and common pre-trauma assumptions often include "'the world is benevolent,' 'the world is meaningful,' and 'the self is worthy'" (p. 6). These assumptions are frequently shattered by trauma (at least temporarily).

Trauma can also arrest hope and freeze meaning-making, as noted by Levi and colleagues (2012): "When you undergo a trauma, you fall apart. . . .

It's the feeling that your hope has been arrested. . . . That you're stuck and can't build on it" (Levi, Liechtentritt, & Savaya, p. 1158). Traumatic experience can often dis-integrate the person or pull apart coherent meaning, identity, and holistic functioning. Trauma has been described as "an assault to the self" (Kerig & Becker, 2010, p. 24), and numerous theorists have noted the need to help clients deal with the existential and meaning-making aspects of trauma that can penetrate the core of personhood, identity, and basic beliefs about security in the world (Park, Currier, Harris, & Slattery, 2017; Rambo, 2010; Schnyder et al., 2015; van der Kolk & McFarlane, 2007). Nevertheless, the existential aspects of trauma generally receive very limited attention in clinical treatment literatures.

Second, the concept of a trauma matrix highlights the importance of diverse cultural, existential, spiritual, and communal meanings and coping processes related to trauma, anxiety, and suffering in differing social contexts. Yansen (2016) explained:

> Trauma is a process; it is created—shaped in the intersection of the extreme events, the individual/group realities, and the social contexts in which trauma arises—the *trauma matrix*. . . . As a consequence, different individuals and collectivities work through trauma in very different ways. (p. 70)

Reductionist clinical approaches to trauma tend to reduce trauma to the biological and psychological "levels." In contrast, the concept of a trauma matrix suggests the need for clinicians to seek to understand the interrelated dynamics of culture, religiosity, community, and other worldview systems of meaning involved in clients' experiences of coping with suffering and trauma. In describing collective trauma, Saul (2014) also pointed to the important differences in communal and institutional patterns and resources related to collective responses to trauma, which can impact suffering and resilience for generations. Chronic systemic problems such as poverty, racism, and other forms of oppression are often chronic traumatic stressors that can serve to perpetuate communal difficulties in trauma responses that go well beyond individual functioning.

Relational Trauma

The trauma matrix brings together collective, sociocultural dynamics of relationality and meaning-making in the process of suffering, yet interpersonal dynamics are also influential in trauma (Park et al., 2017). We have just referenced the existential dynamics of trauma, and our relational framework also leads us to focus on relational development dynamics associated with trauma or what is sometimes called *relational trauma*. While much discourse about trauma focuses on extreme trauma events or the chronicity of trauma, we are here referencing the relational dynamics that emerge and become ratified within the trauma matrix. Herman (2015) defined relational trauma as "violations of human connection" (p. 54), which can arise developmentally in relationships where a child or adult encounters dysregulating patterns that violate the safety and support of secure and trustworthy relationships (attachment), the healthy intimacy of being known and recognized (intersubjectivity), and warm curiosity and respect for differences in perspectives, values, and decisions (differentiation). Parts of the self may be ignored, attacked, or humiliated, and these can be experienced as threats to the existence of these self-states. Contingencies about vulnerability are communicated through interpersonal dynamics, such as an implicit rule in some family systems like "help will only be given if I admit I am defective" or "receiving support requires that I completely submit to your superior knowledge and value system." Some learn the only pathway to help is through personal agency, so a "solo survivor" script develops that jettisons turning to others for assistance.

Bromberg (2011), a leading theorist of the relational trauma perspective, suggested that "we look at trauma not as a special situation but as a continuum that commands our attention only when it disrupts or threatens to disrupt the continuity of self-experience" (p. 13). Developmental or relational trauma exists on a continuum (DeYoung, 2015) and is not to be equated with PTSD but frequently generates PTSD-level symptomatology. Two key clinical assessment questions about relational trauma are: (a) During times of powerful emotional and existential dysregulation in life, to what degree has the person experienced the healthy and responsive relational dynamics that cultivate mindfulness and mentalization? and, (b) When those relational resources have not been available, what relational strategies has the person learned to use for psychological, existential, spiritual, and physical survival? Bromberg went on to explain the developmental process of relational trauma this way:

> A person's core self—the self that is shaped by early attachment patterns—is defined by who the parental objects perceive him [sic] to be and deny him to be. That is, through relating to their child as though he is "such and such" and ignoring other aspects of him as if they don't exist, the parents "disconfirm" the relational existence of those aspects of the child's self that they perceptually dissociate. This makes the disconfirmed aspects of the child's self relationally nonnegotiable because the subjective experiences that organize those self-states can't be shared and compared communicatively, with how they appear in another mind. The main point is that "disconfirmation," because it is relationally non-negotiable, is traumatic by definition and I believe accounts for much of what we call developmental trauma, or as it's sometimes named, "relational trauma." (p. 57)

Bromberg's emphasis on the impact of the disconfirmation of relational existence on a developing sense of selfhood has profound implications for the developmental systems that impact relational spirituality and capacities for meaning-making. Schore (2018), another leading theorist of relational trauma, has emphasized the role of early attachment dynamics with parents and caregivers in developing capacities for affect regulation and right-brain symbolic processing of experience. Disorganized attachment experiences of abuse and neglect serve to cultivate relational trauma that is "affectively burnt in" (Schore, 2018, p. 245) to the developing right brain and shapes implicit relational expectations about dynamics like conflict, basic safety, repair, trust of others, and one's own "lovability." Relational trauma sets up a vicious loop of interpersonal neurobiology—the person does not feel secure in the world or in their connections to others, and their own relational style might contribute to a range of vulnerabilities to further suffering and trauma while also making it difficult for the person to take in new and more constructive relational experiences. The circular dynamics of relational trauma have powerful implications for existential and spiritual development and bring us back to the need to understand existential levels of anxiety and suffering (Rambo, 2010).

EXISTENTIAL THEMES OF ANXIETY AND SUFFERING

As suggested in the existential perspectives above, symptoms of anxiety emerge not just from surface-level fears but also deeper sources of existential threat related to death and finitude. As humans, we generally seek to maintain existential security primarily through meaning-making, relational attachments, and self-esteem (Sullivan, 2016), but these security systems for existential anxiety management will periodically break down in what Jaspers (1970) called *limit situations*. These are situations of existential dysregulation that rupture our taken-for-granted assumptions about our security, our worth, and our connection to the world (Loder, 1989). Awareness of death is the ultimate limit situation and challenges multiple forms of existential security about nonbeing (Tillich, 1952). We could say that death is the ultimate narcissistic injury or threat to self-esteem (Becker, 1973). Experimental studies of death anxiety in the field of terror management theory have shown that priming awareness of death can intensify a person's psychological investment in their cultural or religious beliefs and activate attempts to reinforce self-esteem, as Becker predicted, and these effects are sometimes delayed (Burke, Martens, & Faucher, 2010). In other words, experiences that prompt death awareness make mortality salient, and this can prompt psychological efforts to buffer existential anxiety by trying to reaffirm belief systems or self-esteem over the coming weeks and months. In some cases, particularly following trauma, those efforts may not work because of shattered assumptions or shame about the self, shame about key relationships, or even shame about one's larger community or social environment. From a terror management theory framework, psychopathology is thought to result, in part, from difficulties effectively buffering and managing the impact of existential anxieties.

Existential philosophy came to prominence in Western Europe following the trauma of World War II and strongly emphasized individualistic cultural themes, which is a limitation within much of the classic existential literature. Following Sullivan (2016), we prefer an intercultural perspective on existential themes that values attention to cultural differences, including more collectivistic forms of existential process (considered below). Theorists of Black existentialism, such as Fanon (1963, 1967), offer valuable contrasting insights to White existentialist authors for understanding the impact of racialized violence, colonization, and oppression in the complicated dynamics of human liberation and empowerment necessary for meaning and identity *re*-construction (Vereen, Wines, Lemberger-Truelove, Hannon, Howard, & Burt, 2017). Vereen et al. (2017) noted that Fanon emphasized the problem of existential deviation for Blacks where "all recognized notions of language, culture, and identity are imposed by the dominant culture" (p. 76) and that Black experience is too often "overdetermined from without" (Fanon, 1967, p. 116). Whereas individualistic forms of existentialism focus on individual suffering and flourishing, Black existentialists invite more social and communal understandings of both suffering and flourishing along with systemic deconstruction of barriers to enacting freedom. Thus, existential questioning is not only about individual subjective interiority but requires an awareness of intersubjective aspects of social and cultural identity (powell, 2012).

Existential themes are ubiquitous in the struggles described by psychotherapy clients. Table 4.1 depicts some taxonomies of existential themes or predicaments highlighted by existential theorists Paul Tillich (1952), Victor Frankl (1959), Irvin Yalom (1980), and Robert Neville (2014). A quick review of these themes shows points of convergence with Exline and colleagues' categories of spiritual and religious struggles reviewed in Chapter 3 (e.g., struggles with morality, meaning, the divine, interpersonal relations, and doubt), and with our research finding that spiritual and religious struggles predicted clients' psychosocial functioning over and above their mental health symptoms. This finding offers some support for the general thesis of existential theorists that certain ontological anxieties and ultimate concerns can often be latent or "depth" dynamics that influence psychological symptoms and functioning (and vice versa).

Tillich's (1952) existential taxonomy has also received empirical support in the research of Carl Weems (Weems, Costa, Dehon, & Berman, 2004), who validated a measure of existential anxiety based on Tillich's (1952) three dimensions of absolute concern (death, meaninglessness, condemnation) and their corresponding relative concerns (fate, emptiness, guilt). Weems and colleagues have found these existential concerns are so prevalent even among nonclinical adolescent and adult samples that they can be considered a "normative phenomenon" (p. 395) but are also correlated with struggles in identity development (S. L. Berman, Weems, & Stickle, 2006). Existential anxieties have also been found to be more salient following trauma and to be positively associated with PTSD symptoms (Chung, Chung, & Easthope, 2000; Pyszczynski,

TABLE 4.1. Existential Taxonomies

Tillich Concerns		Frankl	Yalom	Neville
Absolute	**Relative**	**Existential Themes**		
Death	Fate	Suffering	Death	Guilt
Meaninglessness	Emptiness	Guilt	Freedom	Disintegration
Condemnation	Guilt	Death	Isolation	Estrangement
			Meaninglessness	Destruction

Greenberg, & Solomon, 1999; Scott & Weems, 2013; Weems, Russell, Neill, Berman, & Scott, 2016).

How Existential Themes Can Emerge During Therapy

We suggest that existential themes often emerge in the process of psycho-therapy, although it can be easy to miss the existential dynamics of certain client struggles. For example, a client in couple therapy shows a recurrent pattern of dysregulation during certain interactions with her partner, typically following situations in which her partner is very late getting home without any communication (i.e., not responding to calls or texts). At a surface level, there are symptoms of physical and psychological anxiety and anger. Psycho-logically, this pattern could also be linked to the client's preoccupied attach-ment style and her fears of abandonment. But further mindful exploration by the therapist in collaboration with the client ("What else do you notice comes up for you in that situation?") eventually led the client to this awareness: "I guess I start to ask, 'What's the point!' What's the point!'" As the client recounted this, she was crying but also voicing anxious desperation or angst that seemed much deeper than the situation at hand. With further exploration, the client and therapist came to realize it reflected a kind of wrestling with despair about being connected to people one cannot control and could lose at any time. It was not total despair because the client was still subconsciously asking the question, albeit partially as a form of protest, in those situations. While anxiety-provoking and painful to tolerate, this client was voicing a profound and important existential question that has riddled humans for millennia—namely the meaningfulness of loving others given the unavoidable risks of loss.

Another client describes confusion, insecurity, and reactivity to coworkers in a new workplace. After unpacking the related feelings, thoughts, and embodied sensations, the client declares, "I don't know if I have a right to exist there." This existential feeling of angst is more general than the particular emotions or automatic thoughts and reflects a question about the nexus of justice, self-worth, and existence. As the only person of color in that particular area of the organization, there was a racial basis for the client's existential anxiety tied to larger systemic dynamics of racism in U.S. society and the client's prior personal experience of exclusion by Whites which Fanon (1967) called "existential deviation" (p. xviii). Importantly, further exploration revealed the client was implicitly asking the question of whether his coworkers thought he had a right to exist there, but he had also internalized racism in ways that caused him to be unsure about his own right to exist in certain social spaces. The fact that he was now conscious of and troubled by this existential ques-tion was a sign of developmental growth, yet he was confused about how to work with this question and new to the process of relating with others around this form of seeking. While the therapist was tempted to provide immediate reassurance of self-worth to the client, it became evident to both that the existential questions ran deeper, and the systemic realities were broader than could be quickly resolved through a single therapeutic statement.

Existential perspectives also tend to highlight "the dialectical nature of human psychological processes" (Sullivan, 2016, p. 8), which fits our dialectical emphasis within the RSM. For example, clinical and developmental theorists have described versions of the "twin terrors" in intimate human relationships—abandonment and engulfment—or the fear of losing a loved object and the fear of losing one's self through merger with another (see Alperin, 2001). Numerous existential theorists have pointed to a ubiquitous existential dialectic of anxiety and guilt or "uncertainty versus inadequacy" (Sullivan, 2016), and this can be related to the relational spirituality dilemmas of dwelling and seeking. When individuals maintain stable patterns of spiritual and interpersonal dwelling in communal bonds, there is a risk of periodically struggling with guilt over failures in obligations or possibly a nagging sense of not taking fresh risks to develop the self. As suggested in Chapter 3, when individuals do engage in seeking and take risks of prioritizing personal development or new experiences there will often be a rise in anxiety due to the ambiguity and uncertainty in the process. The existential theme of control is also typically in play in this dialectic, as guilt is tied to feeling one should have been able to control certain actions, whereas anxiety often comes from uncertainty about control in life. Shame is another related moral emotion that goes beyond distress about certain actions (guilt) and involves feelings of worthlessness about the self and failures to live up to one's ideals.

As a clinical example of these existential themes in tension, a conservative Christian client described this set of existential dilemmas as he came to realize he had lived his whole life in both shame and guilt based on the conflicts between his sexuality and the theology of his religious community. As he began to differentiate his own theological understanding in ways that differed from his family and church, he felt some reduction in guilt but an increase in anxiety, explaining, "What if it doesn't work out? What if I don't find anyone to love? Who is going to be my support?" Note the anxiety in seeking that comes prior to new forms of dwelling. As this client engaged in new forms of relationship and meaning construction, he also traded one form of shame for another—shame for being gay shifted to shame for overstaying in the closet for so long. This reflects a powerful human tendency to hold on to a sense of personal control even if it means painful feelings of inadequacy, because it maintains an illusion of dwelling with an ego ideal. The anxiety-provoking alternative involves the reduced control of grieving and moving toward humble acceptance of the limits and existential riskiness involved in human development and decision-making.

We have only touched upon a subset of the rich array of existential "big picture" themes that interact with the microrelational dynamics that unfold in therapy. Orange (2011) described the therapy dialectic of attending to developmental work at "the local level" and with "big picture" themes (pp. 192–201). By local level, she had in mind the moment-by-moment, in-session, and intersubjective dynamics between therapists and clients involving the sloppy processes of connection, rupture, and repair that have been highlighted, for example, in the work of the Boston Change group and Jeremy Safran. In referencing the "big developmental picture," Orange meant keeping in mind larger developmental themes and processes that are often beneath or intertwined with these momentary points of relational process in deeply meaningful ways. Orange cited the clinical sensibilities of Kohut and Winnicott as theorists who focused on the "forest over the trees" (p. 201) or the larger gestalt of a person's development. We agree with Orange's argument for the importance of attention to both local-level and big picture dynamics in psychotherapy.

In Table 4.2, we offer a heuristic list of big picture existential themes or existential predicaments that are related to primal fears and may be involved in developmental transitions or episodes of developmental "stuck-ness." As a heuristic, we recognize the list is not comprehensive and the connections between specific existential predicaments and primal fears can be contested and should not be held tightly. It would also be a mistake to impose these themes on a given client in a way that was not responsive to their own local level subjectivity and meaning-making process. Yet these are widely recurring existential themes related to predicaments within human experiences of suffering and trauma, and we have found them to offer clinically useful thematic reference points within therapy dialogue. Clients will seek to negotiate or contend with these predicaments in differing ways, depending upon their worldview frameworks and particular beliefs about suffering (discussed later). But we find it helpful to be familiar with a multifaceted set of existential themes, in part to avoid a more limited existential focus that can be found in certain models of psychotherapy. We return to these themes in the clinical chapters to follow.

TABLE 4.2. Relational Spirituality Model (RSM) Heuristic of Existential Predicaments and Primal Fears

Existential predicament	Primal fear
Death	Annihilation or disintegration
Isolation or loneliness	Abandonment
Freedom or choice	Ambiguity or anomie
Meaninglessness	Absurdity or emptiness
Injustice	Oppression
Guilt	Condemnation
Estrangement	Shame or hatred
Control	Powerlessness
Intimacy	Engulfment
Tragedy	Unpredictability
Alterity or abjection	Exclusion
Achievement	Failure or destruction
Invisibility	Lack of intersubjectivity or human recognition
Defilement	Contamination

Suffering Narratives and Theories of Illness Causation

Entering into a client's trauma matrix involves seeking to understand their underlying beliefs about suffering, which are often tied to cultural and SERT belief systems that take a narrative structure we liken to Kleinman's (1988) concept of illness narratives (see Chapter 1, this volume). Awareness of these differing suffering narratives is a key part of cultural, existential, and spiritual or religious diversity competence and respect for clients' values and perspectives. At many points in history, and presently in many parts of the world, humans have tended to assume (a) life universally involves suffering, and (b) supernatural forces or other ultimate realities cause suffering, most frequently due to human immorality or excessive attachment to illusions. However, in contemporary postindustrial and pluralistic contexts where humans have greater degrees of technological control over pain and suffering and greater exposure to worldview diversity, suffering increasingly tends to be viewed as a problem that invites existential awareness of finitude and spiritual and/or existential questions about ultimate realities and the meaning of life and death (Geniusas, 2013; Wildman, 2018).

Some approaches to psychotherapy actually recommend *not* giving attention to beliefs about the causes of suffering, which are viewed as a distraction that risks self-blame, and such psychotherapies focus solely and pragmatically on solutions to symptoms of surface-level anxiety and suffering. However, such approaches convey cultural and SERT insensitivity and may perpetuate colonizing approaches to treatment. A lack of any meaningful belief system related to suffering risks nihilism (Sullivan, 2016), so therapeutic approaches will likely impose an implicit set of beliefs about the meaning of suffering if not foster intentional sensitivity for relating effectively to client diversity. A well-paced process of seeking to respectfully understand clients' particular beliefs about suffering, should clients be open to this, can also deepen the therapy relationship in ways that often facilitate healing and meaning-making. For these reasons, it is important for clinicians to familiarize themselves with how different worldviews interpret suffering and suggest mechanisms for healing, thus providing therapists with some differentiated background knowledge for engaging clients in this domain. There are many ways to approach developing a more differentiated stance, but we will offer a couple of frameworks we have found helpful.

George Murdock's (1980) global survey of illness causation theories offers a useful heuristic that continues to inform contemporary public health research and the field of ethnomedicine (Erickson, 2008). His work fits with Kleinman's (1988) illness narratives perspective and attention to the interpretive worldview frameworks that shape understandings of suffering. Murdock started by noting several theories of natural illness causation, such as infection, stress, organic deterioration, accident, and overt human aggression. These natural or biopsychosocial theories tend to be dominant assumptive frameworks within Western mental health care and models of psychotherapy based on a biomedical disease model and, notably, do not necessarily require existential and spiritual considerations. In other words, many Western psychotherapists probably implicitly or explicitly assume natural illness-causation theories and minimize or negate other worldviews. But Murdock's cross-cultural research found supernatural illness-causation theories were much more frequent across the globe than were natural theories, and it is important to note that throughout history and around the globe the majority of people have attributed illness and suffering to supernatural forces that control human life and the cosmos. Murdock grouped the supernatural theories of illness causation into three categories: mystical, animistic, and magical (see Table 4.3).

Theories of mystical causation assume illness is due to impersonal spiritual forces, such as fate (e.g., bad luck, astrological influence), ominous sensations (e.g., potent dreams, sights, sounds, smells), contagion (e.g., contact with a polluting substance or person), or mystical retribution or karma (e.g., violation of a taboo or moral injunction). It is worth noting that the theme of fate is a concern in existential theories (Tillich, 1952) and also a prominent causal mechanism in the suffering narratives of certain worldviews. For example, some collectivistic cultures view illness and suffering as a fate resulting from personal immorality, and this view of suffering serves to socially control or repress deviance in contexts that require high degrees of social inter-dependence. Yang and colleagues found this "repressive suffering construal" (Yang, Liu, Sullivan, & Pan, 2016, p. 67) was more common in rural and lower-SES environments characterized by large family size. In such collec-tivistic settings, there is often a cultural emphasis on spiritual dwelling and maintaining a moral order, so suffering is often interpreted through an exis-tential lens focused on moral emotions of guilt and shame. This emphasis on fate or suffering that is morally "deserved" is quite different from the way individualistic cultures and western psychotherapists often frame suffering as related to uncertainty and trauma in a chaotic world (Sullivan, 2016).

Theories of animistic causation attribute illness or suffering to personalized spiritual entities, such as deities, spirits, souls, or ghosts. This can include soul loss or suffering attributed to the separation/exile of the soul from the body (Fadiman, 2012), or what Murdock (1980) grouped together as theories of spirit aggression (i.e., hostile or punitive action by a malevolent and offended supernatural being). Soul loss is particularly interesting for our considerations in this book because it is often thought to be generated by fear over traumatic events. Belief in spirits and ghosts may also be more common than typically recognized by mental health professionals, as psychology of religion research

TABLE 4.3. Murdock's (1980) Supernatural Theories of Illness Causation

Theories of mystical causation	Theories of animistic causation	Theories of magical causation
Fate	Soul loss	Sorcery
Ominous sensations	Spirit aggression	Witchcraft
Contagion		
Mystical retribution		

to date has tended to show a bias toward measures of God as a personal deity or more generalized themes of spirituality (Laird, Curtis, & Morgan, 2017).

Theories of magical causation ascribe illness to covert action by an envious, offended, or malicious human being. Sorcery is aggressive use of magical techniques (e.g., spells, prayers, curses) by a layperson, and witchcraft involves the same by a group with special dark powers and trait levels of envy. Witches and shamans can both use spiritual powers to cause suffering and these spiritual figures are part of belief systems that integrate the human and spiritual realms. I (SJS) worked with a client who was praying that his wife's emotional distress would increase so she might join him in couple therapy, and I was judgmental of this practice until I came to understand it fit within his worldview. In addition to Murdock's (1980) categories, many cultures view illness as resulting from various forms of body imbalance (e.g., humors, energies, hot–cold, emotions), and these imbalances are often understood as related to spiritual dynamics (Erickson, 2008).

Murdock (1980) found spirit aggression to be the most widespread illness theory and nearly universal, followed by sorcery (second most common) and mystical retribution for taboo violations (third most common). He found every society that depended primarily on animal-based agriculture for its economic resources considered spirit aggression a predominant or important secondary cause of illness. Murdock offered the intriguing "pastoral relationship" theory that an emotional connection of "mutuality" (p. 85) with large animals and the need to protect them for communal survival might lead to projecting a similar relationship onto supernatural beings as potentially offering (and withdrawing) protection from danger. This idea fits with more recent cognitive science research on the evolution of religion suggesting that the historical development of settled agricultural societies required bigger and more complicated gods understood as personal beings (anthropomorphized agents) who regulated patterns in nature, structured morality in large social groups, and provided protection from enemies (Norenzayan, 2013; Wildman, 2017). This understanding also has resonance with our limbic-based relational spirituality framework and the important role of relational dynamics (e.g., perceived aggression versus protection) in interpretations of spiritual experience. Across many regions of the world, illness is thought to involve some imbalance or disorganized relations between the individual and their social and/or spiritual environments.

In Western contexts, sorcery might be relatively uncommon as an explicit illness-causation theory, but perhaps shades of this theory are more common than recognized. For example, a client reported being haunted (at a level that sounded traumatic) by her father-in-law's statement some two decades earlier that his son (client's husband) would "prove to fail in life if he went ahead with the marriage." The client experienced this statement as similar to a prophetic spiritual curse that was causally related to their subsequent marital problems and to the husband's ongoing difficulties maintaining consistent employment.

Theories of mystical retribution for taboo violations tap into the complicated dynamics of morality and guilt. Murdock (1980) noted the ways in which internalization of a community's moral standards can promote self-regulation, and how violations can potentially be dysregulating and, therefore, immune suppressing. Since spiritual and religious traditions are often associated with morality, it is common for violations of moral codes to promote anxiety about relational spirituality and the potential consequences of those violations. In some contexts, violations of a certain taboo in areas such as sexuality, gender, or forming relationships outside one's cultural or religious tradition might represent a threat to one's communal standing and can risk exclusion. In many different worldviews, healing involves seeking forgiveness from other humans or from deities and spirits through ritual practices of atonement, but this might not seem feasible for clients who have differentiated themselves in certain ways from their families and communities of origin.

Spiritual and Religious Beliefs About Suffering

Spiritual and religious traditions offer a plethora of different sets of beliefs about the causes and meanings of suffering that supplement Murdock's (1980) categories. Yet specific beliefs about suffering have received very little empirical research attention in the psychology of religion, which led to the development of the Views of Suffering Scale (VOSS; Hale-Smith, Park, & Edmondson, 2012; Park et al., 2017) that engages numerous theological and religious views not considered in Murdock's research. In theistic religious traditions that posit a personal God, *theodicies* are sets of beliefs that contend with the seeming discrepancies between God's goodness and the realities of evil and suffering in the world. More broadly, most philosophical and religious traditions suggest frameworks for understanding the problems of evil and suffering, while it is also important to recognize that some traditions (e.g., Buddhism) view suffering as inevitable and universal.

The VOSS offers another useful heuristic for considering differing spiritual and religious views of suffering and has received initial validation through confirmatory factor analysis with multiple samples resulting in nine subscales reflecting different beliefs about suffering, including theistic and nontheistic views (Hale-Smith et al., 2012; see Table 4.4). The research on the VOSS shows nine distinct factors, but the subscales can be correlated, which means individuals can hold a combination of these views of suffering.

A review of Table 4.4 summarizing VOSS dimensions suggests it is a useful assessment heuristic, but it differentiates several monotheistic views while offering limited engagement of other spiritual and religious worldviews. We cannot do a comprehensive survey of views of suffering, but we will offer a few points to supplement the heuristics offered by Murdock and the VOSS. First, there are different accounts of karma within the many traditions of Buddhism, Hinduism, Jainism, and the singular VOSS dimension of Retribution (Karma) does not do justice to these suffering narratives. Buddhist traditions,

TABLE 4.4. Dimensions for Views of Suffering Scale (VOSS)

Subscale	Description
Random	There is no way to predict suffering and no underlying reason for suffering.
Karma (authors use term *Retribution*)	Based on Buddhist and Hindu beliefs in suffering as part of a cycle where prior individual deeds impact subsequent experiences of suffering
Limited knowledge	Open theism beliefs of God's limited knowledge and control over suffering
Suffering God	Jewish and Christian beliefs of God's compassionate presence amid suffering, or God suffering with humanity
Providence	Belief that God controls suffering
Overcoming	Based on Pentecostal beliefs that one can overcome suffering through prayer or faith
Soul-building	Belief that God always uses suffering as a challenge or personal growth experience
Encounter/Divine responsibility	Beliefs about suffering as a divine encounter
Unorthodox	Beliefs about suffering that include a divine being without characteristics of omnipotence, beneficence, or perfection

for example, assert that suffering is universal and results from misperception and attachment to the illusory, which can be liberated through enlightenment. Karma is a universal self-regulating moral law of cause and effect, often based on relational treatment of others, which generates productive suffering within the quest toward ultimate spiritual goals. The VOSS scale label (Retribution) for karma also fails to convey broader aspects of this spiritual view (see Jennings, 2010).

The VOSS measures an open theism view (which considers God to have limited knowledge and control over the future) and another grouping the authors call "unorthodox" (which views God as not completely benevolent), but this overlooks the varieties of process theism that have been particularly prominent in contemporary theology over the past century (Wildman, 2017). Versions of process theology typically view God as benevolent but also differentiated from some aspects of ultimate reality that cause suffering. Many forms of process theism suggest the divine relationally suffers along with humanity, and these views often promote suffering narratives that emphasize human responsibility and social-justice activism to participate in the transformation of suffering. Liberation approaches to theology and spirituality often rest on these process assumptions and specify social structures of systemic evil and injustice (e.g., racism, sexism, homophobia, poverty, eco-pollution) as key sources of suffering over and above other sources of ontological suffering (see powell, 2012).

Finally, ground-of-being theism represents a set of views that may roughly correspond to what the VOSS authors have in mind for their "unorthodox" view. Ground-of-being theologians do not view the divine as personal or as "good" and caring in a humanly recognizable way (Wildman, 2017, 2018). They regard suffering as ontologically part of divine creativity and also part of the evolutionary fate of humans and all creatures in the world, not as a side effect of other processes that are good. Ground-of-being understandings can be found in religious naturalism and some traditions of Buddhism, Hinduism, Chinese philosophy, atheism, and mysticism, and these views often place total responsibility on human agency for the alleviation of suffering.

From a relational spirituality perspective, there are several questions related to these existential and relational themes that are important to consider across these views and can serve to differentiate clients' suffering narratives. It is also valuable as clinicians to be aware of our own views about suffering and ways this may influence our approach to therapy, particularly in cases of extreme suffering and trauma. For example:

1. Does suffering have a growth-oriented or moral meaning and purpose we should seek to understand, or is it random?

2. If suffering is intended for growth, does that make God or the sacred cruel, loving, or impersonal/pragmatic?

3. Does God or the sacred actually control suffering, or is suffering more a result of (a) natural processes and human freedom, and/or (b) other sources of spiritual, ancestral, or interpersonal malevolence or retribution?

4. Is it acceptable to express anger, disappointment, or confusion with God or the sacred related to suffering, or is it more mature to suppress or repress such feelings and prioritize dwelling over seeking?

5. Does God or the sacred actually suffer along with humanity or remain beyond the experiential realities of suffering?

6. Is suffering always intended to achieve some type of justice (i.e., it is morally deserved), or do the vicissitudes of suffering sometimes unfold in a tragic fashion outside of any moral ledger?

7. Is it important to seek healing or liberation in the present life, or should the focus rather be on transcending this life and finding transformation in a future life?

Note the implicit themes in these questions: presence versus distance, meaning versus randomness, cruelty versus love, justice versus tragedy, control versus freedom, and authentic expression versus suppression or repression. Based on the RSM, we expect these differing existential and relational beliefs about suffering will not only influence coping strategies and assumed pathways toward healing but may also surface in important ways within the therapy relationship and in client assumptions about the therapist. Clients may also have had formative interpersonal experiences and responses to their relational spiritual dynamics involving suffering; for example, a parent or religious leader disapproving of their questions about God's role in their trauma. Exline and Grubbs (2011) found that among those who are angry at God, supportive and empathic relational responses tend to promote spiritual approach behaviors (i.e., engaging their spirituality) whereas unsupportive and shaming responses tend to be associated with continued anger, suppression, distancing from spirituality, and substance abuse.

RELATIONAL SPIRITUALITY AND THE SUFFERING–TRAUMA MATRIX

We have covered several complex topics in this chapter—anxiety, trauma, existential themes, and suffering narratives—and we integrate these ideas in the clinical chapters to follow; however, we will summarize some key points here. Figure 4.1 depicts our RSM conceptualization of the suffering–trauma matrix, which extends the trauma matrix concept to more broadly include suffering narratives. Anxiety and trauma symptoms emerge within a triangle of influence that includes (a) deeper existential anxieties, (b) suffering narratives, and (c) relational spirituality dynamics. Too often, clinical approaches to anxiety and trauma fail to assess client perspectives on the suffering–trauma matrix and thus neglect potentially important dynamics related to diversity, meaning, and ultimate concerns. We have seen other cases where clinicians have imposed particular narratives about suffering, meaning, and spirituality that do not fit client worldviews, and this runs the risk of retraumatizing some clients. Several other summary points follow from the material in this chapter.

First, the Western concept of *trauma* seems to have emerged in 19th-century British discourse about the psychological impact of railroad accidents and introduced an implicit "accident cosmology," or the notion that certain traumatic events happen due to chaotic natural forces without culpability by the victim (Luckhurst, 2008). The diagnostic categories related to trauma took further shape and medical legitimation during the 1980s and following both the Vietnam War and increasing social consciousness of sexual abuse and rape.

FIGURE 4.1. Relational Spirituality Model (RSM) Suffering–Trauma Matrix

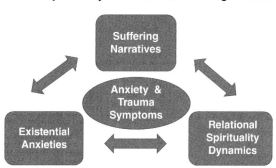

Trauma has become a crucial mental health concept. Yet it is also important to be cognizant that the language of trauma will be unfamiliar to some clients, and the associated accident cosmology may also diverge from the suffering narratives of certain clients. It is important to engage in relationally sensitive assessment of client's understandings of anxiety, suffering, and healing. We believe therapists should start by working from clients' worldviews and traditions (i.e., their suffering and healing narratives) while also beginning to dialogue about clinical perspectives and interventions that could prove helpful. This requires clinicians to begin to develop multilingual capacities related to suffering; that is, the ability to utilize and integrate different forms of language for suffering and healing (e.g., clinical, existential, sociocultural, spiritual, religious; Dueck & Reimer, 2009).

Second, some clients will be focused on spiritual dwelling or trying to regain the sense of community and orientation offered by attachments to sources of dwelling to cope with their suffering. If prior sources of dwelling have been lost due to factors such as migration, relational conflicts, or threats to their worldview, these clients will often struggle with some combination of guilt, existential or spiritual disorientation, ambiguity about norms and values, and anxiety about abandonment or isolation. They may unconsciously (or consciously) long to return to a well-ordered experience of community and reconciled relationships. Other seeking-oriented clients may struggle with a risk of despair if their personal pursuits for meaning and significance seem to be proving vulnerable or unsuccessful (Sullivan, 2016). Whereas dwellers tend to fear negation of their worldview and community, seekers tend to be anxious about the existential negation of the self and threats to self-agency in trying to develop a meaningful life. These anxieties are not mutually exclusive; for example, seekers may also feel both the loss of familiar sources of community as they differentiate and engulfment anxiety as they reengage former relationships.

Finally, with our RSM we are advocating clinician respect for clients' particular relational spirituality orientations while also advancing the idea that healing in response to suffering and trauma typically involves growth in balancing dwelling and seeking in safe, socially just holding environments. In addressing Black existentialism, Vereen and colleagues, drawing on the work of hooks (1989, 1990) and others, have identified the existential need among Blacks for "homeplaces" (Vereen et al., 2017, p. 79) or safe and secure relationships and decolonized communities that can hold the anxiety-provoking process of meaning construction and reconstruction in the face of profound suffering and racialized trauma. This can be particularly challenging to find for individuals from many different nondominant and oppressed groups, since social systems frequently lack sufficient awareness and sensitivity to the chronic traumatic impact of oppression. In the chapters that follow, we describe an approach to psychotherapy that uses the therapeutic relationship and other relational resources to help clients develop healthy capacities to balance dwelling and seeking in their ongoing process of healing and growth.

CONCLUSION

In this chapter, we have argued that anxiety and trauma always have existential dimensions. Understanding these existential dimensions of anxiety can illuminate key themes within what we call the suffering–trauma matrix, but this also requires clinician diversity sensitivity and openness to the varieties of views of suffering and illness narratives (see Chapter 1). We have also further emphasized the role of relational dynamics in anxiety, trauma, suffering, and growth consistent with our RSM emphasis on relational factors in psychotherapy. In Part II (Chapters 5, 6, and 7), we consider three core relational development systems—attachment, differentiation, and intersubjectivity—as they integrate with our RSM approach to psychotherapy.

II

THREE RELATIONAL DEVELOPMENT SYSTEMS

5

Attachment and Relational Spirituality

Intimate attachments to other human beings are the hub around which a person's life revolves, not only when he [sic] is an infant or a toddler, but throughout his adolescence and his years of maturity as well, and onto old age.

—J. BOWLBY, *ATTACHMENT AND LOSS* (1980, P. 442)

As described in Chapter 2, our relational spirituality model (RSM) attends to three developmental systems—attachment, differentiation, and intersubjectivity—that impact human thriving, human struggles, and potential pathways for healing and growth. We use the term *developmental system* to highlight complex relational dynamics in context over time, and ways that prior experience affects subsequent capacities and possibilities in relation to key goals and motivations. The goal of the attachment system is security. In the face of threats and challenges, humans instinctively seek connection with attachment figures who are or who seem to be stronger or more competent (Bowlby, 1988b). In ideal circumstances, these relationships provide immediate assistance—refuge, comfort, and protection—and support development in critical areas such as affect regulation, exploration/assertion in the world, mentalization, and skills in relational rupture and repair. Less than ideal attachment relationships may hinder development and result in relational patterns characterized by anxiety, avoidance, or disorganization (Costello, 2013).

Contemporary attachment theory draws from an extensive research base in developmental studies, social psychology, neuropsychology, intercultural

http://dx.doi.org/10.1037/0000174-006
Relational Spirituality in Psychotherapy: Healing Suffering and Promoting Growth,
by S. J. Sandage, D. Rupert, G. S. Stavros, and N. G. Devor

research, and clinical practice to address a range of concerns including "emotion, close relationships, vulnerability and resilience, and personality development" (Fraley, 2019, p. 23). This chapter focuses on a few key ideas and debates about attachment theory, highlights developmental implications for psychotherapy, and identifies points of connection with RSM themes of dwelling and seeking. We then discuss general strategies for cultivating secure attachment and addressing insecure attachment in psychotherapy. First, however, consider how the following clinical vignette illustrates the potential impact of attachment.

A man in his 60s who suffers from chronic depression starts his 30th therapy session by stating, "It's been terrible week." He goes on to describe several difficult events, including being diagnosed with a failing hip that will require surgery, and hearing that one of his children just lost a full-time job. The therapist offers empathic acknowledgment and some framing comments that mix acceptance with staying in the present. Near the end of the hour, the client smiles and says, "Whew, I feel better. Thanks for hearing me." A minute later he adds, "I guess I will start journaling again." In this scenario nothing circumstantial changed, but the client feels relief and accesses coping strategies. Attachment dynamics may explain why.

FOUNDATIONS OF ATTACHMENT THEORY

John Bowlby and Mary Ainsworth are generally recognized as the founders of Western attachment theory (Wallin, 2007). Bowlby was a British psychiatrist and psychoanalyst affiliated with the Tavistock Clinic in London (Vaillant, 1996). Ainsworth was a developmental psychologist who held faculty positions at the University of Toronto, the Tavistock Clinic, Johns Hopkins University, and the University of Virginia (Bretherton & Main, 2000).

Bowlby's work with children and families included delinquent boys, children who became homeless after World War II, and children who were separated from their caregivers through institutionalization. Through these experiences, Bowlby came to emphasize the impact of primary caregiving relationships on childhood development (Bowlby, 1988b; Costello, 2013; Wallin, 2007). He saw caregiving instincts in parents (especially mothers), and care-seeking behaviors in infants and children, as evolutionary attachment patterns that promote survival. In the most basic sense—a sensibility shared with other mammals—human children seek physical proximity with their caregivers for physical care and protection. However, human attachment involves more than proximity. For human infants and children, attachment security emerges when primary caregivers are sufficiently available, attuned, and responsive (Costello, 2013). The quality of communication/interaction is critical, and essentially teaches the child what to expect and how to adapt to the world.

Bowlby (1988a) referred to these learned expectations and patterns of relating as *internal working models* (p. 4). In secure attachment, attachment figures function as a safe haven—a source of comfort and protection in difficult moments—and as a secure base: a dependable, supportive presence that encourages exploration and engagement of novel experiences (Wallin, 2007). Unfortunately, children do not always have this sort of support. One of the ways Bowlby came to recognize the importance of emotional availability and connection was through observation of children who had lost, or never had, responsive attachment figures. Even if they had their physical needs met, children in these circumstances struggled and typically progressed through stages of protest, despair, and finally detachment.

Ainsworth provided empirical confirmation and further elaborated attachment theory through her research in Uganda and Baltimore, United States. She conducted rigorous observations of infants and mothers in their homes and ran what came to be called the "Strange Situation" experiments (Bretherton & Main, 2000; Wallin, 2007). This research involved mothers and infants (approximately 12 months old) coming to a pleasant but unfamiliar laboratory room filled with toys. The dyads went through several 3-minute episodes involving time together in the room, two separations, two reunions, and exposure to a stranger. These sequences provided opportunities to observe aspects of secure base functioning (e.g., exploration and engagement in the new environment) and safe haven functioning (e.g., seeking and utilizing mother's comfort when distressed). Through these observations, Ainsworth classified the infants as securely attached, avoidant, or ambivalent. Table 5.1 describes behavioral patterns and associated maternal behaviors for each classification. Ainsworth's

TABLE 5.1. Ainsworth's Attachment Classifications With Associated Infant and Maternal Behaviors

Attachment classification	Infant behavior in the strange situation	Maternal behavior during home observations
Secure	Infants actively explored and played.	Mothers were generally sensitive and attuned in responding to their infant, and made adjustments when misattuned.
	Infants became upset and protested when mother left.	
	Infants sought consolation and were comforted by mother when she returned.	
	Infants resumed exploration and play after reunion.	
Avoidant	Infants explored continually.	Mothers tended to reject infant's bids for attention and were often preoccupied with their own concerns.
	Infants seemed indifferent to mother initially, during her absence, and when she returned. (Later research confirmed that despite appearing detached, these infants have high physiological distress.)	
Ambivalent	Infants appeared preoccupied with mother and do not explore/play much.	Mothers tended to be inconsistent in responding to infants and were often misattuned in their response.
	Infants were upset when mother left.	
	Infants were not receptive to soothing upon mother's return: some appeared angry and rejecting, others appeared helpless.	

work offered clear and powerful illustrations of how interactions between mothers and infants shaped the infants' sense of security and subsequent patterns of relating to attachment figures and to the environment.

Mary Main was one of Mary Ainsworth's students at Johns Hopkins University, and she went on to have a distinguished career at the University of California, Berkeley. Main advanced attachment theory in several ways. First, she introduced a strong focus on one's "state of mind with respect to attachment" (Wallin, 2007, p. 28, citing Main). Her research demonstrated that relational experiences with key attachment figures have enduring impacts upon a person's mental state regarding attachment, and that these mental states affect subsequent functioning. She conducted longitudinal studies that found impressive correlations between a parent's state of mind regarding attachment, an infant's strange situation behavior and classification, and the child's state of mind and behavior at 6 years old (Costello, 2013; Wallin, 2007). Main also offered a more nuanced understanding of the internal working model as a set of procedural rules that direct or shape attention, organization of experience, and emotional/behavioral patterns. This is highly relevant for therapists who may mistakenly focus on episodic memories and explicit representations rather than recurrent, often unconscious patterns of perception and response.

Another contribution involved defining a fourth broad attachment category, disorganized attachment, characterized by inconsistent and seemingly chaotic attachment strategies. In Main's original work, participants could be coded "unresolved" and one of the other attachment categories because unresolved patterns were seen in certain moments (typically when discussing abuse or loss), whereas other patterns prevailed at other times. I [DR] would add that some clients—typically those who had earlier or more extensive abuse/neglect—characteristically function in an unresolved/disorganized fashion, whereas other clients only become disorganized periodically or in certain contexts. Main hypothesized that disorganized attachment resulted from caregivers who were (at least sometimes) experienced as a threat, creating "fright without solution" (Hesse & Main, 1999, p. 484) because the attachment figure who was supposed to offer safe haven was also the source of distress.

Finally, Main developed an adult assessment tool, the Adult Assessment Inventory (AAI), that evaluates adults' mental state regarding attachment through analysis of speech patterns. The AAI is a structured interview that inquires about attachment experiences and primarily codes how respondents speak. Main found that different mental states regarding attachment produced different speech patterns; e.g., secure attachment tended to manifest in clear, collaborative communication, whereas forms of insecure attachment were associated with less clear, coherent, or balanced speech patterns (Table 5.2 provides brief descriptions of attachment behaviors and AAI speech patterns, and possible intervention strategies). Relevant history, current relational patterns including ways of relating to the therapist, and patterns of discourse can all be useful for informal clinical assessment of attachment. Attachment dynamics are particularly important in situations that tend to active limbic-based internal working models of relationships, such as situations involving

TABLE 5.2. Attachment Behaviors, Adult Assessment Inventory (AAI) Discourse Patterns, and Intervention Options

Attachment behavior	AAI discourse patterns	Possible interventions
Secure	Flexible attachment behaviors: accesses attachment figures for safe haven, demonstrates secure base through exploration, curiosity, and tolerating anxiety. AAI: coherent, collaborative discourse about attachment.	Assist clients to balance dwelling and seeking as needed, and to utilize existential and relational dilemmas as crucibles for growth. Look for RSM resources that speak to growth areas.
Preoccupied	Hyperactivated attachment behaviors: Anxious relational style and may exhibit relational spiritualities that are reactively angry, fearful, shame-prone, passive, hard to soothe, and showing limited secure base behaviors. AAI: long, elaborate discourse, may be preoccupied with the past, fearful, or angry when talking about attachment experiences.	Help clients increase capacities for self-regulation, self-confidence, mentalization, and differentiation. Crucible work may involve risking more seeking/secure base behaviors and working through (a) disappointment in others and/or in self, and (b) past losses. Look for RSM resources that utilize relational sensitivity but reduce abandonment anxiety and guilt, and support self-regulation, groundedness, and reflective functioning.
Dismissive	Hypoactivated attachment behaviors: Minimizing stance to emotions and relationships and exhibit relational spiritualities that are dismissive of vulnerability, rigid/legalistic, intellectualizing, compulsive, or overly self-reliant. AAI: discourse tends to be brief, generalized, may have contradictory elements (e.g., idealistic about family of origin but describing mostly negative memories when asked for examples).	Help clients increase capacities for self-awareness, self-regulation, and intimacy. Crucible work may involve risking more dwelling/safe-haven behaviors and relational commitments and growing in compassion, humility, and forgiveness. Look for RSM resources that utilize self-reliance but reduce relational avoidance/dismissal and engulfment anxiety and increase connection and collaboration.
Unresolved or disorganized	Chaotic or inconsistent attachment behaviors: may shift quickly between hyper- and hypo-activated strategies; may be chronically dysregulated with relational spiritualities exhibiting paranoid, extremely fearful, and/or chronically dissociative behaviors. AAI: discourse about loss or abuse often involves sudden shifts, lapses in reason or self-monitoring, and intense or absent emotion.	Help clients increase capacities for self-regulation, grounding, and accessing strengths and resources. Crucible work may involve processing trauma/neglect and risking more engagement in life. Look for RSM resources that use awareness of suffering, acknowledge trauma/neglect, and provide meaning and support while remaining (somewhat) open or flexible to account for state shifts.

Note. AAI developed by Main and Goldwyn (1994). Descriptive data derived from Costello (2013) and Wallin (2007).

fear, vulnerability, transitions or separations from familiar people and places, illness, and loss. Clients often present with these sorts of concerns. Granqvist and Main (2017) have been developing a Religious Attachment Interview, and Hall (2014; Bailey et al., 2016) has been developing the attachment-based Relational Spirituality Interview, both of which could be promising assessment tools once validated in clinical contexts.

COMPLEXITIES IN ATTACHMENT THEORY

With this brief background in place, it may be useful to clarify some terms, current understandings, and areas of debate within attachment research and attachment theory. First, the attachment system involves motivations and behaviors related to security-seeking through relationship with attachment figures. It is a complex developmental system that shows patterns of continuity and change in different contexts and across the lifespan (Fraley, 2019). Moreover, and this is a critical point, attachment security affects and is affected by many critical developmental processes and capacities—including neural pruning and other aspects of brain development, affect regulation, mentalization, collaborative/intersubjective communication, rupture and repair dynamics, and coping strategies—and thus the reach and implications of attachment include but go beyond attachment relationships (Costello, 2013; Mikulincer & Shaver, 2016; Ogden & Fisher, 2015; Schore, 2017; Wallin, 2007). Secure attachment is profoundly facilitative, and insecure attachment may undermine development in important and cumulative ways.

Second, attachment styles may be defined and assessed in different ways—for example, observing interactions with a particular attachment figure in a particular context as in the Strange Situation research, assessing one's state of mind with respect to attachment through interviews and other means (e.g., the AAI), or reflecting on relational patterns more generally (typically through self-report attachment scales or card-sort ratings; Fraley, 2019; Wallin, 2007). These assessments are not measuring identical constructs or processes—for example, some evaluate attachment to a specific person while others probe for state of mind regarding attachment based on one's history—and they do not always correlate. However, in some cases they correlate in profound ways; for example, AAI assessments of parents have predicted their infant's strange situation attachment behavior with 75% accuracy (Wallin, 2007, p. 32).

Third, persons may have multiple attachment relationships, and the salience of these relationships may change over time and across different contexts. Examples include contexts with multiple caregivers, adolescents' increasing reliance on peers, and adult relationships with partners and friends. There are ongoing questions about how to best understand multiple attachments. Some researchers argue for attachment hierarchies in which certain persons are more prominent attachment figures and there is some convergence in attachment patterns across different relationships. Others emphasize multiple, variable attachment styles that pertain to specific persons and/or contexts (E. B. Davis, Granqvist, & Sharp, 2018; Fraley, 2019; Wallin, 2007). Rigidity may be the distinguishing characteristic of insecure attachment, in contrast to the flexibility evident when securely attached people adjust their stance in helpful ways depending on the situation and relationship at hand.

Fourth, attachment styles can be defined by categories or along dimensions. Categorical assessments typically involve the basic attachment categories of secure attachment, anxious or preoccupied attachment, avoidant or dismissive attachment, and disorganized or unresolved attachment (Costello, 2013, p. 80; for applications to relational spirituality and forgiveness, see Worthington & Sandage, 2016). However, some researchers have suggested more fine-grained distinctions. For example, Crittenden, Farnfield, Landini, and Grey (2013) offered 13 attachment categories organized around different "self-protective strategies" (p. 240), and Bartholomew and Horowitz distinguished four quadrants reflecting high or low levels of trust of self and trust in others (Harris, 2004).

Dimensional assessments typically plot people along two orthogonal axes, one representing anxiety and one representing avoidance (Fraley, Hudson, Heffernan, & Segal, 2015; Mikulincer, Shaver, & Berant, 2013). In the anxiety-avoidance framework, secure attachment reflects low anxiety and low avoidance, while insecure attachment may involve differing degrees of anxiety and/or avoidance, including "preoccupied" (high anxiety, low avoidance), "fearful avoidance" (high anxiety, high avoidance), and "dismissing avoidance" (low anxiety, high avoidance; Fraley et al., 2015, p. 355).

Fifth, attachment styles and/or behaviors may change over time (Fraley, 2019; Fraley & Roisman, 2019). While early experiences with primary caregivers may have significant and lasting effects (Costello, 2013; Schore, 2017), multiple factors can influence attachment in adults, including becoming parents, ending romantic relationships, trauma related to war, relational conflict or support, "the meaning or construal of life events," "stable vulnerability factors," and psychotherapy (Fraley, 2019, p. 12).

Despite these complexities and uncertainties, a great body of research has shown attachment to be an important factor in human well-being. For example, Fraley (2019) reported that

> those who are secure are more likely than those who are insecure to (a) communicate effectively in their relationships, (b) resolve interpersonal conflict appropriately, (c) recall and discuss painful experiences in a competent manner, (d) feel satisfied and committed in their relationships, (e) regulate their emotions effectively, and (f) report low susceptibility to symptoms of psychopathology and poor physical health. (p. 8)

Schore (2017), a psychoanalyst and neuroscientist, added that attachment experiences impact not only behavior but also more fundamental brain capacities that support or limit adaptation.

CULTURE AND ATTACHMENT THEORY

Our RSM values and attends to cultural differences including the intercultural contextualization of attachment theory. Ainsworth's original research involved dyads from Uganda and from the United States, an early inclusion of different cultural contexts, but like all psychological theories, attachment theory includes cultural presuppositions and limitations. International attachment researchers have warned against "deficit" models that posit universal truths about attachment and then compare cultural groups against these standards (Farkas, Olhaberry, Santelices, & Cordella, 2017, p. 214). Instead, they have suggested that we "approach these differences from a model that recognizes cultural differences and specificities . . . attachment styles may be related to parenting practices that follow distinct cultural guidelines" (Farkas et al., 2017, p. 214).

It is beyond the scope of this chapter to offer a comprehensive review of culture and attachment, so we will focus on several key points. First, there is considerable evidence that when children without severe neurological difficulties "are given the chance" (Mesman, van IJzendoorn, & Sagi-Schwartz, 2016, p. 854), they will become attached to one or more specific caregivers. There are many cultures and contexts in which children have multiple caregivers who may assume different roles, and different studies find different patterns of attachment in these contexts. For example, the Efe people of the Ituri forest in northern Zambia use multiple nonmaternal caregivers during the day, but children sleep with their mothers at night. Researchers noted that during the second half of the first year, children "began to show preference for the care of their own mothers, were more likely to protest against their own mothers' leaving, and wanted to be carried by their mothers on trips outside the camp" (Mesman et al., 2016, p. 855). In contrast, in the Hausa tribe in Nigeria, a society in which mothers provide physical care but all other forms of care are shared with an average of four caregivers, children showed attachment behaviors toward one adult (the person holding or interacting with them most often), but not necessarily the mother.

Second, there are many research examples that caregiver sensitivity—"sensitive and prompt response to infant attachment signals" (Mesman et al., 2016, p. 854)—correlates with secure attachment in children across different cultures, including contexts with multiple caregivers. However, there are cultural variations in how sensitivity is expressed. For example, "in some cultures appropriate responding to infant vocalization may consist of touching or stroking the infant, whereas in other cultures it may be to imitate the sound that the infant made or to smile at the infant" (Mesman et al., 2016, p. 870). This highlights how "different parental behaviors can have the same function in different cultural contexts" (Mesman et al., 2016, p. 869).

Third, there are many examples of cultural and contextual factors altering or shaping attachment patterns. For instance, researchers examining Puerto Rican and Anglo mother–infant dyads found that a predicated association between insecure attachment and high maternal control was not present for Puerto Rican dyads but was present for Anglo dyads (Brown, Rodgers, & Kapadia, 2008). In another study that compared urban/nonindigenous dyads with rural indigenous (Mapuche) dyads in Chile, the Mapuche children were coded with more avoidant interaction styles, a finding the authors interpreted as reflecting Mapuche cultural values of promoting "early independence of young children" (Farkas et al., 2017, p. 212). Finally, and importantly, there are indications of compromised attachment (less secure attachment) across cultures when families and/or primary caregivers lack socioeconomic and relational support (Mesman et al., 2016). Each of these points suggests the need for cultural and contextual sensitivity in assessing the attachment systems of clients.

DWELLING, SEEKING, AND ATTACHMENT

The two primary functions of the attachment system are safe haven and secure base: safe haven refers to comfort and protection in times of distress; secure base refers to dependable support for exploration and assertion in the world. These attachment modes map onto core RSM constructs of dwelling and seeking (see Chapter 3, this volume, for a thorough discussion of dwelling and seeking). Dwelling refers to experiences of abiding and drawing strength from some sort of home, refuge, or resource. In attachment, one finds refuge in the presence and attuned responsiveness of one (or more) attachment figures. In spiritual dwelling, one may find home in various sources such as the divine, spiritual community, or spiritual practices that provide emotion regulation. Notice how both safe haven and dwelling convey a sense of groundedness and protection in safe places: there is somewhere to go, someone or some sacred dimension to be with, for solace and security. In contrast, seeking and secure base functioning are more strongly associated with growth and reaching outward. Seeking has to do with exploration and integrating novel or more complex experiences, themes that can apply to spiritual growth or questing. Secure base functioning involves similar sorts of behavior; for instance, infants exploring and engaging the world around them, or adults taking steps to expand their lives in various ways.

Safe haven and secure base functions have a reciprocal and dialectical relationship. Too much safe haven functioning without secure base functioning can be limiting and/or enmeshed, whereas too much secure base functioning without safe haven functioning can become barren and lonely. Securely attached individuals are generally able to seek support from others and to assert themselves and negotiate novel circumstances, including conflicts (Costello, 2013; Fraley, 2019). Spiritual dwelling and seeking also have a dialectical relationship. Although the balance may vary between persons and/or between moments or seasons of a person's life, the RSM posits that vital living requires some mix of spiritual dwelling (grounding and sustenance for well-being) and spiritual seeking (ongoing exploration and growth). Chapter 3 offers detailed exploration of the balance and interplay between dwelling and seeking.

Attachment patterns can help or hinder spiritual dwelling and seeking, and vice versa. The "correspondence" hypothesis suggests that there are often similarities and parallels between persons' religiosity and/or spirituality and aspects of their limbic-based internal working model of relationships (Granqvist & Kirkpatrick, 2013, p. 144). In the most straightforward sense, persons with secure attachment tend to be more open to closeness and to new experiences, and this sets a good stage for balanced and flexible patterns of spiritual dwelling and/or seeking that are generally conducive to psychological and spiritual well-being (E. B. Davis, Granqvist, & Sharp, 2018). In contrast, persons with preoccupied attachment styles may seek or report an entangled and anxious relationship with God or spiritual leaders and community members, whereas persons with a dismissing attachment style may view God or spiritual leaders and community members as distant or untrustworthy. Consider, for example, a Jewish client who had a distant relationship to her mother and a conflictual and sometimes abusive relationship with her father, and who finds herself in therapy at age 58 saying, "I guess I don't really trust anybody, and that includes God. I'm afraid of God's judgment, so I obey the commandments. . . . I don't go to synagogue too often. I prefer to handle things on my own." This brief disclosure alludes to the correspondence between this client's attachment style with both God and other humans in her relational network.

Spiritual and religious resources may also potentially help people cope with poor attachment experiences, a pattern referenced as "compensation" (Granqvist & Kirkpatrick, 2013, p. 147). Clinical examples include persons who grow up in abusive families and later turn toward religious or spiritual practices (often different from what was espoused in the family of origin) to find meaning, comfort, and connection, or persons who restart troubled lives reflecting childhood difficulties (problematic attachment, adverse events) after a spiritual conversion. However, compensatory attachment styles may involve taking up spirituality and religion in ways that reinforce anxiety and insecure relational patterns; for instance, persons prone to see others as cold and uncaring may be drawn to spiritual or religious perspectives or practices that encourage intimacy with the sacred, yet the person continues to suffer the same insecure relational patterns in interpersonal realms. Compensatory forms of spiritual attachment can be similar to the notion of spiritual bypass discussed earlier (Fossella, 2011). Readers interested in the relationship between attachment, spirituality, and religion will find a rich literature (too much to review here) that includes studies of religious attachment, God representations, and attachment and spirituality related dynamics, and empirical support for both correspondence and compensation effects (Augustyn, Hall, Wang, & Hill, 2017; Davis et al., 2016; Granqvist & Kirkpatrick, 2004, 2013, 2016; Griffith, 2011; Hall, Fujikawa, Halcrow, Hill, & Delaney, 2009;

Kirkpatrick, 2005; Mikulincer & Shaver, 2016; Sandage, Jankowski, Crabtree, & Schweer, 2015; Worthington & Sandage, 2016). Overall, we find it is important to struggle against psychologizing or spiritualizing attachment. The former minimizes or overlooks spiritual, existential, or religious factors to focus solely on psychological aspects of attachment, and the latter privileges spirituality in a way that minimizes or bypasses bio-psycho-sociological dimensions, including attachment.

ATTACHMENT AND A DEVELOPMENTAL APPROACH IN PSYCHOTHERAPY

Different therapeutic orientations and modalities focus on different mechanisms of change. Attachment theory focuses on facilitative relationships that promote developmental capacities for vital, adaptive living (Costello, 2013; Holmes, 2001; Lewis, Amini, & Lannon, 2000; Wallin, 2007). We discuss several clinical implications of an attachment-informed, developmental approach to psychotherapy next.

(Enough) Interaction Over Time

Facilitative relationships generally take time to develop and matter. We respect the possibilities for influence and change in powerful moments or brief but meaningful exchanges. At the same time, attachment research highlights the impact of sustained availability and attunement (Costello, 2013; Wallin, 2007). Clinical research on the therapeutic alliance (Flückiger, Del Re, Wampold, & Horvath, 2018), relational bond (Wampold & Imel, 2015), therapist responsiveness (Stiles & Horvath, 2017), and rupture and repair (Safran & Kraus, 2014) suggests similar contributions from sustained availability and attuned interaction in relational psychotherapy with adults. Attachment-informed psychotherapy generally requires significant interaction over time. For example, transference-focused psychotherapy, a psychodynamic treatment (originally) created to address borderline personality disorder that has demonstrated personality-related changes (including attachment style), recommends twice a week therapy for "at least 12–18 months" (Yeomans, Levy, & Caligor, 2013, p. 2). This is still far less contact than caregivers have in childhood. We suspect that attachment dynamics may become active (and potentially malleable) relatively quickly in adult psychotherapy in part because therapeutic conversations tend to address difficulties, threats, and struggles, topics that are likely to activate the attachment system. Nevertheless, therapists do well to consider how they can help clients access and utilize attachment relationships and communities of support in their lives, and to utilize relational modes of treatment (couples, family, group) when possible to harness the power of multiple relational experiences.

Cultivating Capacities

In contrast to kinds of change that may occur in a moment by utilizing existing resources differently—by, for example, making a different choice or seeing a new option—expanding or developing new capacities requires a sequence of growth-oriented investments and experiences, something akin to growing a plant, learning a language, or increasing physical fitness. Developmental capacities associated with attachment include affect regulation, mentalization, emotional attunement, and interpersonal coordination or negotiation (these capacities are described in more detail in Chapter 7). Attachment-informed psychotherapy often involves promoting personal growth in one or more of these areas. Along this line, Summers (2005) suggested strategies for promoting new ways of being in psychoanalytic therapy, including creative struggle, playing and practicing, and recognition/support for nascent expressions or initiatives.

Individualized and Flexible Therapeutic Stances

Facilitating developmental change requires flexible and personalized interactions. I [DR] believe most parents recognize that good parenting requires a varied repertoire, including relating to different children differently (i.e., according to their particular strengths, vulnerabilities, and preferences), recognizing that different moments and contexts call for different responses, and adjusting to account for ways children have grown or changed (Siegel & Hartzell, 2013). Attachment research has linked growth-enhancing parenting with parental capacities for attunement, intersubjective coordination, and emotional regulation (Beebe, Rustin, Sorter, & Knoblauch, 2003; Knox, 2013; Lyons-Ruth, 2007; Schore, 2012). Parents who lack these capacities may respond rigidly, reactively or inconsistently, patterns associated with insecure attachment and developmental disruption. In parallel fashion, attachment-informed psychotherapy requires individualized and ongoing treatment planning, and flexible, attuned interventions (Costello, 2013; Slade & Holmes, 2019; Wallin, 2007).

From this perspective, inflexible stances by therapists—even around generally helpful treatment strategies—may be less helpful than fitted, collaborative, and adjustable stances. Psychodynamic theorists have long argued for nuanced, fitted responses to clients (Bromberg, 2011; Orange, Atwood, & Stolorow, 1997; Weiss, 1993), and there is also a growing body of psychotherapy research along this line, including recent reviews of therapist flexibility and responsiveness (Owen & Hilsenroth, 2014; Stiles & Horvath, 2017), effective psychotherapy relationships (Norcross & Lambert, 2018), and treatment monitoring approaches that emphasize adjustment based on client feedback (Brattland et al., 2018). Of course, no therapist is attuned and optimally responsive at all times, so rupture and repair processes are critical. In addition, more fluid or flexible approaches may become sloppy or incoherent if therapists do not have an overarching framework and mechanisms for feedback, consultation, support, and accountability (see Chapter 11 for more on this).

ATTACHMENT-INFORMED CLINICAL STRATEGIES

Clinical and attachment researchers have made some progress in identifying relational patterns and stances that tend to promote secure attachment and related functions in adult psychotherapy (Berry & Danquah, 2015; Costello, 2013; Mikulincer et al., 2013). Nevertheless, more research is needed to further clarify (a) how attachment changes in psychotherapy, (b) how attachment relates to other desired therapeutic outcomes, (c) how cultural and contextual factors shape or supplant attachment dynamics, and (d) how attachment dynamics in psychotherapy may differ from other attachment relationships (e.g., caregivers, partners, friends, elders). Next, we review general strategies for strengthening secure attachment in adult psychotherapy, and then discuss strategies for addressing insecure attachment in treatment. The latter is especially relevant for clinicians, as many clients enter treatment with insecure attachment styles and compromised capacities for affect regulation, mentalization, and intersubjectivity. For these clients, working with attachment means encountering and working with insecure attachment patterns, and attachment security is a treatment outcome as much as a treatment resource, at least in the early phases of treatment.

General Strategies for Secure Attachment

Attune to Emotions and Coordinate Communication

In general, secure attachment results from attuned responsiveness by attachment figures. Developmental researchers have highlighted maternal/caregiver "sensitivity" (Beebe, Rustin, et al., 2003; Costello, 2013; Lyons-Ruth, 2007), which involves awareness and empathy, and an ability to respond in fitting, helpful ways, including making adjustments as needed. Costello (2013) framed these dynamics as "coordinated communication" (p. 96). He argued that communication is critical because caregiver sensitivity depends on the caregiver recognizing and responding to the child's communications (verbal and nonverbal), and because attachment behaviors can be viewed as attempts to establish a coordinated state in which an infant or child feels in sync with the caregiver to gain confidence that help is available if needed. Also, in the attempt to establish coordinated communication with an attachment figure, a child learns to adjust communications to account for the response patterns of the other, and these accommodations become part of the child's internal working model and attachment style. With regard to communication in psychotherapy, Wallin (2007), utilizing the ideas of Lyons-Ruth (1999), described four key principles for "collaborative" communication:

- Be receptive to the whole range of emotions and experiences. This includes sharing and enhancing positive affect as well as acknowledging the full range of negative emotions.

- Initiate efforts at repair if the relationship is strained or disrupted (see Chapter 7, this volume, for more on rupture and repair).

- Scaffold the client's efforts (e.g., lend a hand when needed, only as much as needed).

- Be willing to engage and struggle together through difficulties, including setting limits and tolerating protests.

Balance Individual and Dyadic Affect Regulation

Beebe and colleagues encouraged therapists toward what she called a "mid-range balance model" of coordination and bidirectional regulation (Beebe, Rustin, et al., 2003, p. 833). In her microanalyses of mother–infant inter-actions, Beebe clarified that overly close tracking (mother and infant are overly or anxiously attentive and synchronized) and overly loose tracking (mother and infant are not coordinated) correlate with insecure attachment; midrange tracking allowed for coherence and feeling connected, but also for variability and a mix of dyadic regulation and self-regulation (Beebe, 2010). Therapists struggle with insecurity too, and the client–therapist dyad can easily slip into overly tight or loose tracking through misguided attempts to manage their anxiety. Therapists must avoid polarized positions and instead make ongoing adjustments to balance joining (dwelling) with giving space for self-organizing (seeking) within a given interaction. Balance here does not refer to an ideal, static midpoint, but to making adjustments as needed within an unfolding inter-personal process. For example, after an intervention that did not land well, one client needed silence and brief open-ended questions to recover voice, but later in the session became withdrawn until the therapist engaged more actively.

Support Affect Regulation and Mentalization

Affect regulation and mentalization are two key developmental capacities that influence, and are influenced by, the attachment system (Ogden & Fisher, 2015; Schore & Schore, 2014; Wallin, 2007); these capacities are also critical for the differentiation system and the intersubjectivity system (see Chapters 6 and 7, this volume). *Affect regulation* refers to ways that persons may individually or relationally modulate emotional intensity to stay in a useful range that some call the "window of tolerance" (Ogden & Fisher, 2015, p. 227). Emotions that are too powerful (hyperarousal) or muted (hypoarousal) are overwhelming or ineffective, while emotions operating within the window of tolerance have adaptive functions like directing attention, providing information, generating motivation, and evoking adaptive responses (Costello, 2013; Ogden & Fisher, 2015). Affect regulation is a key component of safe haven and secure base expe-riences with attachment figures and has significant impact on a child's brain development (Schore, 2017).

As described in Chapter 3, *mentalization* refers to "the capacity to under-stand other people and oneself in terms of possible thoughts, feelings, wishes, and desires" (Fonagy, Campbell, & Luyten, 2017, p. 373); or in other words, reflecting on one's own mind and the mind of the other. Mentalization affects and is affected by attachment in multiple ways: (a) a caregiver's capacity for mentalization enables attunement and coordinated communication, promoting secure attachment; (b) mentalization-aided safe haven functioning by attachment figures provides dyadic affect regulation for children, which in turn helps children to develop their own capacity to mentalize (mentalization is hindered by dysregulation); and (c) mentalization facilitates secure base functioning by enabling openness, curiosity, and an ability to learn when encountering differences or novelty (Fonagy, Campbell, & Luyten, 2017; Wallin, 2007). We consider stances and strategies for mentalization and affect regulation in the following section because both are essential for addressing insecure attachment in psychotherapy.

Strategies for Working with Insecure Attachment

Recover Empathic Presence

A first and foundational strategy for working with insecurely attached adults is to work toward (and recover) an open, empathic, mentalizing stance (Fonagy, Campbell, & Luyten, 2017). Individuals who present with insecure attachment have adapted to problematic relational patterns, and often suffered in other ways as well. These clients may be difficult to collaborate with precisely because their capacity for collaboration was compromised or distorted in prior relationships. For example, I [DR] have several long-term clients who often seem allergic to direct conversation about change (even though they emphatically state that they need to change), a stance I mostly attribute to prior relational experiences of expectation/demand, control, disappointment, or abuse. However, these same clients often make initiatives on their own (often announced afterwards) when feeling secure and supported, so a key intervention is trying to be present and reduce "the sense that one's mind is alone" (Fonagy, Campbell, & Luyten, 2017, p. 373). Even this can be challenging with clients who have experienced attachment figures as unhelpful or trustworthy, so the work often involves acknowledging and tolerating critique/rejection of efforts to be present.

Listen for What is Absent

Another strategy involves attending to excluded affect and constricted communication patterns (Costello, 2013; Wallin, 2007). This requires broadening attention beyond what is consciously presented by the client to also consider what might be absent, muted, implied, unformulated, dissociated, or perhaps unspeakable, and engaging these experiences as possible. There are different ways to recognize what has been left out, including noticing gaps in the narrative, attending to small incongruities and surprises in the interaction, and noticing one's own intuitions, associations, and emotions. On emotional knowing, Schore (2012) pointed out that a therapist's intuitive feel for and attention to a client's dissociated affect may intensify the affect and help the client to subjectively register it. When therapists help clients to access previously inaccessible emotions or perspectives, clients gain access to additional information, motivation, and action tendencies that may assist them toward their goals, and they may feel empowered to continue with more expansive or inclusive communication that might include disclosures about spiritual and existential dynamics.

Adjust Interpersonal Distance

Several authors have highlighted strategies for engaging insecure clients in familiar, tolerable ways while slowly asking them to stretch beyond their familiar ways (Mallinckrodt, 2015; Slade & Holmes, 2019; Wallin, 2007). For example, Daly and Mallinckrodt (2009) identified a core strategy of regulating therapeutic distance. This means meeting and engaging clients at their preferred interpersonal distance early in treatment, and gradually introducing more or less distance over time. For dismissive clients, emotional distance, minimizing/devaluing needs for others, or self-reliance may predominate early in the treatment, while the therapist works toward greater immediacy, emotional depth, and safe-haven behavior over time. For preoccupied clients, there may be many bids for closeness, validation, and reassurance early on, with gradual efforts to introduce greater differentiation, self-direction, and secure base behavior. The art lies in finding the right timing and ways of adjusting interpersonal distance in session in order to promote growth without overwhelming the client or provoking retrenchment. Reynolds, Rupert, and Sandage (2019) offered a detailed case study that illustrates how one therapist negotiated therapeutic distance with a dismissively attached client.

Assist With Affect Regulation

Affect regulation is a critical and often difficult issue for insecurely attached clients, especially those who have experienced disturbed or abusive attachment relationships leading to unresolved or disorganized attachment (Lyons-Ruth, 2007; Schore, 2012; Wallin, 2007). Developmental/relational trauma can be profoundly painful and disruptive, and persons who suffer developmental trauma may struggle when facing difficulties later in life (Bromberg, 2011; Knox, 2013; Schore, 2012). Treatment must address relational influences on the resulting patterns of hyperarousal (e.g., overwhelm, reactivity, rage) and hypoarousal (e.g., dissociation, numbness, shame, disgust).

Component-based psychotherapy (Grossman, Spinazzola, Zucker, & Hopper, 2017) and sensorimotor psychotherapy (Ogden & Fisher, 2015) are two helpful approaches that explicitly consider ways that trauma (especially developmental trauma) and attachment interrelate, and both offer helpful strategies for affect regulation for clients with disorganized or other highly insecure attachment styles. With these clients, the therapeutic relationship is "a primary medium for healing" (Grossman et al., 2017, p. 88) and a critical factor facilitating or hindering other interventions. Therapists are encouraged to demonstrate the core qualities of good enough attachment figures; for example, sensitivity, warmth and presence, responsiveness, collaboration, and flexibility. However,

> because of the extreme sensitivities and vulnerabilities clients may bring to therapy, nuanced aspects of the therapeutic relationship are required, such as the development of gently and empathically humorous rituals, careful use of

confrontation, responses to shifts in state, and thoughtful use of self-disclosure. How therapists are in the room is more important than what regulation techniques they use. (Grossman et al., 2017, pp. 89–90)

Within an attuned therapeutic relationship, there are many specific interventions that may be helpful for dysregulation including the following:

- Collaboratively identifying, building up, and utilizing personal resources and strengths. Resources may be emotional, somatic, relational, cultural, spiritual, religious, artistic, psychological, intellectual, material (physical/economic), and so on. Examples include journaling, exercising, coloring, meditating, praying, being with friends, participating in services or rituals, having a pet, etc. The RSM includes attention to ways that spiritual/religious practices and communities that may (or may not) be helpful resources for some clients (see Chapter 3). Ogden and Fisher (2015) presented an extensive, nuanced discussion of specific resources in their book on sensorimotor psychotherapy.

- Utilizing somatic, body-focused experiences and exercises to promote sensory/motor awareness, regulation, and expression (Grossman et al., 2017; Ogden & Fisher, 2015). This includes structured somatic practices (e.g., breathing exercises, movement, rituals, imagery, sensory experiences) and spontaneous interventions that might be integrated with clients' relational spirituality. Knox (2013) provided a simple and powerful example of a spontaneous intervention that consisted of inviting a traumatically dysregulated client to pass a pillow back and forth in the session, thereby activating her motor system and implicitly redirecting the focus back to their safe relationship.

- Using the therapeutic relationship as a container for recognizing and engaging dissociated self-states and working through enactments that involve dissociated states in the therapist (Benjamin, 2018; Bromberg, 2011; Grossman et al., 2017). It is important to keep in mind that spiritual experiences can sometimes be part of dissociative self-states, which might serve protective functions but also limit the development of attachment security when compensatory. See Chapter 7 for further discussion of self-states and enactments.

- Working to access, hear, and construct narratives and systems of meaning. This includes efforts to frame past suffering but also to situate clients' lives and identities within larger relational stories that reflect their values, commitments, and preferences (Freedman & Combs, 1996; Grossman et al., 2017). These conversations often touch on spiritual, religious, or existential themes. Potential interventions include exploratory and experience-generating questions, creating or accessing metaphors and stories, and elaborating emotionally evocative moments. For example, one client struggling with shame about childhood abuse and what he saw as subsequent personal failures found solace and self-respect as we identified and discussed his social justice commitments and two resonant personal metaphors: "living bravely" and "bringing light into the world." These metaphors subsequently proved spiritually generative for the client, and this validating coconstruction was a new experience of relational spirituality.

Work Through Cycles of Activation and Regulation

Schore (2012, 2018) also spoke extensively about helping clients regulate intense emotion and expand their capacity for affect regulation, but he focused on implicit "right-brain" processing and communication. He encouraged therapists to (a) use intuition and unconscious right-brain processing to *feel with and "be with"* clients in moments of intense dysregulation, because being recognized and joined is regulating (Schore, 2012, p. 103); and (b) expand capacities for regulation by working at the edges of the windows of tolerance through cycles of activation and regulation of intense emotions (Schore, 2012; Schore & Schore, 2014). Schore preferred the phrase *windows of tolerance* to account for variability in brain hemispheres and different affect states. Importantly, he did not see midrange arousal as ideal, and instead suggested that expanding one's capacity for affect regulation requires working at the edges of what can be tolerated with dyadic support. Repeated cycles of distress followed by dyadic regulation promote implicit brain capacities for self-regulation (Schore, 2012). Working near the edge of capacity is intense, as suggested by the RSM metaphor of the crucible, and therapist–client dyads must negotiate these tensions. In some moments and with some clients, sustained empathic acknowledgment and recognition (e.g., "That is so painful!") is best. Other moments call for some additional response or perspective from the therapist, such as the following:

- "How do you bear it?"
- "I see your intentions, and I know its hard but try to stay with that, what does [your intention] mean in this moment?"
- "Where is God [or some other SERT language] in this?"
- "You are showing so much courage and honesty."
- "And all this on top of what you already face every day as a woman of color."
- "It's so messy and confusing and painful now . . . but I am still here and so are you."

Help Clients Rebuild Trust so They Can Learn

A final strategy for assisting insecurely attached clients comes from Fonagy and colleagues through their recent work on rebuilding "epistemic trust" (Fonagy, Luyten, Allison, & Campbell, 2017, p. 1). Fonagy, Luyten, et al. (2017) argued that most mental health problems reflect a fundamental lack of resilience caused by loss of trust and negative appraisal tendencies. Essentially, repeated or severely negative social experiences create distrust that precludes social learning. Rigid and problematic patterns persist because clients cannot distinguish different contexts or sources, learn from experience, or receive assistance from others. Fonagy and colleagues outlined three systems of communication for rebuilding epistemic trust (Fonagy, Luyten, et al., 2017).

First, the therapist must communicate ideas about treatment and an understanding of the client that somehow perk the client's interest despite preexisting distrust. To do this, therapists must communicate that "they see the patient's problems from their perspective, recognizing them as an agent, and with the attitude that the patient has things to teach the therapist" (Fonagy, Luyten, et al., 2017, p. 9). This is a form of respectful joining with the client.

Second, the therapist builds upon and deepens the client's experience of collaboration and mentalization. This involves (a) consistently recognizing the client as a subject and agent, and negotiating with the client from that position; (b) noticing and acknowledging the client's emotional states, which helps to regulate arousal and model a mentalizing stance; and (c) helping the client to consider possible links between mental states and life events.

Third, the therapist facilitates the client's engagement and learning from the larger social world. This involves helping clients utilize their growing capacity for mentalization to make better judgments about who/what is trustworthy and resume social learning outside of therapy. Fonagy, Luyten, and colleagues (2017) noted that this process requires a reasonably benign social environment; it may be neither possible nor useful to build trust in an unsafe context. From an RSM perspective, psychotherapy can help to rebuild epistemic trust by offering a good enough therapeutic relationship (as described earlier) and by helping clients access additional spiritual, cultural, and relational resources that support openness, awareness, wisdom, and agency.

CONCLUSION

Attachment is an innate developmental system that enables enable humans (and other mammals) to negotiate fear, threat, loss, and distress by obtaining support from dependable attachment figures. In addition, secure attachment facilitates the development of other vital capacities such as mentalization, affect regulation, flexible coping, and openness to social learning. Attachment dynamics of safe haven and secure base functioning interact and overlap with relational spirituality constructs of dwelling and seeking. While therapists can only provide modest attachment support compared with what clients may experience from caregivers, lovers, friends, or communities, they may nevertheless help clients alter problematic attachment patterns and expand relational capacities. In this way, attachment-informed psychotherapy may facilitate resilience, human connection, and vital living.

6

Differentiation and Relational Spirituality

Differentiation is about how life forms evolve and gain new abilities.
—D. SCHNARCH, *INTIMACY AND DESIRE* (2009, P. 86)

This chapter focuses on the second of the three developmental systems we assess and clinically engage in the relational spirituality model (RSM): the differentiation system. As Schnarch noted in the volume referenced above, the differentiation system includes *species differentiation*, or the ways members of a species evolve over time through interaction with their own and other species. At the human level, *personal differentiation* refers to individual growth in the complexity and integration of selfhood in interaction with key relationships and social contexts. As we noted in Chapter 2, this volume, the differentiation system focuses on the relational dialectics of (a) self and other, and (b) emotion and thought and the associated challenges of managing anxiety about differences or relational alterity (i.e., "otherness"; Sandage & Brown, 2018; Sandage, Paine, & Morgan, 2019). Kerr and Bowen (1988) also described ways the differentiation system evolved from the need for humans to cooperate across complex social differences, and challenges in human cooperation remain a consistent clinical concern.

The dynamics of relational spirituality can influence the developmental processes of the differentiation system by facilitating or discouraging the acceptance of difference and the positive sacred meaning of cooperating across differences. For example, spiritual or religious traditions sometimes encourage

http://dx.doi.org/10.1037/0000174-007
Relational Spirituality in Psychotherapy: Healing Suffering and Promoting Growth,
by S. J. Sandage, D. Rupert, G. S. Stavros, and N. G. Devor

compassion and respect for those of other traditions even while acknowledging important differences, but spiritual and religious traditions can also define such differentiated relational stances as dangerously compromising, impure, and even heretical. In reciprocal fashion, the developmental pull toward differentiation can lead individuals and communities toward changes in their relational spirituality templates or "rethinking" their spiritual–existential–religious–theological (SERT) worldviews. As we described in Chapter 3, such change processes sometimes unfold in the context of psychotherapy and can be destabilizing and anxiety-provoking of spiritual and existential tensions between the contrasting pulls toward individual freedom and relational obligations. These tensions often shape powerful developmental dilemmas related to differentiation and the meaning of *integrity* for an individual or relational system.

Consider the following clinical scenario. Seo-yun (age 28, Korean American) asks her parents to come to a session with her therapist because of their refusal to attend her wedding ceremony. Seo-yun is marrying Ray (age 34, German American), who self-defines as atheist. Her parents are conservative Christians and deeply value the New Testament instruction to "not be unequally yoked with unbelievers," which they take to mean that it is immoral to marry someone who is not a Christian. This conflict is so hurtful and anxiety-provoking for Seo-yun and both her parents that they cannot communicate about the issues without intense, painful feelings of anger, shame, and sadness that exacerbate their existential experience of alienation and loss. The three of them are each struggling to develop the differentiation necessary to be able to even communicate about the issues, much less resolve the conflicts. Her parents experience Seo-yun's decision to marry someone outside their faith tradition as a desecration or violation of spiritual principles. It feels insulting and embarrassing to them and ruptures their sense of spiritual generativity as they envisioned her life course. Seo-yun knew her parents would struggle with her decision given the particular theological beliefs of their church community, but she is hurt and angry that they do not seem able to put their own beliefs to the side and respect her need to define her own beliefs as an adult. From one angle, we could say that Seo-yun is prompting a crisis of differentiation in this family system by forming an intimate relationship outside her religious community. But we could also note that her grandparents on both sides converted to Christianity as immigrants in the United States as an act of differentiation from their prior religious background, which facilitated their acculturation process but now leads to further intergenerational challenges of differentiation. Furthermore, Seo-yun's therapist, Ivan (age 47, Puerto Rican and African American, humanistic spirituality), is also challenged toward the differentiation to both support his client and relate respectfully with her parents amid this set of spiritual, existential, religious, and theological tensions in the family system and their wider social contexts. Ivan has his own beliefs about these issues, but he will need to stay focused on how to help Seo-Yun manage her conflicts with her parents rather than resolve it for her.[1]

In this chapter, we first define differentiation as a concept and developmental system, and we then review key theoretical perspectives that inform our understanding of differentiation. We then consider cultural dynamics and differentiation and describe the role of differentiation in relating to clients across spiritual and religious diversity. Next, we highlight relational spirituality dynamics that interact with the differentiation system. Finally, we offer clinical strategies to facilitate differentiation in psychotherapy.

DEFINING DIFFERENTIATION

The concept of *differentiation* is multidimensional and involves capacities for self-regulation of emotions (intrapsychic dimension), interpersonal balancing of connection and autonomy (interpersonal dimension), and effective relating across sociocultural differences (intercultural dimension). We will explain each of these dimensions below in relation to key theoretical influences. Whereas the attachment system orients primarily toward security and the balancing of safety and exploration, the differentiation system deals with self-identity and the flexibility of selfhood to balance cooperation and boundaries amidst differences. The family systems literature uses the term *differentiation of self* (DoS) to emphasize the idea of different levels of differentiation within an individual's sense of self. The term can also refer to how we hold onto our sense of self in close proximity to others (see Schnarch, 1997), with the manner or degree to which we do this ranging widely from reactive violence to grounded openness. We will build upon this understanding of DoS but also use the broader term *differentiation* when referencing dynamics beyond relational selfhood.

Attachment and differentiation are somewhat overlapping concepts with *healthy development*, defined as including the abilities to both function autonomously (self-regulation) and connect with others (relational regulation). However, the attachment literature places a stronger emphasis on relational regulation or drawing support from others to manage emotions, whereas the differentiation literature tends to highlight capacities for self-regulation or self-soothing of emotions. The few empirical studies using measures of both attachment and DoS validate this understanding that these developmental systems are correlated but also distinct (Hainlen, Jankowski, Paine, & Sandage, 2016; Lampis & Cataudella, 2019; Skowron & Dendy, 2004; Xue et al., 2018).

---

[1]If this were family therapy, Ivan would have the ongoing challenge of developing a working alliance with each family member without letting his own views lead him to side with one member or part of the system.

At the larger social systemic level, differentiation also involves the ways individuals and groups manage the evolutionary tensions between cooperation and competition, dialogue and boundaries (Sennett, 2012). Systems that rely heavily upon social hierarchy (i.e., structured authority) and homogeneity need less of the kind of differentiation we are describing because roles define appropriate behavior. And the need for differentiation may remain relatively dormant as long as individuals avoid social and relational differences. However, systems (e.g., families, congregations, clinics, societies) that move toward more egalitarian relations of power sharing and greater diversity will require individuals to develop more differentiated capacities to dialogue, relate effectively, and cooperate across differences. These systemic contexts will present greater ambiguity about appropriate boundaries and behavior, and interpersonal differences will need to be negotiated. Thus, the differentiation system will become increasingly relevant as individuals transition into unfamiliar and diverse contexts and engage in new identity development processes in those contexts.

THEORIES OF DIFFERENTIATION

We draw on several interdisciplinary streams of influence in understanding differentiation in clinical practice, including theories from family systems, psychoanalysis, neurobiology, human development, intercultural relations, and spirituality.

Family Systems

Murray Bowen (1978; Kerr, 2019; Kerr & Bowen, 1988) was a seminal figure in applying the concept of differentiation from evolutionary biology to relational dynamics within family systems and family therapy. In Bowenian theory, DoS is a dialectical construct that involves an intrapsychic capacity to integrate emotions and cognitions (or limbic and neocortical brain functioning), as well as the interpersonal flexibility to engage in both connected and independent functioning in relationships. Some theorists have preferred the term *individuation* or use it as a synonym for differentiation (e.g., Jung); however, our dialectical view of differentiation means we understand individuation or autonomous functioning as one pole that is balanced by movement toward connection and communion with others (Bakan, 1966; Kegan, 1994; Schnarch, 1997).

As mentioned in Chapter 4, this volume, Bowen (1978) emphasized the role of anxiety in families and other relational systems and the need for differentiation to manage the anxieties of personal differences and conflicts and changes in systems over time. Individuals and systems with low levels of differentiation tend be very emotionally reactive to differences and changes with limited coping skills. This can lead to either rigid patterns of behavior that work against needed changes in systems, or at the other extreme, chaotic patterns of behavior when individuals or relational systems lack a coherent sense of identity for decision-making.

At the interpersonal level, Bowen (1978) described *fusion* and *cutoff* as opposing problems of differentiation. In fusion, anxiety promotes movement toward relational enmeshment and a need for similarity with little tolerance for difference. This reflects abandonment anxiety. In cutoff, anxiety promotes distancing, thicker boundaries, and drawing out distinctions between self and other. Cutoff can reflect underlying anxiety about engulfment. Relational patterns of fusion are higher among those with an anxious–ambivalent attachment style, whereas cutoff is more common among those with an avoidant attachment style (Hainlen et al., 2016). It is important to note that fusion and cutoff can be problematic; however, systemic thinking suggests we also try to understand the functionality of those relational stances in certain contexts and their normality in some cultures. For example, movement toward fusion in a family or religious community might be temporarily adaptive during a crisis in which intense levels of support and solidarity are needed. Cutoff can also be an adaptive response to experiences of abuse in a family or religious congregation (Sandage, 2010). The key clinical questions based on the RSM for a given case are (a) whether relational patterns formed during a crisis or traumatic experience have limited the present capacity for greater differentiation, and (b) whether patterns of fusion or cutoff (i.e., limited differentiation) have impacted the development of healthy and mature relational spirituality among these clients.

Bowen also introduced the concept of *triangulation*, or the ways relational dyads can rely on a third party for stabilization (Kerr & Bowen, 1988; Titelman, 2008), such as when a conflicted couple approaches their religious leader for help with their relationship. Triangulation is a ubiquitous dynamic in human systems and not always problematic. However, some forms of triangulation can limit relational development because of power dynamics or the chronicity of use; for example, if the same couple relied on one of their children to try to arbitrate all their conflicts or if they found they could not resolve any of their conflicts without a third party. Extremely stressful or traumatic events can prompt overuse of intergenerational triangulation in ways that limit the development of DoS (Peleg, 2014). Triangulation can also occur in nonhuman forms, like the reliance on substances, work, spirituality, or various hobbies and diversions to distract from or compensate for problems in an unstable relationship (Guerin, Fogarty, Fay, & Kautoo, 1996). When people are triangulated, the key question is whether they have sufficient DoS to relate effectively and equitably to all parts of the relational system they are recruited to help. As mentioned in Chapter 3, there is some evidence that high levels of family triangulation among emerging adults may limit their own spiritual development (Heiden-Rootes, Jankowski, & Sandage, 2010), and this is likely due to limiting their emotional freedom for the development of their own differentiation.

Rabbi Edwin Friedman (1985) applied Bowenian theory and the concept of DoS to dynamics within religious congregations and noted the parallels between the ways therapists are triangulated with conflicting interests of family members in family therapy and the ways clergy are triangulated amid the varied agendas of congregants. God or the sacred can be invoked in poorly differentiated systems as triangulating power moves against accepting differences, or control moves to prevent needed changes in the system (Sandage & Brown, 2018). This family-systems tradition of differentiation also places a strong emphasis on self of the therapist formation (or self of the leader) and the ongoing need to manage one's own anxiety and continue to grow in differentiation to navigate the dynamics of frequent triangulation (Grosch & Olsen, 2000; Olsen & Devor, 2015). A common understanding in this tradition is that, as a therapist, I can only help people to a level of differentiation that I have personally achieved. Given the stress of working intensely with people amid suffering and profound change, it is crucial for clinicians to cultivate and maintain their own highly differentiated personal and professional relationships to provide both support and stimulation for self-confrontation and growth.

David Schnarch's work on DoS from the couple therapy and sex therapy fields is discussed in-depth in Chapter 3 and is a key influence on our RSM understanding of differentiation. Schnarch's (2009, p. 72) particular crucible model of therapy posits "four points of balance" as part of DoS: (a) a "solid flexible self" (self-identity dimension), (b) a "quiet mind—calm heart" (self-regulation dimension), (c) "grounded responding" (interpersonal flexibility dimension), and (d) "meaningful endurance" (distress tolerance dimension). This latter dimension of meaningful endurance is implied in some other models but is a relatively unique SERT-oriented contribution to the differentiation literature with Schnarch's emphasis on "tolerating discomfort for the sake of growth" (p. 72). Numerous views of suffering (Chapter 4) could be embraced for distress tolerance, as the differentiation system pulls for one's deepest values, hopes, and desires to generate meaning for the endurance, grit, and seeking processes needed to grow through suffering.

Elizabeth Skowron (Skowron & Schmitt, 2003) developed a widely used multidimensional measure of DoS (Differentiation of Self Inventory—Revised [DSI–R]), and studies using versions of this measure have established empirical evidence of positive associations between DoS and numerous indices of mental health, relational functioning, marital adjustment, healthy parenting, problem solving, resilience, and physical health with a wider literature rapidly developing (Rodríguez-González, Schweer-Collins, Skowron, Jódar, Cagigal, & Major, 2018; Skowron, Van Epps, & Cipriano-Essel, 2014). The four dimensions assessed on the DSI–R are (a) I-position (self-identity), (b) fusion with others, (c) emotional cutoff, and (d) emotional reactivity ([b], [c], and [d] are negative indices of DoS). There is also a growing body of empirical literature on DoS in relation to various mental health problems, such as depression (Rodríguez-González et al., 2018; Sandage, Jankowski, Bissonette, & Paine, 2017), eating disorders (Buser & Gibson, 2014), schizophrenia (Peleg & Arnon, 2013), trauma (Giladi & Bell, 2013; Halevi & Idisis, 2018), and child maltreatment perpetration (Okado & Azar, 2011). DoS has also been negatively associated with shame-proneness and accounted for the relationship between shame and reduced social connectedness in an adult sample (Williamson, Sandage, & Lee, 2007). Chronic shame can be debilitating to the agency, endurance, and relational supports needed to cope with suffering and trauma, and DoS can be particularly important for maintaining relational connections and healthy communication patterns when going through significant struggles (Giladi & Bell, 2013). DoS has also been negatively correlated with symptoms of vicarious trauma and ruptured cognitive schemas (related to self, safety, trust, intimacy, and control) among therapists (Halevi & Idisis, 2018), supporting the understanding that DoS represents an important suite of resilience factors that may be protective for those with heavy exposure to suffering and trauma.

Psychoanalysis

Numerous psychoanalytic theorists have also emphasized differentiation as part of the healthy development of self-identity. For example, Hamilton (1990) utilized object relations theory (ORT) and ego psychology to describe differentiation and integration as complementary ego functions that serve to both divide and unite mental objects, and Hamilton agreed with numerous developmental theorists in positing that differentiation and integration each play important dialectical functions in shaping how an individual relates with others and manages the tensions of interpersonal differences. Kernberg (2012) also articulated an ORT perspective on differentiation as part of reflective functioning and individuals' abilities to conceptualize both self and object representations with complexity and an awareness of differing affective experiences of self and other (i.e., the ability to mentalize). Self–other differentiation has also been described as essential to developing capacities for intersubjectivity, the focal topic of Chapter 7 (Auerbach & Blatt, 2001; Benjamin, 2018). Thus, differentiation helps prevent projection of one's own feelings onto others and enhances the capacity to understand others as distinct from self.

Kohut's (1971, 1972, 1977) self psychology offered an important contribution to understanding connections between differentiation, spirituality, and relational trauma with his theory that the cohesive self has "differentiated psychological functions" (Kohut & Ornstein, 2011, p. 62), which develop in relation to an individual's ideals, values, and guiding principles. Kohut also believed that "traumatic frustrations" in idealization during self-development can lead to problems in differentiating from others, and this might show up in spiritual and existential problems forming one's own guiding beliefs, values, and goals (ideals) and sustaining those in the face of interpersonal differences and disappointments (Kohut & Ornstein, 2011, p. 357; see also Patton, Connor, & Scott, 1982). Jones (2002) related Kohut's self psychology understanding of idealization to spirituality based on the idea that what we consider sacred or ultimate necessarily converges with developmental dynamics influencing our ideals in life. For Kohut (Kohut & Ornstein, 2011), low levels of differentiation mean strong cathexis with narcissistic libido and a lack of transformed grandiosity within self-identity, and this contributes to vulnerability for conflict with others, a lack of humility, and a risk for self-depletion and depression. Sandage and colleagues found empirical support for these associations in a sample of graduate students in the helping professions in a Christian training context (Sandage, Jankowski, et al., 2017), and this highlighted the importance of integrating self-development, ideals, and humility.

Neurobiology

Researchers within the field of interpersonal neurobiology have also described the connections between healthy relational development, mental health, and differentiated and integrative brain functioning. For example, Siegel (2007a) noted that "mental well-being is created within the process of integration, the linkage of differentiated components of a system into a functional whole" (p. 288; see also Cozolino, 2017). He went on to explain how neurobiological coordination occurs through the differentiated growth of prefrontal fibers in the brain, which are formed in response to relational processes of intrapersonal and interpersonal attunement. Intrapersonal attunement involves the vertical integration of the brain and body and the "differentiation of distinct streams of awareness" (Siegel, 2007b, p. 259), and this mindfully differentiated way of relating to one's self can be cultivated by contemplative practices and highly-attuned relational experiences such as those that can be provided in psychotherapy.

Intercultural Relations

Differentiation has also emerged in the field of intercultural relations as a key characteristic in the development of intercultural competence or the ability to understand and respond effectively to cultural differences (Bennett, 2004). Ethnocentrism can be viewed as a problem of cultural differentiation and a tendency to project one's own cultural orientation as the standard for all other cultures. Skowron's (Skowron & Schmitt, 2003) measure of DoS has been positively associated with higher levels of intercultural competence among graduate trainees in the helping professions (Paine, Jankowski, & Sandage, 2016; Sandage & Jankowski, 2013). Intercultural differentiation consistent with intercultural competence involves the capacity to balance awareness of similarities and differences across cultures, and this requires cognitive complexity and well-differentiated perceptual abilities. Cultural differences can be anxiety-provoking, particularly in unfamiliar contexts and experiences of alterity or "otherness" (Sandage, Paine, & Morgan, 2019), so the emotion regulation dimension of DoS is important for managing the stress of such encounters without emotional reactivity or defensive reactions that lead to denigrating or idealizing others.

CULTURAL DYNAMICS AND DIFFERENTIATION

There are important considerations about cultural differences related to differentiation. Certain construals of differentiation that emphasize the autonomy or individuation pole of the dialectic are weighted toward Western individualism and the emphases on personal boundaries, subjectivity, and agency. However, we have framed differentiation as dialectical and involving a flexible capacity for both autonomy and connection. Extremes of individualism undervalue this capacity for connection and may promote excessive use of emotional cutoff.

It is also important to note that there is recent empirical research on DoS in various cultural contexts beyond the United States, such as China (Lam & Chan-So, 2015; Xue et al., 2018), Hong Kong (Ng, 2014), Iran (Amanelahi, Tardast, & Aslani, 2016), Israel (Peleg, 2014), Italy (Lampis, Cataudella, Agus, Busonera, & Skowron, 2019), Portugal (Ferreira, Narciso, Novo, & Pereira, 2016), Spain (Rodríguez-González, Skowron, & Jódar Anchía, 2015), Taiwan (Chang, 2018), and Turkey (Işik & Bulduk, 2015). A review of this cross-cultural research on DoS is beyond the scope of this chapter, but the general picture that is emerging suggests the dimensions of DoS may tend to hold up across cultures but with different meanings and different cutoff points on measures to indicate health versus pathology. For example, in highly collectivistic cultural contexts fusion with others will generally be less pathological than in individualistic cultural contexts, whereas cutoff will tend to be problematic (Rodríguez-González et al., 2015). Individualistic contexts might reinforce cutoff in a greater number of situations than would occur in collectivistic contexts, although research indicates cutoff tends to generally correlate with negative psychological and relational effects across contexts. Different cultural contexts may pull for somewhat differing aspects of DoS (Peleg & Messerschmidt-Grandi, 2018).

Beyond differing cultural expressions of differentiation dimensions, DoS appears to be consistent with healthy cultural identity development and the ability to relate flexibly and effectively across cultures (i.e., intercultural competence), as referenced above. There is some evidence DoS is also consistent with integrative bicultural identity among first-generation immigrants or the ability to hold onto traditional cultural values and also effectively adapt to a host culture (Lee & Johnson, 2017). DoS has also been positively related to a sense of ethnic group belonging among persons of color in the United States (Skowron, 2004), which also validates the thesis that DoS involves an ability by nondominant group members to maintain cultural connections and cultural identity. DoS, as we understand it, is consistent with Choi's (2015) notion of postcolonial selfhood formed among Korean immigrant communities of a hybrid identity that fluidly integrates a sense of being an individual ("I"), being part of ethnic communities or collectives ("We"), and being connected with others who are perceived as both culturally different and similar ("with others" in radical hospitality). Forming a differentiated self-identity in this fashion is much more difficult for those facing racism and other types of prejudice and oppression than for those with greater social privilege, which is relevant for understanding systemic factors that force the identity challenges for some clients who feel unable to integrate certain "split off" aspects of their experience. But this postcolonial model of differentiated-yet-related aspects of self-identity (personal, communal, alterity) can have wide applicability. Clinically, we have found it useful to assess and dialogue with clients about points of connection and/or dissonance between these aspects of identity and their associated self-states.

Higher levels of DoS have also been associated with a greater commitment to social justice across four studies from our lab with graduate students in the helping professions (Hainlen, Jankowski, Paine, & Sandage, 2016; Jankowski, Sandage, & Hill, 2013; Sandage, Crabtree, & Schweer, 2014; Sandage & Jankowski, 2013). In these studies with predominantly Euro American students in a Christian university context in the United States, social justice commitment was operationalized in terms of concerns to work against racism, sexism, and poverty. More research is needed in other contexts and with other justice concerns, but this research is suggestive that DoS may help individuals differentiate their own values and goals from dominant forces of systemic oppression and to sustain hope for change in the face of seemingly intractable social problems. Many social-justice scholars (e.g., Martin Luther King, Jr., Paulo Freire, bell hooks, James Cone, Cornell West) have developed this important connection between hope and social justice, which also has empirical support (Sandage, Crabtree, & Schweer, 2014; Sandage & Morgan, 2014). For those suffering oppression, differentiating their sense of self-identity from hostile and shaming images in the surrounding systemic forces may be liberative, and this will require positive and affirming relational and cultural self-object experiences to counter the oppressive (Sheppard, 2011).

SPIRITUAL AND RELIGIOUS DIVERSITY AND DIFFERENTIATION

DoS can also play a constructive role in relating effectively across spiritual and religious diversity, and this is central to spiritual and religious competence among clinicians (Vieten et al., 2016). Our RSM understanding of clinicians' spiritual and religious diversity competence is informed by a conceptual model of interreligious competence (Morgan & Sandage, 2016; Sandage, Dahl, & Harden, 2012) that builds upon Bennett's (2004; see also Hammer, 2011) model of intercultural competence. These models tease apart differing ways individuals orient toward differences (spiritual/religious or cultural), and we find these orientations provide a helpful heuristic for ways we as clinicians approach spiritual, religious, and other diversity dynamics. All clinicians will have a personal perspective on spiritual and religious issues whether they consider themselves spiritual and/or religious or not, and self-awareness about these perspectives is critical for spiritual and religious competence (Richards & Bergin, 2014; Strawn et al., 2014; Tummala-Narra, 2016; Vieten et al., 2016).

Our focus here will be on spiritual and religious differences and orientations among clinicians, but these models can also apply to clients and certain strengths and challenges related to spiritual and religious diversity.

Denial

When operating from *denial*, a clinician is largely unaware or even avoidant of giving attention to spiritual and religious dynamics among clients and in the larger world, in what represents a kind of undifferentiated cutoff. They may be dismissive of the relevance of spiritual and religious experiences if they are unimportant to them personally, or they may tend to operate with the fused perception that everyone shares their particular spiritual and religious worldview. Denial tends to require limited exposure to spiritual and religious diversity and can be endangered in diverse settings.

Polarization

Clinicians can also operate from spiritual and religious *polarization*, which can take two different forms. Spiritual and religious *defensiveness* is an orientation in which a clinician perceives their own worldview to be superior and other worldviews to be inferior and often threatening. This can promote loyalty toward one's own spiritual or religious traditions and communities, but also grandiosity, anxiety, and hostility toward other perspectives. This could lead clinicians to a dismissive and attacking stance toward a client's spiritual or religious perspectives or practices, such as a clinician who actually interpreted her client's report of speaking in tongues[2] in session as "an obvious attempt to redo your infancy."

Spiritual and religious defensiveness can also be detected in clinicians who implicitly or explicitly seek to proselytize clients toward a fusion with the clinician's own perspective, such as a Christian therapist in a community mental health setting who gave some of his clients an evangelistic booklet on how to become a Christian when he found they were struggling with spiritual and existential ambiguity. Another example is an atheist clinician with some appreciation for Buddhist philosophy who gave an adolescent client an unsolicited book on Buddhism because he perceived the client's struggles with anxiety and perfectionism were rooted in the Orthodox Judaism of the client and her family and thought Buddhism would offer a better worldview. This might have been a legitimate area of exploration in therapy if the client had initiated it, and if the therapist could have been more differentiated about his

---

[2]Speaking in tongues, or *glossolalia*, is an ecstatic spiritual practice in Pentecostal branches of Christianity and some other religious groups involving speaking in unknown languages. Some psychoanalysts have interpreted this kind of spiritual behavior as representing pathological regression toward infant babbling (Wulff, 1997). However, this type of reductionistic psychological interpretation misses the complexity and potential adaptive value of these kinds of spiritual experiences.

own and other perspectives. These very explicit examples are less common than more subtle expressions of spiritual and religious defensiveness, such as when a client mentions spiritual or religious issues and the clinician shifts the conversation in another direction because those issues are perceived as unimportant or unhelpful.

Spiritual and religious *reversal* is the second form of polarization, and the opposite of defensiveness, in which a person perceives their own spiritual or religious orientation to be inferior to that of others with a tendency to idealize those other perspectives or traditions. As with defensiveness, reversal is also a relatively undifferentiated template for spiritual and religious differences and lacks complexity or a nuanced understanding of various perspectives. Reversal can involve chronic negative emotions about one's own spiritual and religious background or perspectives, including shame and fear, along with difficulty perceiving both the strengths and challenges within other perspectives and traditions. For example, a therapist frequently referred to himself as a "recovering Catholic" in a joking manner with clients who raised spiritual and religious issues, and this therapist came to realize these jokes belied some unresolved shame and anger at the Catholic Church for dynamics he experienced as dysfunctional in his early family and religious experience. He also tended to idealize the spirituality of a series of clients from minority religious traditions in the United States, even appropriating certain symbols and artifacts from those traditions into his office space. Through some spiritual and religious diversity training and personal therapy, he was able to self-confront about his limited accurate understanding of these other traditions and the ways this idealization was driven by painful relational spirituality ruptures in his own background.

Minimization

Spiritual and religious *minimization* involves focusing on similarities between various spiritual and religious traditions and minimizing attention to differences. This is different from denial, as those working from minimization may state a general interest in and respect for diversity; however, in practice they will tend to fall back on a focus on presumed similarities with their own perspectives and a neglect in engaging differences. In some cases, focusing on similarities can be effective for building trust and collaboration. For example, a therapist providing dialectical behavior therapy drew a connection between principles of mindfulness practice and her client's mention of the importance of compassion in her Islamic faith. However, when the client expressed reverence for divine compassion as the source of all human compassion and uncertainty about how mindfulness would fit with his own prayer practices the therapist abruptly interjected, "All religious traditions value meditative practices like mindfulness." While this universalizing point by the therapist about meditation might be a useful consideration as part of a broader conversation, it was asserted in a relational dynamic that not only overpowered sensitivity to actual spiritual and religious differences but also implied that the therapist understands these concerns better than the client. In supervision, the therapist became aware that she became anxious about possible differences between herself and the client and also about her limited knowledge of Islam, so she tried to emphasize universal similarities (ironically, in a manner that was not very relationally mindful) to preserve the treatment plan. This move did not facilitate trust or alliance-building with the client; nor did it convey humble curiosity about the client's beliefs, values, and practices that is essential to spiritual and religious competence (Vieten et al., 2016). As we suggested in Chapter 4, there are important differences among various spiritual and religious worldviews on the nature and meaning of suffering, and minimization will tend to prevent clinicians from becoming knowledgeable, respectful, and skillful about these dynamics.

Acceptance

Spiritual and religious *acceptance* is a more differentiated and open orientation to spiritual and religious diversity that involves active interest and curiosity about differences with a tendency to view other worldviews as equally complex. This does not mean the person views all worldviews as equally valid or beneficial, and it is fine to prefer one's own spiritual or religious perspective over others. But those in spiritual and religious acceptance do not feel a need to reduce the complexity of other worldviews and are more mindful of and interested in diversity than those in the other orientations described above, which include growing self-awareness about the impact of their own spiritual, religious, and theological backgrounds and traditions on their clinical perspectives and ethics (Strawn et al., 2014; Wright et al., 2014).[3]

However, those operating from acceptance may lack well-developed skills for working effectively within other spiritual and religious perspectives. For example, a therapist who identified as Evangelical Christian was open to exploring and trying to better understand a particular client's Sikh faith and how it influenced their stated values about family obligations. The client seemed to appreciate the interest and opportunity to share in depth some of his religious beliefs and values as they shaped his concerns in therapy. The conversation itself felt somewhat helpful to both, although the therapist was unclear about how to make use of that information in the subsequent therapy process. The therapist's self-awareness and openness (i.e., DoS) led her to seek out consultation with a therapist with greater spiritual and religious competence and experience, and they considered clinical strategies for continuing the conversation with the client and exploring ways to integrate his

---

[3]Clinicians who want to increase their knowledge and awareness of spiritual and religious diversity in relation to clinical practice might access McGoldrick and Hardy (2019); Richards and Bergin (2005, 2014), and Walsh (2010). Several conference presentations on spiritual diversity and psychotherapy from differing perspectives and traditions are also available for free viewing on our Danielsen Institute website: http://www.bu.edu/danielsen

specific beliefs and values into the treatment plan. Acceptance highlights the developmental difference between awareness of diversity and the skills to work effectively within diversity.

Adaptation

Spiritual and religious *adaptation* combines cognitive openness to spiritual and religious frame-shifting (i.e., seeking to understand other perspectives in depth) and behavioral skills in code-switching (i.e., adapting one's behaviors to fit a different worldview). This involves the highly differentiated relational capacities necessary to actually relate effectively across spiritual and religious differences, which can also necessitate skills in repairing ruptures of misunderstanding. For example, a therapist who identified as agnostic had worked with a client for approximately two years without much discussion of the client's religious faith, which he had perceived as fairly peripheral to the client's identity. The client related in a serious tone that his daughter had started attending a well-known conservative Christian megachurch in that city, and in a moment of sloppiness and misunderstanding the therapist said, "So I gather you are worried about her joining that church?" The client, rather surprised by the comment, replied,

> Oh . . . no, I am so relieved. I have been afraid she would not become a Christian. I am so grateful for this . . . (pausing and starting to tear up) . . . I have wanted to be sure God would watch over her and protect her and feared that wasn't going to happen due to my inconsistency about my own faith. I know God drew her there and now she will be all right.

The therapist experienced the momentary disorientation that came with realizing he had not only misunderstood that situation but had also not been aware of this part of his client's internal world (we would say, "relational spirituality"). Moreover, the therapist had an initial strong countertransference reaction of negative feelings about that theological form of conservative Christian belief in a personal God who determines all events and protects (some) people from suffering. It might often take some time to recover from this rupture; however, this therapist described taking a deep breath and then humbly leaning into the difference as part of the repair by saying,

> Hey, I'm sorry I misunderstood how you might feel about your daughter going to this church. I realize I haven't learned much about you in this area of your faith and the struggles you are referencing, and I would value knowing more about that if you want to talk about it.

By the end of the session, the therapist had internally metabolized his own countertransference and found ways of wrapping the client's own relational spirituality perspectives about divine providence and protection back into the clinical dialogue. This resilience and flexibility showed the clinician's resilient level of differentiation and capacity to engage and make use of the client's own religious framework in the therapeutic process. This example also highlights the point that spiritual and religious competence is less about avoiding mistakes and ruptures than about the ability to regain attunement, respect, and clinical wisdom in working with clients' relational spiritualities.

Our RSM approach to spiritual and religious diversity within the therapy process is also informed by the multicultural orientation (MCO) framework developed by Owen and colleagues (Davis, DeBlaere, et al., 2018; Owen, Tao, Drinane, et al., 2016) and the growing literature on cultural competence (Tummala-Narra, 2009, 2016) and cultural humility among clinicians (Hook, Davis, Owen, & DeBlaere, 2017). In short, our application of this MCO framework to spiritual and religious diversity suggests clinicians should seek to (a) develop a humble, open, and interested stance toward spiritual and religious differences with clients that includes ongoing education, training, and consultation on diversity; (b) look for clinically relevant opportunities to engage spiritual and religious issues in the therapy process in ways that fit particular clients; and (c) increase their comfort with initiating and dialoguing about spiritual and religious dynamics in therapy with a widening range of clients (Vieten et al., 2016). This framework is consistent with our emphasis on DoS in this chapter, as described previously, as it takes solid DoS to practice humility (Jankowski, Sandage, Bell, Ruffing, & Adams, 2018; Jankowski, Sandage, & Hill, 2013; Paine, Sandage, Rupert, Devor, & Bronstein, 2015), engage opportunities to discuss spiritual and religious issues in ways that fit particular clients (rather than the therapist's own preferences), and develop affect regulation strategies to become more comfortable engaging differences in therapy. Thus, in our RSM framework growth in spiritual and religious competence requires the integration of dwelling and seeking, connecting with others and tolerating ambiguity to explore new and more complex understandings. We have also found it important to maintain awareness that clinicians and clients who are spiritual and religious minorities in a given context may find it harder to access resources that support and inform their perspectives (i.e., dwelling), which can make perpetual seeking highly stressful and even traumatic. This raises systemic issues we return to in Chapter 9.

RELATIONAL SPIRITUALITY INTEGRATED WITH DIFFERENTIATION

Individual differences in relational spirituality also interact with the differentiation developmental system in complex ways. Just as differentiation needs to be understood along a continuum, forms of relational spirituality will vary in the extent to which they are integrated with the differentiation system (Schnarch, 1991; Shults & Sandage, 2006; Worthington & Sandage, 2016). Empirically, DoS has been positively associated with numerous indices of spiritual health and virtue, such as spiritual well-being, realistic acceptance (a measure of spiritual maturity based on ORT; Hall & Edwards, 2002), meditative prayer practices, daily spiritual experiences, intrinsic religious motivations, hopefulness, gratitude, and interpersonal forgiveness (Jankowski & Vaughn, 2009; Ng, 2014; Worthington & Sandage, 2016). The integration of relational spirituality with the differentiation system can be assessed across the three major dimensions of DoS described above: (a) self-regulation of emotions, (b) relational flexibility balancing connection and autonomy, and (c) relating effectively across differences.

Self-Regulation Aspects of Differentiation

As mentioned in Chapter 3, healthy forms of relational spirituality should contribute to capacities for self-regulation of emotions, which is one reason DoS is positively correlated with the markers of spiritual health and virtue described above. This means spiritual beliefs and practices need to be internalized over the course of development and integrated into a person's embodiment and overall holistic functioning. Forms of relational spirituality that are more defensive than authentic tend to be characterized by spiritual bypass (the tendency to "overspiritualize" in attempts to avoid difficult emotions or painful experiences; Fox, Cashwell, & Picciotto, 2017) and sometimes also occur with narcissistic symptoms (e.g., personal superiority, lack of empathy, chronic needs for attention or validation; Sandage & Moe, 2011). When an individual engages in spiritual dwelling and seeking in highly differentiated ways, there will generally be expressions of internalization and intrinsic motivation, mindful embodiment, authentic processing of emotions with a balancing of self-confrontation and self-soothing, and distress tolerance for the suffering that can be part of purposeful growth.

Relational Spirituality Internalization and Intrinsic Motivation
Forms of relational spirituality that are meaningfully internalized by an individual and become part of their set of intrinsic motivations are more differentiated and generally more healthy and life-enhancing than relational spirituality orientations that are based on conformity or the introjection of others' expectations (Bravo, Pearson, & Stevens, 2016; Ryan, Rigby, & King, 1993; Strunk, 1965). This is because internalized beliefs, values, and practices that are intrinsically motivated are more effective resources for self-regulation, and this becomes particularly important for adult development and in sociocultural settings where communal supports are not always readily available. Intrinsically motivated forms of relational spirituality also have greater existential vitality and intentionality for meaningful growth in differentiation, which Tillich (1952) described as the "courage to be" (p. 79) and "the power to create beyond oneself without losing oneself" (p. 81). Allport (1960), the seminal psychologist of religion in theorizing the importance of intrinsic motivation for religious experience, explained, "When we say that the mature religious sentiment is differentiated we are calling attention to its richness and complexity" (p. 57). In contrast, introjection involves taking in the beliefs or practices of others in relatively concrete or undifferentiated ways without making those beliefs or practices "one's own," so introjected forms of relational spirituality do not tend to facilitate self-regulation under stress.

This emphasis on self-regulation is particularly important for adaptation in highly individualistic contexts such as the United States, and it is important to note that extrinsic spiritual motivations are often valued in collectivistic contexts in which interdependence and concern for others' perceptions are highly adaptive (A. B. Cohen & Hill, 2007). Nevertheless, self-regulatory capacities are necessary, at least for adults, in most contexts. So the internalization of spiritual beliefs and practices is a valuable aspect of differentiated relational spirituality, and clinicians can help clients with this through dialogue about relational spirituality dynamics that can facilitate integration in this area (e.g., "What are your thoughts about this [belief or practice]? What feels important to you about this? What does it mean to you?").

Mindful Embodiment

Self-regulatory aspects of differentiation involve RS forms of dwelling that promote mindful embodiment (discussed in Chapter 3), which reflects the ability to integrate one's bodily experience with spirituality. Shame and dissociation are two psychological states of low differentiation that work against mindful embodiment. Sexuality is one key aspect of embodiment that can be difficult for some clients to integrate with relational spirituality in well-differentiated ways due to shame or dissociation, which can be prompted by certain spiritual and religious influences or traumatic experiences involving a loss of a sense of the sacred (i.e., desecration; Pargament, 2007; Park, Currier, Harris, & Slattery, 2017). It is important that clinicians remain sensitive to diverse client perspectives on sexuality and sexual desire, including asexuality.

Yet it is also worth noting that DoS has been positively associated with sexual desire, intimacy, and couple satisfaction in couples research (Ferreira, Narciso, Novo, & Pereira, 2014), and Schnarch (1991, 1997, 2009) is particularly helpful in illuminating the need for high levels of DoS to help individuals experience and responsibly own their sexual and spiritual desires, since authentic desire can be so anxiety-provoking in both realms. Clinicians' level of DoS has also been positively associated with their level of comfort in communicating openly and respectfully about client sexuality in a study using case vignettes, and higher levels of DoS appeared to help clinicians contain the influence of personal bias on their assessments of clients' sexual behaviors (Heiden-Rootes, Brimhall, Jankowski, & Reddick, 2017). These findings also underscore the potential significance of relational interactions between client and therapist levels of DoS in clinical dialogues about sexuality, as well as other sensitive topics.

Balancing Self-Confrontation and Self-Soothing

Differentiated self-regulation involves the authentic processing of emotions with a balancing of self-confrontation and self-soothing. Some clients will struggle to integrate the experience of difficult emotions (e.g., shame, fear, guilt, anger, pain, envy, despair) with their relational dynamics with the sacred. Difficult or "negative" emotions may be dissociated or compartmentalized from spiritual engagement or practice. Put differently, these clients have not experienced the ability to relate with the sacred while feeling negative emotions; therefore, their relational spirituality has not become a well-developed resource for self-regulation. Integrating the differentiation system with the client's relational spirituality in this kind of case involves using the therapeutic relationship to help the client reflect on how their spirituality relates to these difficult emotions. The idea is not to make the feelings immediately disappear (a defense of reaction formation) but to explore connections, seeming disconnections, and possibilities for engaging their spirituality in the midst of difficult emotion states. This kind of relational and reflective processing can lead to greater differentiation as the client internalizes this way of mentalizing and their relational spirituality becomes more accessible for self-regulation.

Developing the ability to balance self-confrontation and self-soothing is another important self-regulatory aspect of the differentiation system (Schnarch, 1997, 2009; Schnarch & Regas, 2012). *Self-soothing* is essentially the calming or "cooling down" of anxiety and other difficult emotions. *Self-confrontation* involves a person's ability to wrestle with important questions about discrepancies between their integrity and their behavior. Schnarch is unique among differentiation theorists with his clinical emphasis on inviting clients to reflect on their integrity, which involves core values or what is "near and dear to their hearts." This clinical attention to integrity, values, and one's heart brings the differentiation process into the moral and spiritual dimensions of a person's self-identity and serves to integrate the DoS process with relational spirituality.

Tolerating Distress

Self-regulatory aspects of differentiation can also cultivate capacities to tolerate the distress and suffering that is sometimes necessary for developmental growth (Schnarch, 2009; Schnarch & Regas, 2012). As described in Chapter 4, many spiritual traditions and theorists of psychotherapy concur in the understanding that growth will involve certain experiences of suffering, including the loss of illusions and idealizations about life. Developmental progress in DoS will require the self-regulatory capacity to "see the bigger picture" and to activate motivations to tolerate the distress that comes with growth. It is interesting to note the ways many of us have been in situations in which we found it easier to tolerate the distress that comes with maintaining familiar but dysfunctional patterns of behavior than to tolerate the anxiety and unfamiliarity that comes with changing our behavior. We have found this dilemma about "familiar versus unfamiliar distress" to be very useful to raise with clients to provide a frame for understanding the process of differentiation.

Promoting Flexibility Between Autonomy and Connection

The integration of relational spirituality and the differentiation system should also promote relational flexibility and the ability to balance autonomy and connection. Spiritual writers have described the formative value of both solitude and community, and this indirectly speaks to differentiation-based spirituality and the benefits of learning to deal with existential anxieties about loneliness and interpersonal enmeshment. Developing the differentiation system involves resisting the urge for chronic or rigid use of either fusion with others to avoid abandonment anxiety, or cutoff from others to avoid engulfment anxiety. Although we must be careful with generalizations, clients struggling with tendencies toward fusion and ambivalent attachment may move toward growth in differentiation when RSM clinicians emphasize self-regulation, self-identity development, trusting one's own resources and ideas, metabolizing shame and guilt, and learning to regulate existential fears about loneliness and abandonment. Clients struggling with tendencies toward cutoff and avoidant attachment may find the work of differentiation involves relational spirituality emphases on relational regulation and trusting others, cultivating empathy and compassion for others, metabolizing repressed anger and unforgiveness, and learning to regulate existential fears about loss of self through relating with others.

Connections between differentiation and relational spirituality also frequently emerge in seeking cycles representing the individuation side of the differentiation developmental system. Firestone and colleagues (R. Firestone, Firestone, & Catlett, 2013) offered an excellent chapter on "Death Anxiety and Differentiation" in their therapeutic model of differentiation. Building on numerous existential and depth theorists (Becker, 1973; Fromm, 1941; Piven, 2004; Rank, 1941; Schnarch, 1991; Tillich, 1952), they suggested death anxiety often increases as clients take steps toward individuation or expressing and developing their authentic self. This is because movement toward pursuing personal goals and authentically expressing one's self begins to stir existential themes related to finitude, mortality, and anxieties about whether one's contributions will be sufficiently meaningful and lasting (see Chapter 4, this volume). Defense mechanisms mobilize to reinforce conformity to others' goals and patterns of living, which can seem to provide security about an externally validated life project (Becker, 1973). Research in the field of terror management theory has shown that conformity to the worldview beliefs of one's society can be used to mitigate death anxiety (McCoy, Pyszczynski, Solomon, & Greenberg, 2000). In addition to conformity, Firestone et al. (2013) described "microsuicidal" behaviors that are self-defeating, self-harming, and self-silencing forms of what they called "death of the spirit" and withdrawal from authentic living that may reduce the anxiety of individuation and existential choice (p. 139). Therapeutic approaches that encourage clients to individuate, pursue their personal goals, and express their "true self" often underestimate the spiritual and existential anxiety that will arise in this process, particularly for those from oppressed groups whose sense of selfhood has been traumatized by systemic injustice.

Relating Effectively Across Differences

We have already described the role of differentiation in intercultural competence and spiritual and religious competence, but a few other key dimensions of relational spirituality often surface with clients who are struggling with relating across sociocultural differences. Terror management research has also suggested that reminders of mortality (death anxiety) can prompt some individuals toward biased or hostile reactions to those who are perceived to belong to out-groups, which terror management theory researchers view as a form of negative other-validation or a feeling of superiority in comparison to an inferior "other" (Sullivan, 2016; see also Schnarch, 1997). Clients who have experienced extreme stress or trauma will sometimes manifest this pressure to denigrate out-groups when existential anxieties are activated, although individuals who are high in DoS may feel less need for this kind of self-esteem enhancement. Therapists who can empathize and nonjudgmentally explore these perspectives and their underlying existential dynamics can help foster greater differentiation.

Differentiation-based forms of relational spirituality are characterized by alterity virtues such as humility, compassion, and gratitude. Humility includes a differentiated openness to other perspectives, a tendency to view others as equal to self, and an ability to accept human limitations in knowing. Compassion involves caring for the suffering of others, and differentiated forms of compassion move beyond immediate social and kinship networks toward an ever-widening circle of concern for humanity and the cosmos. Gratitude has been associated with intercultural competence and involves a tendency to appreciate others and their contributions (Jarrett, 2003; Sandage & Harden, 2011). Evolutionary psychologists have suggested gratitude likely evolved to promote reciprocal altruism or the upstream reciprocity of passing on benefits to others beyond one's kin network (McCullough, Kimeldorf, & Cohen, 2008), which fits with the sociocultural dynamics of differentiation and cooperation discussed in this chapter.

CLINICAL STRATEGIES FOR ENCOURAGING HEALTHY DIFFERENTIATION

We further illustrate dynamics of therapeutic engagement with the differentiation system in the clinical applications chapters (8, 9, and 10) of this book, but in this section we briefly describe key RSM clinical strategies that can facilitate growth in differentiation.

Negotiating the Differentiated Alliance

As stated throughout this volume, our relational approach to psychotherapy means the working therapeutic alliance is viewed as a central source of gain for therapeutic change (Wampold & Imel, 2015). The development of a securely attached working alliance can promote reflective functioning, a secure base for collaboration on goals and exploring new ideas and behaviors, and corrective relational experiences and "limbic revision" of internal working models of relationship (Lewis, Amini, & Lannon, 2000, p. 142; see also Schore, 2012; Wallin,

2007). However, we agree with Doran and colleagues that the literature on the therapeutic alliance emphasizes cooperation and agreement to the neglect of negotiating differences and repairing ruptures between client and therapist, which is a key dimension of differentiated relatedness (Doran, 2016; Doran, Safran, & Muran, 2016, 2017). Doran et al. (2017) noted the importance of this therapeutic alliance dynamic of negotiating differences, which can impact client perceptions that their therapist (a) can handle discussion of negative feelings and experiences in the alliance (i.e., ruptures) and (b) values their autonomous functioning, which they found to increase in significance over the course of therapy and to predict clinical outcomes. Timing is important in this regard, as well as the therapist's attunement to the level of difference or conflict a client can seem to handle at a given time even if clients initiate these discussions. When clients are working on developing DoS, they may engage the therapist around perceived differences as a way of practicing differentiation, which is different than avoiding attachment with the therapist.

As discussed in Chapter 2, the relational ecology of the overall therapeutic context will often involve multiple providers or clinical administrative staff involved in treatment (Kehoe, Hassen, & Sandage, 2016; Sandage, Moon, et al., 2017). Differentiated alliance negotiation in this regard means the therapist needs to pursue a collaborative communicative stance with other providers (to the extent clients approve) and administrative staff. Differentiation can be difficult if providers disagree about treatment decisions and strategies, or if stressful ruptures occur between clients and administrative staff over insurance, billing, or other aspects of the health care experience. These are underrated challenges in the therapy process, and it will be difficult for clients to grow in differentiation if the relational ecology of treatment is chronically conflictual and poorly differentiated.

Differentiated alliance negotiation also involves consideration of therapeutic positioning in light of what we call the *relational spirituality triangle*: (a) client's prior relational history and patterns, (b) client's ways of relating with the sacred, and (c) client's approach to developing a working alliance in therapy. By *positioning*, we mean the degree to which the therapist promotes connection or autonomous functioning with a given client, which is more complicated in relational modalities of treatment (e.g., couple or family therapy). Therapists need high levels of DoS to be flexible in their own relational functioning in the therapy process and to assess client relational tendencies to determine what will be both therapeutic and a well-timed corrective experience to potentially revise relational templates. As suggested in Chapter 3, therapists need to attend to our own anxiety responses and relational patterns when exposed to client suffering and avoid tendencies to either "rescue or run away."

Helping Clients Mentalize Key Integrity Dilemmas

Another clinical strategy to encourage differentiation involves the therapeutic use of questions that are not aimed at information from clients as much as inviting awareness and self-confrontation of key SERT-related dilemmas and their associated choices. As mentioned previously, Schnarch (1997, 2009) has poignantly described the power of helping clients wrestle with integrity dilemmas about core values, personal identity, and existential choices when clients might prefer the fantasy that there is some way around making a choice. Of course, as therapists it is not our role to tell clients what their integrity requires, but it can be helpful to ask clients the question and to invite personal reflection. Once a solid working alliance has developed, one form of the question we have found helpful is to ask (while remaining sincerely open and curious) is, "Was that your integrity or your anxiety acting in that situation?" Clients will sometimes want clarification about what we mean by integrity and may also give a mixed answer, but when clients are starting to work on differentiation, this is the kind of reflective question they often find helpful for wrestling with what is most important to their core beliefs and values. As a clinical strategy, this is using the therapy relationship to help clients develop reflective functioning about SERT dynamics and core values.

Managing Intensification

As mentioned in Chapter 3 in relation to the metaphor of crucible process in therapy, it is important for therapists to stay attuned to the level of emotional intensification for clients at a given point in therapy and to seek to make wise clinical judgments about the appropriate level of "heat." Differentiation is unlikely to develop for clients without some intensification of personal challenge, self-confrontation, and spiritual and existential seeking, but overwhelming levels of intensification in the absence of regulatory skills and resources will activate retraumatization rather than differentiation. We have found it helpful to utilize the metaphor of therapy as "cooking." in that too much or too little heat and inattention to timing can be problematic. Again, therapists need high levels of differentiated self-awareness of their own tendencies for imbalances of intensification (e.g., withholding support, being too provocative, rescuing), and this is best discerned relationally in an ongoing process of professional consultation with close colleagues.

Considering Relational Modalities of Treatment

As mentioned in Chapter 2, our RSM emphasis on relational development systems and systemic perspectives leads us to strongly value relational modalities of treatment (e.g., couple, family, and group therapies). Some cases are not a good fit for relational modalities at a given point in time, such as when there are safety concerns or traumatic experiences have been unprocessed for an individual, and affect regulation and perspective-taking skills are minimal. But we think it is important to consider whether a client might be ready for deliberate work on the differentiation system, and a relational modality of treatment can offer (or even necessitate) growth in DoS in ways that may be more limited in individual therapy. In certain cases, a client might tend to use individual sessions to process their complaints about a spouse/partner or family member, and the individual therapy modality may offer a limited opportunity for the client to develop more differentiated responses to the other person. Engagement of SERT issues in relational modalities of treatment is almost certain to require the development of differentiation, because SERT dynamics are so highly personalized, and therapists can help clients contain or redirect their anxious responses to interpersonal differences in these treatment modalities.

Detriangling in Context

Triangulation of third parties can be adaptive in some contexts or situations, but a clinical assessment of triangulation patterns can suggest certain contexts in which triangulation has been unhelpful or overutilized (Guerin et al., 1996). In such cases, the therapist might invite the client(s) to reflect on these patterns with respect to the helpful and unhelpful consequences of triangulation. From a dialectical and systemic perspective that encourages differentiation, we find it important to consider both the helpful and unhelpful aspects of triangulation. This kind of reflection can prompt anxiety and reactivity in some clients, and it often surfaces SERT dynamics embedded in the client's relational spirituality. For example, one partner (Sheila) in a couple regularly consults her mother about major life decisions but does not trust her partner (Maria) with these conversations. Sheila has found Maria to seem either uninterested or too opinionated and judgmental. Maria complains of being "left out" of major decisions that impact both of them, which feels unfair and like they are "not a real adult couple."

When the couple therapist raises the detriangling question—"What would it be like for each of you to work on collaborating as a couple on these decisions prior to you talking to your mom about them, Sheila?"—it activated existential and even spiritual questions for each of them related to themes of trust, openness, judgment, forgiveness, and respect for boundaries and the other person's wisdom. The therapist framed the question in a differentiated manner that invited each person to awareness of their own challenges and possibilities in that relational process. Again, it is important to assume detriangling will typically increase anxiety and require affect regulation and collaboration skill development that is consistent with healthy spiritual development. In some cases, detriangling may also mean at least a temporary loss of connection, however healthy or unhealthy, with a previously idealized parent, other family member, friend, or mentor who has been a source of guidance. Thus, detriangling is at times part of a developmental deidealization process that can be existentially and spiritually turbulent (Jones, 2002), so these losses may need to be processed with attunement to those SERT dynamics.

Cultivating Self-Identity Development

Self-identity development is another expression of the differentiation system and often emerges for clients when appropriate levels of relational security are cultivated through a solid working alliance. Many systems approaches to therapy emphasize the use of genograms with clients to facilitate DoS through understanding relational histories and patterns (McGoldrick, Gerson, & Petry, 2008), and resources are available for integrating cultural, spiritual, and religious dynamics into genograms (Hardy & Laszloffy, 1995; Hodge, 2001, 2005; Walsh, 2010). While some Bowenian therapists have tended to do formal genogram sessions with clients early in the therapy process, we have found it more helpful to initially form the working alliance around presenting problems and concerns and later do genogram sessions when clients reach a point of significant readiness for self-identity work.

From an intersectional perspective on differentiation, it is important to ask questions and invite awareness of various intersecting aspects of a client's self-identity and the roles of SERT dynamics in how they relate to these aspects of themselves (Tummala-Narra, 2016). In some cases, there will be painful or even traumatic associations between SERT dynamics and aspects of one's identity, so this clinical strategy also requires sensitive attunement, compassion, and flexibility by therapists. Clients may need help being patient with the self-identity development process and recognizing small gains, such as one of our clients who realized he experienced a "warm sacred presence" when listening to a certain musician. Owning this realization about himself and his preferences and working to counter other internalized voices telling him this was not "real spirituality" was an initial step of growth in DoS for this client, which he was able to build upon.

Working on Diversity Competence

As we suggested earlier, *diversity competence*, or the ability to relate effectively across differences, is an expression of healthy and adaptive functioning of the differentiation system; therefore, we view both client and therapist growth in diversity competence as key goals within our RSM. We recognize that diversity competence is not an initial therapy goal for many clients, just as those clients would likely not initially articulate growth in "differentiation" as a reason they sought treatment. The negotiation of treatment goals with clients is an essential aspect of therapeutic alliance formation and requires that therapists can explain how their approach to therapy integrates with clients' goals and concerns. We find it important to be clear about the assumptions of our therapy model, which include the belief that diversity competence is not simply a developmental skill for professionals but also an expression of healthy relational and spiritual development. And we also understand that some clients will not share that assumption, and we will need to try to negotiate a level of fit between clients' and therapists' perspectives. In many social contexts, it is increasingly easy to identify the need to develop relational capacities to relate well across differences, and most of our own clients recognize this need even if they continue to struggle with certain forms of bias, prejudice, and wounds or trauma effects related to oppression.

Clinically, developing the differentiation toward diversity competence starts with normalizing differences. This requires sensitivity to hurt, fear, anger, and other intense emotions that a client may have about differences, while not engaging in simplistic reframes. Rather, we suggest careful empathic pacing of client perspectives and building toward lead moves that invite awareness of differences and possibly some brief psychoeducation about certain differences that clients describe. For example, a Euro American client was describing his resentment toward a coworker who raised her voice at him in front of others over a conflict and continued to intensely question him about the matter for several minutes before he walked away. The client was distressed by his inability to forgive the coworker despite repeated efforts to pray about it over several weeks, as forgiveness was an important value within his religious faith. He was also bothered that he had previously enjoyed very friendly interactions with this coworker and now felt unable to relate to her. The therapist offered empathy about the impact of this encounter, which proved embarrassing and shaming to the client. Given their prior work together, the therapist was also able to help the client reflect on the parallel between this relational dynamic and a recurring pattern of getting berated by his father in front of his younger siblings for some minor mistake. This was an initial invitation to the reflective functioning to differentiate the experience with the coworker and experiences in his family of origin.

The client had also mentioned the coworker's ethnicity, which was consistent with cultural groups that often value direct communication and affective engagement during conflict as an indication of caring about the relationship. The therapist noted to the client that it can be dangerous and stereotyping to make generalizations about a cultural group, but she wondered if the client had reflected on different cultural conflict styles and assumptions about conflict and went on to describe different cultural preferences about direct versus indirect communication and emotional expression versus restraint during conflict (Hammer, 2005). The client found this helpful not only about this work situation but also because it illuminated some differences in prior dating relationships. This clinical strategy might have proved unsatisfying to some clients who needed longer pacing of their own emotions and perspectives or who lacked curiosity about cultural differences, so therapist flexibility is required and a willingness to drop back into pacing if the stretch toward differentiation seems too great. In this particular case, the client continued to struggle with a level of hurt and embarrassment about this encounter, but he was also able to mentalize the relationship in more complex and differentiated ways that made it less personally offensive and to start to accept the reality of cultural differences for which he had lacked awareness. This kind of progress in differentiation combines aspects of mindfulness and mentalization (dwelling and seeking) and is empirically supported as one pathway that facilitates forgiving others (Worthington & Sandage, 2016).

CONCLUSION

In this chapter, we summarized some of the multiple disciplines, theoretical traditions, and intercultural perspectives that have informed our clinical understanding of the differentiation developmental system and how that system interfaces with relational spirituality and relational dynamics of change in psychotherapy. A well-developed differentiation system is crucial to help individuals and relational systems cultivate clear yet flexible forms of identity and integrity, manage the strengths and tensions of human diversity, and adapt to changes that are inevitable across the life cycle. In Chapter 7, we consider the developmental and clinical implications of the intersubjectivity system.

7

Intersubjectivity and Relational Spirituality

But knowing is not enough; the irreparable must somehow be repaired, and the only way the past-as-present can be repaired is within a relationship that repeats the failure of the past but somehow does more than repeat it. Something new must occur—something that has to emerge out of what the patient and analyst do in an unanticipated way.
—P. BROMBERG, *AWAKENING THE DREAMER* (2006, P. 94)

Intersubjectivity, which may be broadly defined as the interplay and "emergent relatedness" between persons (Orange, 2009, p. 237), offers clinicians a powerful frame to enrich and inform psychotherapy. While attachment focuses on the empowering effects of felt security, and differentiation emphasizes interpersonal and intrapersonal balance, intersubjectivity attends to patterns of interaction and their effects, with particular attention to how interactions may be enlivening and create intimacy. The intersubjectivity system reflects and expresses central aspects of human experience, which are summarized below.

First, we exist in relational webs. Orange (2009) put it this way:

> It seems to me axiomatic, as it does to all relational theorists known to me, that personal experience takes form, is maintained, and transforms itself in relational contexts. . . . I become I—with my characteristic ways of thinking, feeling, believing, and living with others—only within complexly nested and overlapping systems: infant caregiver, family, culture, religion, occidental life-worlds. (p. 241)

http://dx.doi.org/10.1037/0000174-008
Relational Spirituality in Psychotherapy: Healing Suffering and Promoting Growth,
by S. J. Sandage, D. Rupert, G. S. Stavros, and N. G. Devor

Second, subjectivity emerges in and through relationship. From our earliest moments, we are drawn to others and engage in presymbolic interactions that become more complex over time (it is beyond the scope of this chapter to discuss extreme isolation or medical conditions that alter capacities for relationship other than by noting that even in such circumstances people may be significantly impacted by others and express aspects of intersubjectivity). Moreover, the nature and quality of our childhood interactions significantly impacts our state of being and mental/emotional development (Stern, 2004; Trevarthen, 2011; Wallin, 2007).

Third, intersubjectivity is a unique developmental system, distinct from attachment and sexuality. We are innately motivated to seek recognition, responsiveness, and greater or lesser degrees of intimacy/closeness with others (Lyons-Ruth, 2007; Stern, 2004).

Fourth, human relations are dynamic and complex, with great potential for enlivening or disruptive effects. Intersubjectivity studies offer perspective on constructive and problematic relational patterns including interpersonal coordination and synchrony, attunement, affect regulation, and rupture/repair cycles (Aron, 2018; Benjamin, 2018; Bromberg, 2011).

Finally, spiritual and existential struggles related to traumatic suffering may particularly necessitate intersubjectivity for both psychological and spiritual healing, in part because larger relational systems often have trouble recognizing and working with the complex experiential dynamics of severe and/or chronic suffering (Benjamin, 2018; Van Deusen & Courtois, 2015). Trauma assaults subjectivity; attuned interaction and recognition are essential for rebuilding a sense of self, connection to others, and orientation toward whatever one considers sacred or most important.

As a conceptual framework, intersubjectivity applies to topics ranging from infant-caregiver research to philosophical reflections on the interpersonal nature of mind and personhood. This chapter focuses on intersubjectivity as a developmental system and clinical framework, with an emphasis on clinical practice. We review three overarching approaches to intersubjectivity, cultural considerations, and two modes of intersubjective processing. The final sections discuss interpersonal coordination and attunement, rupture and repair, affect regulation, and mutual recognition.

SYSTEMS VIEW OF INTERSUBJECTIVITY

Some authors—for example, Stolorow, Atwood, and Orange (2002)—have emphasized what may be called a macro or systems approach to intersubjectivity. They frame intersubjectivity as an *existential given, the nature of reality*:

> For us, intersubjectivity has a meaning that is much more general and inclusive, referring to the relational contexts of all experience, at whatever developmental level, linguistic or prelinguistic, shared or solitary, it takes form (Stolorow and Atwood, 1992). An intersubjective field is neither a mode of experiencing nor a

sharing of experience. It is the contextual precondition for having any experience at all. (Stolorow et al., 2002, p. 85)

Systems thinkers draw heavily from philosophy, ethical perspectives, and systems theories to inform their clinical stance (Beebe, Knoblauch, Rustin, J., & Sorter, 2003; Orange, 2009). From this orientation, subjectivity exists in and emerges from one's context. Proponents have encouraged "perspectival realism" (Orange, 2009, p. 240), the belief "that no one and no group can take more than a partial view of anything" (p. 241). Experience and understanding are the priority:

> We must attend to truth-as-possible-understanding and not truth-as-correspondence-to-fact. Whatever the facts may be, we must find ways to converse about the meanings, and arguments about reality and the associated insistence that the patient recognize the analyst's perspective are usually the quickest exit from the search for understanding. (Stolorow et al., 2002, p. 119)

Clinicians are encouraged to empathically attend to "emotional convictions (organizing principles) that pattern a person's experiential world" (Orange, 2009, p. 245). Inevitable misunderstandings are not fatal as long as the therapist remains flexible and willing to learn. The systems view aligns well with emphases in many major religious traditions on the sacredness of persons, interconnectedness, and limited human understanding. It promotes dwelling in the sense of empathic joining to create a sense of intimacy or togetherness, and seeking in the sense of embracing uncertainty and open-ended dialogue.

DEVELOPMENTAL VIEW OF INTERSUBJECTIVITY

The developmental approach comes primarily from developmental researchers and neuroscientists who view intersubjectivity as a developmental capacity and/or achievement (Beebe, Sorter, Rustin, & Knoblauch, 2003; Trevarthen, 2011). This perspective has roots in infant and childhood research. Newborns demonstrate intrinsic motivation to communicate with other people and engage in simple, early forms of interaction soon after birth. In the course of normal development, children demonstrate increasingly complex forms of interaction, such as shifting from direct face-to-face sequences with a caregiver (e.g., peekaboo) to games with objects to pretend play (Brugué & Burriel, 2016). Through fine-grain video analysis and other creative strategies, researchers have identified patterns of interaction—such as imitation, coordination, synchrony, attunement, rupture and repair—that embody and facilitate relationships in childhood and across the life span (Beebe, Sorter, et al., 2003; Mesman, van IJzendoorn, & Bakermans-Kranenburg, 2009; Stern, 2004; Xavier et al., 2016). The developmental approach to intersubjectivity focuses on innate motivations and capacities for relatedness, and on developmental trajectories or impacts from different forms of relatedness. This approach most clearly illumines intersubjectivity as a developmental system, and highlights relational spirituality model (RSM) themes of relational dwelling for connection and seeking for growth.

RELATIONAL/CLINICAL APPROACH TO INTERSUBJECTIVITY

A third approach to intersubjectivity, which we will call the *relational/clinical approach*, integrates developmental research with contemporary relational approaches to psychotherapy and psychoanalysis to examine the nature and impact of relational experience in psychotherapy and life more broadly (Aron, 2018; Barsness, 2018; Beebe, 2004; Benjamin, 2018; Bromberg, 2011; Ringstrom, 2010). The relational approach views intersubjectivity as a quality or type of relatedness characterized by authenticity, recognition, and response. From this viewpoint, intersubjectivity represents mutual engagement and intimacy (emotional closeness) and stands in contrast to other forms of interaction, such as reactivity, objectification, manipulation, neglect, or domination.

Relational thinkers emphasize the role of relationships in development and functioning. For example, infants and young children develop expectancies about relationships, an automatic sense of how things will go, how to think, feel, and act in a given relational context (Beebe, 2004; Stern et al., 1998). These patterns, referred to by some as "implicit relational knowing" (Beebe, Knoblauch, et al., 2003, p. 745), reflect adaptations from prior relationships that inform current relationships. These dynamics enter the therapeutic relationship as well, creating here-and-now opportunities to engage and alter problematic patterns. The relational approach focuses on interactive patterns and possibilities for cultivating or recovering intersubjectivity within (and beyond) the clinical hour. Spiritually, it reflects the RSM emphasis on how we relate to one another and to sacred or ultimate concerns.

CULTURE AND INTERSUBJECTIVITY

As with all aspects of human thought and behavior, intersubjectivity theory and research is culture-bound. Intercultural competence, cultural humility, and social justice are key elements of our RSM because we recognize the destructive, colonizing effect of frameworks that ignore critical differences at the individual, group, and systemic level. The views expressed in this chapter are undoubtedly incomplete and culturally limited, and subject to meaningful critique by persons from different locations. The RSM emphasizes dialogue with others—especially dialogue across difference—as an essential source of feedback for growth.

Cultural systems organize fundamental ways of being and moving through the world. The intersubjectivity system creates possibilities for recognition and coordination between persons, but in lived experience, individual and group differences often present profound challenges to recognition and mutuality.

Moreover, social oppression in its many forms is a direct affront to the dignity and subjectivity of nondominant persons. Intersubjectivity requires and reflects a kind of social justice. Practically, attempts at intercultural dialogue often fail if participants fail to acknowledge power imbalances and allow for differentiation (including anger) in the relational process.

Models of intersubjectivity include assumptions about the nature of the self and the basis of subjectivity. Western psychology has been critiqued as overly individualistic and atomistic—for instance, taking an essentialist stance that overemphasizes individual attributes without adequate attention to relational, contextual, and historical variables; minimizing power dynamics; or holding a dualistic view of personhood (Stolorow et al., 2002; D. W. Sue & Sue, 2016). In contrast, collectivist societies often start from different assumptions, including locating the self (in so far as self is even a consideration) primarily and centrally through one's role and relationship to others in the extended family or cultural group (D. W. Sue & Sue, 2016). Intersubjectivity incorporates a relational perspective through its focus on persons-in-interaction (Beebe, Knoblauch, et al., 2003). Nevertheless, Western views on intersubjectivity have considerable room for cultural extension and nuance. For example, much of the psychological literature on intersubjectivity attends to a primary dyadic relationship with limited consideration of larger relational ecologies and contexts. In addition, there is ongoing debate about the best way to conceptualize persons-in-relation, with some authors critiquing "Cartesian" assumptions embedded in attributions of individual characteristics, and others arguing that personal factors are important too (Ringstrom, 2010). We think of personal and systemic dimensions of intersubjectivity as interwoven and dialectical.

A second cultural critique arises around definitions of intersubjectivity that emphasize mutual recognition and knowing the other's mind (Benjamin, 2018; Stern, 2004). Recognition of the other as a like subject whose intentions can be (partially) understood is a critical component of intersubjectivity theory (Benjamin, 2018). This view emerges from multiple sources, including infant research and research on interpersonal coordination and empathy in adults that identifies capacities for synchronized interaction, inferring intentions, and sharing feeling states. These findings are compelling and important. However, they are contextualized and delimited by enthnographic research showing that some cultural groups manifest intersubjectivity quite differently by, for example, holding beliefs about the fundamental unknowability of another's mind while utilizing other mechanisms such as somatic experience to inform social relations (Groark, 2013), deprioritizing mutuality to emphasize shared obedience to the wisdom of ancestors (Danziger, 2013), or utilizing rituals and spirits as intermediaries between persons (Hanks, 2013). These complexities encourage a humble approach to intersubjectivity that leaves room for various forms of coordination and communication and that recognizes how fleeting moments of mutual understanding may be.

IMPLICIT AND EXPLICIT PROCESSING

The intersubjectivity system operates through implicit and explicit processes, and these processes may be more or less integrated. The nature of, and distinctions between, these modes of functioning are complex, and different authors have defined them in different ways (Beebe, Knoblauch, et al., 2003). In a general sense, implicit processes refer to embedded, intuitive, and automatic ways of perceiving and acting, whereas explicit processes are more overt and self-conscious (Beebe, Knoblauch, et al., 2003; Stern, 2004). Implicit processes generally involve one or more of the following:

- nonverbal communication and/or nonlinguistic verbal communication; for example, facial expressions, posture, gestures, gaze, tone, inflection, cadence, volume, sounds such as sighs or chuckles;

- quick, intuitive perception or recognition; examples include intuitively recognizing an unexpressed feeling state or pattern in someone's behavior;

- automatic or nonconscious reactions that link perceptions with emotions and/or actions; for example, becoming entrained with someone in a conversation or making involuntary empathic reactions (e.g., wincing when hearing a painful story); and

- procedural knowledge (i.e., goal-directed action patterns that do not require symbolic thought); for example, riding a bike or automatic (learned) responses to certain situations or emotions.

In contrast, explicit processes generally have to do with verbal communication, formal language, deliberate action, and symbolic thought (Beebe, Knoblauch, et al., 2003). Explicit processes require certain mental and physical capacities that develop over time, including formal language acquisition, symbolic thinking, and mentalization, which is the ability to reflect on one's own mental states and the mental states of others (Liljenfors & Lundh, 2015).

Infants, who lack or are slowly developing explicit processing capacities, interact primarily through implicit processes, and thus infant research offers insights on implicit modes of intersubjectivity. Several examples of implicit processes have been observed in infants and young children. For example, Meltzoff and Moore (as cited in Beebe, Sorter, et al., 2003) documented that as early as 42 minutes after birth, infants may attempt to imitate the facial expressions of persons they observe, and that 6-week-old infants can repeat expressions observed 24 hours earlier when presented with the same person. These findings demonstrate recognition and representation of another's actions, and innate procedural responses to align with the other.

Infants also track interaction patterns and demonstrate preference for coordinated responses and frustration with noncontingent or poorly coordinated responses. For example, when researchers use technology to alter the timing of responses between mothers and 2-month-old infants who were previously interacting through video—effectively disrupting the sense of synchrony and responsiveness—the infants became avoidant and distressed (Beebe, Sorter, et al., 2003). Similarly, when 9-month-old infants were briefly separated from their mothers and then reunited, they ceased to be upset but remained solemn, and preferred to look at a sad face rather than a happy face (Beebe, Sorter, et al., 2003). This experiment highlighted affective attunement; that is, sensing and preferring congruence between their own emotional state and the expression on the other's face (Stern, 2004). Finally, at 18 months, children watched actors who tried to pull an object apart but repeatedly let their hands slip off the ends. The infants then successfully pulled the object apart on their own without repeating the failed attempts, demonstrating that they inferred the intention of the actor and did not simply copy the motion (Meltzoff et al., 2009).

The implicit processes used by infants do not fade away or become completely superseded by later perceptual and cognitive capacities, but instead "continue to be an important part of social understanding in adult life" (Liljenfors & Lundh, 2015, p. 52). Intersubjectivity in adults is more complex than for infants, as adults may participate in and process interactions on implicit and explicit levels simultaneously, and these modalities may be more or less integrated and coordinated. Intersubjectivity theory invites therapists to attend to implicit processes as well as explicit processes, and to the relationship between these different modes of perceiving and acting. "From a clinical point of view, any implicit knowings about the relationship will influence the explicit agenda and vice versa. Neither one can be considered independent from the other" (Stern, 2004, p. 121). In RSM terms, dwelling and seeking occur in explicit and implicit ways, and both need attention.

Implicit processes can enrich therapy in multiple ways, including enabling communication of experiences that cannot be (or are not) put into words; promoting intuitive, right-brain to right-brain empathy and regulation; identifying embedded procedural (action-based) and limbic (emotional) patterns; and providing an additional dimension for therapeutic contact and impact (Beebe, Knoblauch, et al., 2003; Schore, 2011, 2012; Stern, 2004; Wallin, 2007). Along these lines, Beebe (2004) wrote,

> Interactions in the nonverbal and implicit modes are rapid, subtle, co-constructed, and generally out of awareness. And yet they profoundly affect moment-to-moment communication and the affective climate. They organize modes of relating, Stern's (1985) "ways of being with." . . . Critical aspects of therapeutic action occur in this implicit mode. . . . We can teach ourselves to observe these implicit and non-verbal interactions simultaneously in ourselves and in our patients, and thus expand our own awareness and, where useful, that of our patients. (pp. 48–49)

Here is a commonplace clinical example: A client with recurrent depressive episodes started the hour by reporting a rough week and reviewing a series of difficulties. The therapist attempted to track the client, offer empathic acknowledgment, and explore the concerns. About halfway through the session, the therapist became aware that the conversation felt flat. This awareness interrupted the therapist's current thoughts and comments. As she quieted, the therapist became aware of feeling confused, and noticed that the client seemed confused as well, which she tentatively mentioned. The client cried, stating that she was confused but did not know why. The therapist shared an association to moments of confusion in the client's family of origin, and the session opened into a vital conversation about confusing relational dilemmas in the client's family and religious community. In this session, the therapist's conscious thoughts and reactions had little impact; her implicit emotional resonance and automatic associations proved helpful. As Schore (2012) suggested,

> Rather than conscious logical reasoning and technical explicit skills, the clinician's intuitive implicit capacities may . . . dictate the depth of the therapeutic contact, exploration, and change process. (p. 137)

Generally speaking, implicit processes are intuitive and nonconscious, and cannot be easily initiated or controlled. However, therapists may identify personal strategies to cultivate states of openness and awareness to facilitate receptivity to and integration of emergent feelings, perceptions, and associations (Barsness & Sorenson, 2018; Rousmaniere, 2019; Wallin, 2007). However, because therapist perceptions, intuitions, and associations are fallible and will not always be aligned with clients, implicit knowing must be balanced and bounded through tentativeness, direct and indirect feedback from the client, reflection, and consultation with colleagues.

INTERPERSONAL COORDINATION AND ATTUNEMENT

Interpersonal coordination refers to ways that behaviors in an interaction become "patterned or synchronized in both timing and form [simultaneous movements or change of postures]" (Xavier et al., 2016, p. 2). From a behavioral perspective, there are two primary forms of coordination: behavior matching or imitation, and synchrony, which refers to "adaptation . . . to the rhythms and movements [of the other]" as well as "degree of congruence between . . . cycles of engagement or disengagement" (Xavier et al., 2016, p. 2). Stern argued for a third form of alignment focused on emotional congruence, which he called *affective attunement* (Stern, 2004).

From infancy onward, humans seek to engage each other in aligned, responsive interactions (Beebe, Sorter, et al., 2003; Trevarthen, 2011). Stern (2005) described these inclinations as "the empathic, participatory, and resonating aspects of intersubjectivity" (p. 80). Resonance manifests in various ways ranging from imitation to complex turn-taking and accommodation. For example, Davidsen and Fosgerau (2015) noted that

> Linguistic studies have shown that interactants automatically imitate each other's actions in several acoustic and bodily aspects. They mirror not only phonetic variables (Babel, 2009; Gallois, Ogay, & Giles, 2005; Trudgill, 2008),

but also sentence grammar (Bock, 1989), and speech rhythm (Cappella & Planalp, 1981). Mirroring has also been shown to take place in relation to physical movements. (p. 441)

Noteworthy facets of interpersonal coordination include recognition of the other as a "like subject" (Benjamin, 2018, p. 4), motivation to engage others and seek aligned responses (Beebe, Sorter, et al., 2003), mutual influence (e.g., responses are shaped by the preceding response[s] as well as history/context; Stern, 2004), and systemic patterns (e.g., emergence of patterns that are attributable to the system rather than individuals in the system; Gallagher, 2014).

Interpersonal coordination highlights the potential impact of resonance or being in sync. Benjamin (2018) called this resonance the *rhythmic third*, and described it as "sharing a pattern, a dance, with another person" (p. 30). She viewed the rhythmic third as one critical aspect of relatedness, an intrinsically beneficial joining that occurs as both participants accommodate to shared patterning and feel a sense of recognition and unity (Benjamin, 2018). The intersubjectivity system can generate positive relational experiences that are satisfying, promote coordination and intimacy, and help to modulate and balance negative emotions. However, these sorts of connections—moments of intimacy and dwelling together—exist alongside differentiation and conflict, as discussed later in this chapter.

Stern (1985) emphasized the emotional dimension of interpersonal coordination in his work on affective attunement. *Affective attunement* refers to sharing feeling states (Stern, 2004). Stern described attunement as "interpersonal communion" (p. 148), which he related to sharing experiences without altering them, and to changing with the other. To share without altering means demonstrating emotional recognition and resonance through corresponding responses. Imagine, for example, a client who happily describes a personal success and sees her therapist's eyes widen and brighten with joy. Note that the mirroring or marking response must be "contingent"—clearly related to the affect being expressed—and "marked"—sufficiently different to show that the response is intentional and expresses recognition (Wallin, 2007, p. 49). With children, marking often involves an exaggerated tone, but in adult exchanges other forms of differentiation are required.

To *change with* refers to "micro-momentary dynamic shifts in each person's behavior" (Beebe, Sorter, et al., 2003, p. 793) to match the contours of emotional experience, or what Stern called "vitality affects" (Stern, 2004, p. 36). *Vitality affects* refer to the shape and temporal shifts of emotional experience, which are "best captured by kinetic terms such as *surging, fading away, fleeting, explosive, tentative, effortful, accelerating, decelerating, climaxing, bursting, drawn out, reaching, hesitating, leaning forward, leaning backward* [emphasis in original], and so on" (Stern, 2004, p. 64). For example, imagine an exchange in which a client bangs his hand on the chair three times, with a brief pause between each movement and more force each time, and then therapist says crisply, "You have had it, Had It, HAD IT!," matching the punctuated, rising complaint.

Affective attunement enables a sense of communing and connection (Beebe, Sorter, et al., 2003), what the RSM posits as a kind of dwelling together.

Developmentally, attunement is essential for dyadic regulation of affect and supporting a child's brain development and capacity for self-regulation (Schore, 2012). Relationally, attunement (or lack thereof) organizes implicit understandings of what may be felt, expressed, and shared with others (Beebe, 2004; Beebe, Sorter, et al., 2003; Stern et al., 1998). These understandings may be reengaged and expanded through attuned interactions in psychotherapy or psychoanalysis (Stern, 2004). Along this line, Schore and Schore (2104) argued that

> the core skills of any effective psychotherapist are right-brain implicit capacities which include empathy, the regulation of one's own affect, the ability to receive and express nonverbal communication, the sensitivity to register very slight changes in another's expression and emotion, and an immediate awareness of one's own subjective and intersubjective experience. (p. 189)

How can therapists increase their right brain, implicit capacities? Clinical experience, other kinds of intentional relational experiences (e.g., personal therapy, group work, consultation, deliberate practice), and practices that cultivate emotional awareness (e.g., meditation, music, journaling, contemplative prayer, dream work) may be helpful. For therapists aligned with a particular spiritual and religious tradition, the tradition may offer experiences and practices to promote awareness or awakening to implicit and symbolic dimensions of experience.

With regard to specific in-session strategies, Stern and colleagues reported deepening the implicit relational dimension of their work through focus on the present moment (Stern, 2004). Stern argued that therapy may be viewed as a series of present moments, brief periods of time that contain and express experience in subjectively meaningful units. He suggested focusing on present moments to promote two types of change. The first involves subtle shifts that occur in the back and forth of conversation:

> As the dyad moves along, linking together present moments, a new way of being-with-the-other may arise at any step along the way. These new experiences enter into awareness but need not enter into consciousness. . . . These moments, each lasting only several seconds, accumulate and probably account for the majority of incremental therapeutic change that is slow, progressive, and silent. (Stern, 2004, pp. 219–220)

More dramatic changes may occur through what Stern (2004) called "now moments" (p. 166). *Now moments* occur unpredictably when some kind of challenge, tension, or disruption arises in the therapeutic interaction (Boston Change Process Study Group, 2013); they represent a minicrucible that may often relate to the larger crucible process of seeking and growth. If the therapist negotiates an affectively charged now moment by making "an authentic response finely matched to the momentary local situation" (Stern, 2004, p. 168), it may become a transformative "moment of meeting" (p. 220).

Stern (2004) offered several suggestions for deepening implicit awareness and engagement in session: (a) Focus on "the local level made up of present moments . . . small events, especially nonverbal and implicit events" (p. 223).

The idea is to stay with the client in the present by attending to what just occurred, however small or subtle. (b) Focus less on finding explicit meanings, and instead try to hear the music (rather than analyzing it). (c) Embrace the creative opportunity of now moments by attempting "well fitted" responses that have your "personal signature" (p. 226).

RUPTURE AND REPAIR

Interpersonal coordination is imprecise at best, and in any given interaction people fluctuate between greater and lesser alignment. Moments of misalignment, which may occur at an implicit or explicit level (or both), may be experienced as a *rupture*, a strain or break in the relationship. Minor ruptures occur frequently in most interactions and are often negotiated implicitly and without great effort (Morton, 2016; Stern, 2004). Major or repeated ruptures may be painful, disruptive, or even traumatic, and typically lead to elevated conflict or withdrawal. The long-term impact of a rupture often depends on whether, and how, it was repaired. *Repair* refers to acknowledgement and/or realignment between participants (Beebe, Sorter, et al., 2003; Benjamin, 2018). Examples of repair include (a) a caregiver recognizes that an infant wants a more boisterous or quieter interaction and adjusts accordingly; (b) a parent hears a child's hurt and apologizes for speaking sharply; (c) a therapist perceives a patient's emotional withdrawal in a session, inquires about it, and owns his participation in the exchange that left the client feeling injured; and (d) civic and religious leaders arrange community witnessing meetings that bring perpetrators and victims together to acknowledge and strive to overcome legacies of violence and injustice.

Developmental research suggests that rupture and repair cycles are critical aspects of human development. When children encounter strain or tension with a caregiver but then experience the caregiver actively working through the strain with them, they learn critical lessons about themselves and relationships (Beebe, Sorter, et al., 2003). It is neither possible nor ideal for a child (or therapy client) to have perfectly attuned and responsive caregivers; a more realistic and helpful goal is good enough responding that includes successful rupture and repair cycles. Potential benefits of rupture and repair cycles include learning that strains occur but can often be repaired, learning to emotionally regulate during ruptures, and learning how to initiate and participate in repairs. Rupture and repair cycles promote attachment security—a sense of trust that breaks can be repaired—and intersubjectivity in the sense of recognizing and responding to differing minds, and thus contribute to both developmental systems.

Contemporary psychotherapy researchers have identified several markers of rupture in therapist-client interactions, and potentially useful strategies for addressing ruptures (Safran & Kraus, 2014; Safran, Muran, & Eubanks-Carter, 2011). Ruptures typically manifest in some form of withdrawal or conflict, and therapists are encouraged to notice these indicators and explore the client's here-and-now experience in a collaborative, nondefensive manner. Safran and colleagues also noted that repair attempts may be more difficult with certain clients, such as insecurely attached clients (Miller-Bottome, Talia, Safran, & Muran, 2017).

Intersubjectivity theories identify several paths for repair in client–therapist relationships. Systems thinkers like Orange have emphasized radical openness and relentless empathy (Orange, 2009). They have suggested that we should not argue for our own view or experience with clients, but rather continue to explore and listen until we find some shared understanding. From their perspective, ruptures may be repaired as therapists return to empathic exploration and joining.

Developmentalists such as Beebe and Stern have focused on possibilities for realignment through close attention and implicit adjustments to interactive patterns. Interactions provide continual feedback to both participants, feedback that can inform ongoing shifts in the therapist's stance or interventions. From this perspective, repair has to do with reestablishing attunement and synchrony (Beebe, 2004) or establishing a new, broadened form of collaboration (Boston Change Process Study Group, 2013; Stern, 2004). For example, if a client struggles with a question in a manner that signals overwhelm or misattunement, the therapist might refocus on the present moment and offer a new experience, perhaps an acknowledgment (e.g., "That wasn't helpful, was it?!") or a question communicating openness (e.g., "Where are you now?").

Relational theorists tend to frame ruptures as enactments that replay old relational failures. Like systems theorists and developmentalists, they believe that ruptures are inevitable, and hold promise for therapeutic gain if repaired. However, relational theorists tend to emphasize the difficulty, complexity, and effort required to work through major impasses. In some cases, these dynamics may become the central therapeutic crucible. For example, Shaw (2010) highlighted how the children of narcissistic parents, in the context of their personal struggle to regain subjectivity and agency, are often highly sensitive to therapeutic missteps and repeatedly press the therapist to own mistakes and limitations. He encouraged therapists to embrace thoroughgoing humility and responsibility-taking:

> The reparative processes—acknowledging fallibility, being accountable for doing harm, apologizing, forgiving, expressing and receiving gratitude—are shame diminishing, "subjectifying" processes. . . . The reparative processes can instill hope, and perhaps even faith, in the possibility that disruptions do not have to be catastrophic or terminal, but can be meaningfully repaired, and that one's badness, and the badness in others, can exist along with, and not override and destroy goodness. (Shaw, 2010, p. 56)

Repair may be particularly poignant and important for persons who have experienced trauma or chronic suffering, as these experiences often shatter trust and hope.

Bromberg (2006, 2011) viewed major ruptures as enactments involving dissociated, "not-me" self-states that hold traumatic, unsymbolized affect. He brought a distinct perspective on rupture and repair through his emphasis on self-states—relatively independent constellations of subjective or felt experience, each having its own typical perspectives, emotions, and behavior patterns—that (he argued) exist in all people. Self-states are somewhat autonomous and dissociated from each other. In normal functioning, people naturally access whatever self-state is adaptive in the current context. Other states are temporarily dissociated and off-line, but available if needed. This degree of dissociation is adaptive (focused, efficient, and flexible) as the mind activates only the most salient self-state for a given moment. Trauma, which may be developmental and/or acute, disrupts this normal functioning by engendering more rigid and inflexible forms of dissociation. When traumatic experience is overwhelming, and traumatized self-states are not relationally acknowledged and regulated, dissociation intensifies to isolate and minimize dysregulated affect. While protective in one sense,

> The person's present and future are plundered by an overly rigid sequestering of "me" and "not me" self-states. . . . No matter how hard one tries, "not-me" self-states are never anaesthetized completely or indefinitely. (Bromberg, 2011, p. 5)

From this base, Bromberg viewed therapeutic rupture as a "collision of subjectivities" that occurs as a client's and the therapist's dissociated self-states interact to produce an enactment, "a shared dissociative event" characterized by confusion and dysregulation in both parties. The therapist

> loses his [sic] bearings. . . . He cannot even find what appears to be a useful way of engaging with the patient in the here and now because the patient's mind is feeling so unfamiliar. He then dissociates, which leads to his disconnecting affectively from his patient. (Bromberg, 2011, p. 110)

Both therapist and client find themselves confronted, simultaneously, with dissociative gaps and threatening affect. Prior forms of interaction no longer work, and the dyad is forced to seek new ways of relating. Bromberg offered several ideas of how this might occur:

> (a) A good analytic relationship also provides what the past lacked—a self-reflective, involved, and caring other who will not protect his [sic] own truth, *indefinitely*, by holding it to be evident. (Bromberg, 2009, p. 357)
>
> (b) Eventually, if the analyst is sufficiently attuned to his own internal experience, he [sic] will emerge from the shared dissociative cocoon and consciously experience the "something else" that is going on, without knowing what it is. As he begins to find a way to address it in the moment, with his patient, the work is then drawn into a potentially productive dialectic between the "here and now" and the "there and then." (pp. 555–556)
>
> (c) During enactments, what LeDoux (1996) calls the fear system is activated under safe (but not 'too' safe) conditions, in which the analytic relationship inevitably repeats the failures of the patient's past but must do more than just repeat it. Something new must occur—something that has to emerge out of what patient and analyst do in an unanticipated way. I've called these unanticipated relational events 'safe surprises,' because it is only through surprise

that a new reality—a space between spontaneity and safety—is coconstructed and infused with an energy of its own. (Bromberg, 2003, p. 572)

(d) In the session, the threatening dissociated affect must be activated to some
degree, but in trace form, regulated sufficiently so as not to trigger new
avoidance, and with some transformation of meaning. The questions of how
much and when to activate or to permit this activation, so as to repair the
dissociation rather than to reinforce it, must be addressed specifically for
each patient. (Bucci, 2002, as cited in Bromberg, 2003, p. 568)

Facilitating repair can be challenging for the therapist. As noted above,
Bromberg (2009) emphasized "affectively alive interpersonal engagement"
(p. 356). Wallin (2007) observed how therapists tend to feel trapped when
involved in an enactment, and he encouraged recovering "freedom to act"
through mindfulness, mentalization, and compassion. Benjamin (2018) highlighted the willingness to own and acknowledge one's mistakes and failures
through "keeping faith with the intention of our connection" (p. 21). From
an RSM perspective, repair requires and expresses some form of integrity and
commitment toward the relationship, and reparative processes often include
spiritual values and practices such as humility, confession/acknowledgment,
acceptance, forgiveness, kindness, and gratitude (Shults & Sandage, 2003;
Worthington & Sandage, 2016).

In one case, an African American man with a history of childhood abuse
reported chronically poor self-care (not getting enough sleep, eating poorly,
little exercise). When his White female therapist reflected this during a difficult session, the client shut down. With inquiry, the client said, "You see me
as another Black man who can't get his act together." The therapist felt
ashamed but worked to stay in the conversation by saying, "I just missed you,
that's on me. Let me listen and try to understand." The client replied, "You'll
never get it, no White woman knows what it's like for someone like me." The
therapist replied, "I'm sure you are right, I don't get it." This honest exchange
opened an important conversation about race and gender that shifted and
informed their discussions on self-care. However, about 6 weeks further into
treatment, the client said, "Don't be so soft on me, I need help moving forward!" This became an opportunity for the therapist to acknowledge that
anxiety about the prior rupture was constricting her, and that they needed a
better balance of attunement and struggling together to make progress. In
processing this rupture, the dyad found that they both valued "Keeping it
real" and "It is what it is, so what are you going to do?" These became trea-
sured, shared aspects of their relational spirituality in the treatment.

AFFECT REGULATION AND INTERSUBJECTIVITY

Affect regulation is a key factor in all three developmental systems discussed
in this book. It is a critical function and outcome of secure attachment and
an essential capacity for differentiation and intersubjectivity. *Affect* refers to
the raw level of intensity, and pleasurable to painful quality, of emotion

(Russell, 2003); affect and emotion are closely related and interchangeable for our purposes. Emotions can be helpful dimensions of human experience, providing information, motivation, and potentially useful action tendencies (Greenberg, 2012). For example, sadness may clarify desire, and often moves people to pause, grieve, seek support, or reorient; anger flags potential problems and provides energy to push back or push away. However, these benefits occur when emotions occur in a certain range that some have called the *window of tolerance* (Ogden & Fisher, 2015, p. 69). The window of tolerance framework suggests that when affect arousal is too great (hyperarousal) or too low (hypoarousal), emotions may not support adaptive functioning. Hyperarousal tends to produce distress and chaotic/disrupted perception, cognition, or action (e.g., fight or flight, flooded), and hypoarousal tends to produce numbness, inaction, dissociative gaps, and lack of vitality (frozen, dissociated; Ogden & Fisher, 2015; Schore, 2012). The window of tolerance is highly idiosyncratic and may vary by person, time, situation, and so forth.

Affect regulation refers to ways that people experience, influence, and express emotion in themselves (self-regulation) or influence emotion experience and expression in others (dyadic or interpersonal regulation). Ideally, persons have capacities and resources for affect regulation that enable them to stay within their window of tolerance most of the time, and to recover from states of dysregulation (being above or below the window) reasonably quickly and effectively. However, many factors impact this, and clients who come to therapy are often struggling with affect regulation in some way. Acute traumatic events evoke extreme emotions that cannot be coded coherently or integrated with other memories (Ogden & Fisher, 2015). Developmental trauma—chronic patterns of intrusion, disruption, nonrecognition, invalidation, or neglect by primary caregivers or other significant figures—may also produce significant and recurring dysregulation (Schore, 2012).

Insufficient affect regulation in infancy and childhood may have lasting negative impacts. For example, chronic states of hyperarousal and/or hypoarousal affect brain development, impairing neurological capacities for affect regulation later in life (Schore, 2012). Children may also develop procedural responses and dissociative patterns that are adaptive in the current system but tend to persist in rigid and problematic ways later in life (Ogden & Fisher, 2015; Wallin, 2007), and they may suffer a lack of positive development in various domains—such as basic trust in self and other, interpersonal skills for collaboration, negotiation, and repair, and affect-regulation strategies—due to the lack of positive interaction and challenging but manageable learning opportunities (Beebe, 2004; Beebe, Sorter, et al., 2003; Lyons-Ruth, 2007; Wallin, 2007).

Affect regulation processes are relational and contextual. *Dyadic regulation* refers to the ways partners in an interaction influence and regulate each other's emotions. For example, when caregivers practice good enough coordination and attunement with their children—"which create[s] states of positive arousal" (Schore, 2012, p. 32)—and good enough interactive repair after ruptures—"which modulates states of negative arousal" (p. 32)—children receive help with emotional regulation and develop capacities for self or autoregulation. Autoregulation refers to strategies that individuals use to regulate their own emotions. This occurs in many ways; for instance, looking away in a conversation, deep or rhythmic breathing, taking a walk, journaling, reframing, repeating a mantra, singing, exercise, practicing mindfulness, refocusing. Of note, Western intersubjectivity theorists write mostly about dyadic regulation and autoregulation; other cultural frameworks may give more attention to communal relationships and contexts that help with emotional regulation, such as families, groups, communities, art, nature, and spiritual experiences/practices.

Beebe and colleagues made a persuasive case that health and development proceeds best when dyads (caregiver and child, romantic partners, client and therapist) find a balance between dyadic regulation and autoregulation (Beebe, Rustin, Sorter, & Knoblauch, 2003). They pointed out that overly close tracking and tight dyadic regulation map onto preoccupation with the other as often found in insecure–preoccupied attachment, while loose and inattentive dyadic regulation maps onto excessive self-regulation, preoccupation with self, and lack of engagement with others as often seen in insecure dismissing attachment (Beebe, Rustin, et al., 2003).

Affect regulation is a key element in relational psychotherapy (Schore, 2012). This includes dyadic regulation and autoregulation in session and accessing resources and strategies for affect regulation outside of session. As noted earlier, dyadic regulation generally means evoking positive affect and modulating negative affect. However, there are many variations and complexities in practice. Some clients need to feel and express more negative emotions. Moreover, clients may fluctuate between dissociative and/or numb states, adequately modulated states (being in the window of tolerance), and overwhelmed, dysregulated states; and thus therapists must assess and adjust to the current self-state and level of arousal throughout the session. Moreover, effective therapy often requires engagement at the edges of the window(s) of tolerance (Schore, 2012). Therapy that avoids working near personal limits may sacrifice growth for comfort; therapy that works near the edge of capacity must avoid overtaxing or retraumatizing clients. Change often requires some degree of destabilization; therapists must attend carefully, collaborate with the clients, and get consultation as they seek to create a therapeutic space and pace that is "safe but not too safe" (Bromberg, 2006, p. 4). In RSM terms, the crucible must have enough heat and intensity, but also enough containment.

Intersubjectivity research and theory highlights multiple possibilities for affect regulation. Empathic synchrony and resonance can be intrinsically regulating, even with painful emotional content. Interpersonal coordination allows for influence—up-regulating or down-regulating arousal—as each response (and pattern of responses) influences the next response. This may involve purposeful influence (e.g., assisting a dysregulated client to ground, helping a minimizing client to express) or coconstructed, emergent processes that involve surprise. An example of an emergent intervention was saying to a suicidal client, "It seems like you are saying something in this story needs to die . . . but maybe it's not you?" In general, relational therapists aspire to "overarching attunement to moment by moment shifts . . . responding affectively and personally. . . . What matters here is the therapist's affective honesty" (Bromberg, 2011, p.106).

Affect regulation in the RSM includes accessing a client's personal values, strengths, or preferences, as these personally salient factors may evoke or alter strong emotions. Salient factors may include personal or communal meanings, intentions/commitments, metaphors, inspiring stories, gratitude, humor, or many other things depending on the person's spiritual and cultural framework. For example, I [DR] have several clients who are often able to soften (regulate) despair or self-loathing if we consider humility or surrender, spiritual values that are meaningful for them.

RECOGNITION, COMPLEMENTARITY, AND FINDING THE THIRD

Jessica Benjamin (2018) offered several distinctive emphases and perspectives on intersubjectivity, perspectives that incorporate ideas presented earlier in this chapter but which she developed in unique ways. She began by positing *recognition* as the core of intersubjectivity. Recognition has two primary dimensions or meanings:

> First, as a psychic position in which we know the other's mind as an equal source of intention and agency, affecting and being affected; and second, as a process or action, the essence of responsiveness in interaction. (Benjamin, 2018, p. 3)

The first aspect of recognition is awareness of the other as a "'like subject,' another mind that can be 'felt with' yet has a distinct, separate center of feeling and perception" (Benjamin, 2018, p. 22). This means seeing others as subjects—not objects or extensions of oneself—worthy of equal consideration. This kind of alterity is a strong focus in the RSM. The second aspect of recognition is "responsiveness in action" (Benjamin, 2018, p.4). Here Benjamin referred to implicit and explicit actions that communicate understanding and care. Recognition is not dispassionate observation, but embodied, heartful engagement.

> Acts of recognition confirm that I am seen, known, my intentions have been understood, I have had an impact on you, and this must also mean that I matter to you; and reciprocally, that I see and know you, I understand your intentions, your actions affect me and you matter to me . . . we share feelings. (Benjamin, 2018, p. 4)

From an RSM perspective, recognition requires a high level of differentiation and seeing the sacredness of the other. For some this may be framed around the image of God or the divine light in each person. Others may see a cosmic interconnectedness or shared humanity. For example, in one moment of intense conflict in a couple's case, both partners looked at the therapist to see what she would say (whose side would she take?). The therapist paused and said, "I feel for both of you. I see two people trying hard, wishing things were different, feeling a lot of hurt and confusion. How can we make a little space, let the dust settle, so you can see each other again . . . see the light in each other and not just the hurt?"

As mentioned earlier, relational thinkers tend to frame intersubjectivity as a certain quality of interaction. For Benjamin (2018), the essence of intersubjectivity is mutual recognition, and her work emphasized "developmentally and clinically, how we come to the felt experience of the other as a separate yet connected being with whom we are acting reciprocally" (p. 22). At the same time, Benjamin was well aware of how difficult and fleeting recognition may be: "recognition continually breaks down . . . thirdness always collapses into twoness . . . we are always losing and recovering the intersubjective view" (p. 39). This is inescapable in a "non-linear system of two subjects, each presumed able to destabilize the other's self-certainty or be destabilized at any moment, so that meanings are emergent" (p. 3).

Benjamin (2018) contrasted intersubjectivity with complementarity, which she also described as "twoness" (p. 39) or "doer-done to" (p. 5). *Complementarity* refers to patterns of interaction that lack mutuality and recognition. In complementarity, both parties typically feel that the other is the problem: *you are the doer* (aggressor or neglectful one) *and I am done to* (the victim, the innocent one). Complementarity involves binary framing, leaving one with a felt sense that there are only two options, submission or resistance, and only one valid position—"Either I'm crazy or you are" (Benjamin, 2004, p. 10).

Benjamin and others have suggested that "the Third" (Benjamin, 2018, p. 26) or *thirdness* is a way out of complementarity (see also Aron, 2018). The Third is not a particular thing but rather "a quality or experience of intersubjective relatedness that has as its correlate a certain kind of internal mental space" (Benjamin, 2018, p. 23). The correlated mental space involves "holding the tension of recognizing difference and sameness, taking the other to be a separate but equivalent center of initiative and consciousness with whom nonetheless feelings and intentions can be shared" (Benjamin, 2018, p. 4). There is no universal expression of thirdness: The Third exists in context in whatever ways people can relate with mutuality and responsiveness. In the deadlock of complementarity, the Third represents *something else*, an alternative to the rigid binary struggle, something discovered through seeking. In this sense, thirdness emerges from and transcends only the preceding form of complementarity; what serves as a Third in one moment may become part of the next struggle and require a new form of thirdness.

Benjamin spoke of three forms of thirdness. The first is the *rhythmic Third* mentioned earlier: "the mutual accommodation that brings about the sense of union or in-sync-ness" (Benjamin, 2018, p. 51). This is initially manifest (ideally) in good-enough attunement and coordination between caregiver and infant, but continues throughout the lifespan through interpersonal coordination and affective attunement. Rhythmic thirdness is primarily implicit and procedural; it involves finding rhythm or resonance with the other.

A second form of thirdness is the *differentiating Third*, which refers to "explicit, symbolic forms of thirdness that recognize one's own and others' distinct perceptions, intentions or feelings" (Benjamin, 2018, p. 21). This dimension reflects differentiation (cf. Chapter 6, this volume), including respect for individual and cultural differences, and capacities for humility and alterity.

A final form of thirdness is the *moral Third* (Benjamin, 2018, p. 51). Here Benjamin (2018) focused on repair of the inevitable ruptures that occur between people. She suggested that there is an element of integrity and fairness in recognition that must be negotiated through "acknowledgment of disruptions, disappointments, violations of expectancy . . . injuries and trauma" (Benjamin, 2018, p. 51).

Within Benjamin's (2018) approach, the key issue is how to create, sustain, or recover the Third, which could also be framed as offering or recovering mutual recognition. As mentioned above, Benjamin warned against concretizing or reifying the Third, as if there were some particular strategy or resource— an insight, theoretical idea, or relational move—that we must grasp. Instead, she suggested that "in the space of thirdness, we are not *holding onto* a Third; we are, in Ghent's (1990) felicitous usage, surrendering to it" (Benjamin, 2018, p. 23, her emphasis). Unlike submission, which involves "*giving in* or *over* to someone, an idealized person or thing," surrender involves "letting go into *being with* them. . . . We follow some principle or process that mediates between self and other" (Benjamin, 2018, p. 24, emphasis in original).

What is the principle or process that mediates, to which we surrender? Broadly speaking, it often involves some movement toward greater honesty and more loving or just ways of relating, but we must be careful about a priori answers. The Third is contextual and relational (Sandage & Brown, 2018). We surrender to what is, and to what is possible toward greater wholeness and integrity within the relationship at a specific moment. For many, Thirdness has spiritual quality, and involves a turn toward God or something transcendent that helps us find the other. Hoffman suggested that surrender may invite us to move through loss to gratitude, a kind of "resurrection" from her Christian perspective (Hoffman, 2011, p. 149). More broadly, one of the values of wrestling with the personal and interdisciplinary tensions that can sometimes be felt between psychotherapeutic theories and our own spiritual–existential–religious–theological (SERT) traditions is the possibility of opening up third space and the cultivation of intersubjectivity (Sandage & Brown, 2018). Thirdness requires courageous seeking but may restore a sense of dwelling together, at least until the next slip into complementarity.

A clinical example involved a client who recurrently complained that I [DR] was not moved or affected by her. We explored what might be happening and what it might represent, and I tried to be more responsive within the hour, all with little effect. Meanwhile the client became increasingly frustrated that I seemed "emotionally untouchable," and we both felt misunderstood. In this case, finding a Third involved becoming able to say, first to myself and then to the client, "Maybe I don't care enough." Surrendering in this way opened a conversation about how there was considerable connection and appreciation between us, and how we "put up with each other" around certain differences and limitations. This frame broke the tension and allowed the work to move forward. Commenting on this later, the client said, "I felt I had not touched you, moved your heart . . . your willingness to be vulnerable made the difference . . . [that] is what I would want therapists to do more."

Realistically, there are times when we cannot find a Third. Clients and therapists must sometimes struggle and bear with one another for an indeterminate period. It's important to tolerate enactments and impasses, to keep faith and allow time to find a Third, while also getting regular consultation to ensure the best possible client care. This includes staying open to the possibility that extended impasses may signal a poor fit. I [DR] have a former client with whom my most meaningful intervention may have been acknowledging that we were stuck and supporting a transfer to a colleague. It appears that the work is going better since the transfer.

Acknowledgment is one important path towards thirdness. Benjamin (2018) emphasized acknowledgment of limitations and failures by therapist and client. Therapists must "witness and . . . admit failure of witnessing." (p. 63). This involves taking responsibility, establishing a realistic balance of goodness and badness (rather than attributing all badness to the other), and sharing struggles rather than denying or avoiding them. When acknowledging failure, therapists seek to manage their own shame and self-criticism to set a tone of acceptance and humility, not humiliation. In this way, therapists may go first in demonstrating that it is possible to survive confrontation with one's own destructiveness and vulnerability, a key aspect of moving from complementarity to intersubjectivity (Benjamin, 2018; Bromberg, 2011; McWilliams, 2011), and an important element in many spiritual traditions.

Such responsibility-taking by the therapist is balanced and nuanced by mutual (but asymmetrical) recognition and participation. For the therapist, mutual recognition means continually eliciting the client's experience and preferences rather than trying to "figure it out on my own" (Benjamin, 2018, p. 93), but also being willing disclose one's own experience in thoughtful and responsible ways. Benjamin (2018) believed that the therapist's subjectivity inevitably enters the process as differences and limitations arise, requiring the dyad to negotiate their differences. Maroda (2018) has added that there may be benefits—such as eliciting and engaging avoided affect, destabilizing problematic/defensive patterns, and sharing authentic feedback—from tolerable levels of conflict in therapy. Many relational writers (Aron, 2018; Bromberg, 2011, 2006) have emphasized the therapist's participation in the struggle to clarify and work through conflicts, impasses, and enactments. Detached observations or interpretations are useful with some clients at some moments, but these sorts of interventions often fail during impasses. Clients may need to experience the therapist as present, willing to struggle with them and for them, and strong enough to survive as a separate but engaged other (Benjamin, 2018; Lyons-Ruth, 1999). Along this line, Benjamin (2018) wrote,

> When the child or patient discovers that the mother/analyst can survive opposition, she becomes a person from whom something real can be received without a price, without sacrificing what feels real to self. Two different realities can thus exist; both minds can live. When the mother/analyst is able to avoid submission without retaliation, can think for and regulate herself, she is neither controlling nor enveloping with weakness; neither a burden nor a puppet. (p. 86)

Importantly, this often requires self-regulation *and* coregulation through sharing feelings, conflicts, and uncertainties (Aron, 2018, Barsness & Strawn, 2018). When, how much, and what kind of disclosure must be discerned and negotiated. Too much of the therapist may distract or overpower the client; too little may leave the client or the therapist alone (without an intersubjective partner) and miss opportunities for coconstruction. For example, in one long-term treatment, the therapist learned to say very little during the hour, and this continued for many sessions. The client commented later, "I needed you to be small so I could become big." Later in the work, the client explicitly asked for more engagement, leading to moments of resonance and coordination as well as rupture and repair.

CONCLUSION

From our perspective, relationships play a central role in human flourishing and human struggle. Intersubjectivity contributes to our understanding by illuminating relational dynamics—patterns of interaction and their effects—that support (or hinder) wellness and intimacy. Key aspects of the intersubjectivity system, such as coordination and synchrony, attunement, affect regulation, rupture and repair, and interpersonal recognition, have a crucial role in healthy development and relationships, at least in certain cultural contexts. Psychotherapy research also highlights the impact of intersubjective relational factors, such as the therapeutic alliance, cultural humility, affect regulation, and rupture and repair (Flückiger, Del Re, Wampold, & Horvath, 2018; Hook, Davis, Owen, Worthington, & Utsey, 2013; Lingiardi, Holmqvist, & Safran, 2016; Schore, 2012). Indeed, it appears that if we are able to hold onto ourselves and connect deeply with one another, something new may emerge, something that may be enough.

CLINICAL APPLICATIONS OF THE RELATIONAL SPIRITUALITY MODEL

8

Relational Spirituality in Individual Therapy

In therapy we find that the ability to recognize and appreciate the complexity and paradoxical nature of life and people is, in fact, one of the crucial components of psychological wholeness.

—E. FRANKEL, *SACRED THERAPY* (2003, P. 211)

Given the complex historical relationship between psychotherapy and religion (Bartoli, 2007; Gonsiorek, Richards, Pargament, & McMinn, 2009), we are often asked, occasionally with a measure of wariness and skepticism, what psychotherapy and psychotherapy training and research look like at the Danielsen Institute, an organization that emphasizes the close connection between spirituality, religion, and mental health. A common response is to say that our staff shares a belief in and commitment to the idea that the provision of the best possible psychotherapy to suffering persons is, in and of itself, an act of sacred responsibility and trust. Depending on one's training and culture, this might be called service, or ministry, or mitzvah, or healing relationship, or a host of other descriptors. Whatever the label, our approach to psychotherapeutic care, training, and research centers on a relational commitment to the person of the client(s) and their particular needs, struggles, and strengths, and to collaborative discernment of possible paths to alleviate suffering and promote growth and change.

The relational spirituality model (RSM) is a developmental, relational, depth-oriented, and systemic way of thinking about the human person in the

http://dx.doi.org/10.1037/0000174-009
Relational Spirituality in Psychotherapy: Healing Suffering and Promoting Growth,
by S. J. Sandage, D. Rupert, G. S. Stavros, and N. G. Devor

context of the relational and cultural webs and experiences they inhabit, along with the intimacy, trauma, loneliness, support, isolation, connectedness, opportunities, and limitations these webs offer. In this chapter, we are choosing to present our work with a particular client, Anthony, and his family because his young life reflects so many of the issues that the RSM emphasizes—and because his life and situation help to illustrate the central commitment of our clinical/training/research enterprise at the Danielsen: effective, ethical, compassionate clinical care within a developmental crucible.

It will become clear that explicit references to religious and spiritual life, tradition, practice, and belief are often not central to the treatment. While this may seem contradictory given our work on a relational *spirituality* model, it is not that unusual in our experience. We hope to illustrate how the psychotherapist respectfully enters into the ways that clients make sense of themselves, others, and the world within and around them; and in this case, as is so often true and necessary, practices hospitality toward the client's needs for both relational security and exploration, for dwelling and seeking, for development and healing. In these ways, relational spirituality is often more implicit than explicit in the clinical process (Tan, 1996). At the same time, the RSM makes ample space for clinically appropriate and relevant engagement with and reflection on more explicit religious, spiritual, or existential concerns in moments or seasons when explicit conversations would be helpful.

CLINICAL VIGNETTE 1: ATTACHMENT SYSTEM FOCUS

Anthony first presented for treatment when he was 16 years old, the younger of two children of professional parents from an intact marriage. Anthony's mother, Karina, is Lebanese American, born and raised near Providence, Rhode Island, and the daughter of two parents who are Lebanese immigrants. Anthony's father, Nick, is Caucasian and of mixed ethnicity, born and raised in Philadelphia by parents who were both children of immigrants. Nick's father has Italian and Irish ancestry, and his mother has Sicilian, English, and Scottish ethnicity. Anthony's parents met when they were both in college in Boston and have continued to live in Boston while starting their careers and family. Karina is a Maronite Catholic Christian who continues to attend church two to three times per year on major holidays. Nick is a nonpracticing Roman Catholic Christian who accompanies Karina to holiday services at a local Maronite parish. Anthony reports attending services with his mother "to make her happy." Anthony had hesitantly come out to his parents as gay just after his 15th birthday, but there had been almost no discussion with his parents of his sexuality, or sexuality in general, since that time. In the 6 months leading up to Anthony's evaluation for intensive outpatient treatment, he had been psychiatrically hospitalized three times for suicidality, including recent episodes of standing on a train platform and threatening to jump and two serious overdoses of his psychiatric medications. At the time of his intake evaluation, he states that all of his problems are "because of my parents" and that he does not want any further treatment. He then adds:

ANTHONY: I'm evil and worthless. I'm a stupid, ugly faggot and everyone hates me, so if I kill myself at least I'll be doing one good thing for the world.

After 4 weeks of group dialectical behavior therapy, a full psychopharmacological evaluation and treatment plan, and 4 weeks of individual therapy, the family was referred to me for a consultation, and they were quite resistant to family therapy, describing multiple family meetings and consultations with previous therapists that were disruptive for the parents and contributed to feeling intense shame about their son's situation. They reported that their son had made the last therapist cry during family therapy. The session begins with this:

KARINA: So, can you tell us where you stand on the idea that kids are suicidal because of their parents?

The intensity of her question and the look in her eyes, which appeared to be one of fear and expectation of punishment, contributed to my taking a few moments in responding.

GSS: I think the reasons for your son's suicidality extend well beyond his relationship with you. What I was hoping you could help me understand is what this past six months has been like for the two of you. How have you been coping and dealing with everything that's happened with Anthony?

Both parents begin to tear up. Within the first few sessions of family therapy, Karina shared that she suffered severe postpartum depression after Anthony's birth and that she had also tried to return to work as a corporate tax lawyer just 6 weeks after Anthony was born. Both parents shared their account of having a succession of three nannies care for Anthony and his older brother when Anthony was an infant and toddler, and how each of the nannies had to leave the position after 6 to 12 months. After 15 sessions of family therapy, the parents, in a session without Anthony, asked if I would consider expanding my role to become Anthony's individual therapist. After multiple consultations with senior colleagues, and agreement by Anthony and both of his parents, I assented to a provisional period of holding both roles, with ongoing evaluation of how treatment was progressing.[1]

Two existential "self and other" dynamics that stand out quickly about Anthony in the context of his evaluation and early treatment are the

---

[1]This stance is more common among systemically oriented therapists than some other theoretical orientations. The advantage can be that the therapist can understand the differing relational dynamics within an overall system and cultivate a therapeutic alliance with various members of the system. It requires working at high levels of differentiation on the part of the therapist and necessitates good consultation, and there are cases in which it would not be an effective clinical strategy.

viciousness of his self-hatred and the intensity of his loneliness and longing for connection, both of which drive his ambivalence about remaining alive. These early clinical observations play a central and interconnected role in the longer-term work with Anthony. The RSM offers developmental frameworks within which to begin formulating hypotheses and questions around this knotty combination of self-destructiveness and desperate relational searching. A good place to start in treatment planning is attachment theory (see Chapter 5), which along with family systems theory and relational psychoanalytic theory form the theoretical, developmental, and relational foundations of RSM. Why is attachment theory a part of the theoretical foundation of RSM? While our earlier chapter on attachment addresses this question in detail, it is worth highlighting the importance of attachment theory for individual psychotherapy in particular with reference to Anthony's case for illustration (see Table 8.1).

Assessment of Early Relationships

Attachment theory is a theory of human development that is focused on relationships, making it possible to connect early relational experiences with their developmental impact downstream on relational templates. In Anthony's life, our clinical assessment would note the combination of his mother's postpartum depression, early return to full-time work, and the losses associated with three nannies departing from the care of Anthony and his brother when Anthony was a toddler and infant. It appears that reliable, consistent

TABLE 8.1. Relational Spirituality Model (RSM) Assessment and Intervention With Attachment System Focus in Individual Therapy

Assessment	1. Identify early relational trauma, loss, neglect, and abuse.
	2. Assess internal working models for relationships through current relationships, relationship with therapist, and ways of talking about relationships.
	3. Assess capacities for emotion regulation, mentalization (perspective-taking), and empathy.
	4. Assess tolerance for negative affect and regulation of relational stress.
	5. Assess attachment style connected with SERT experience and behavior.
Intervention	1. Recognize enactments of family attachment dynamics and seek nondestructive, corrective relational experience.
	2. Emphasize both dwelling and seeking, support and challenge.
	3. Appreciate the confusing, contradictory, and paradoxical content, behavior, and process that accompanies suffering.
	4. Expand vocabulary for suffering and for life-giving meaning.
	5. Identify RSM resources that provide appropriate experiences of dwelling and seeking.

Note. SERT = spiritual–existential–religious–theological.

parental/caregiver attunement and care were tenuous in the relational milieu and conditions of Anthony's early development. Attachment theory suggests that Anthony's emotional suffering and intense self-hatred are connected to this compromised caregiving milieu and are profoundly relational in nature. They are symptoms, if you will, of attachment-based injuries of early development which are now forcefully manifesting themselves in Anthony's transition into adolescence.

Internal Working Models

It is possible for psychotherapists to assess a client's relational hopes, fears, and expectations, their internal working models for relationships (Ainsworth & Eichberg, 1991; Main, 1995), by appreciating how their attachment stories continue to play out in their lives, including in their relationship with the therapist (Fonagy & Allison, 2014; Wallin, 2007). Thus, attachment theory gives psychotherapists a framework within which to consider and better understand the often confusing, contradictory, and paradoxical content, behavior, and process they can experience with suffering clients within the developmental crucible of therapy. For example, in my second individual session with Anthony, I found him in the waiting room with his head in his mother's lap while she stroked his hair. He then entered our individual therapy session and immediately began a profanity-laced description of how his parents had set limits on his time with a friend with whom he had been caught smoking marijuana the previous week. It was hard to imagine that his mother, or anyone else in the clinic, could not hear him, and I [GSS] was caught off guard by this rapid shift in mood and presentation, getting into a struggle of my own in setting limits with Anthony. It took 20 turbulent minutes in session before Anthony and I could enter into anything resembling an early-treatment, alliance-building conversation.

After the session, I felt angry at Anthony, ashamed that I did not anticipate and could not control his outburst, confused about the tender but awkward image of Anthony and his mother in the waiting room, and quietly grateful that I was not the direct target of Anthony's rage. It was only with postsession consultation that I was able to begin untangling my own affective reaction and regain my equilibrium. My supervisor encouraged me to reconnect with the steadiness and resilience within and around me; first, because I would need it to survive these storms, and also because my ability to reestablish my own regulation would be necessary in providing Anthony the containment that his troubled attachment style would require over the course of our treatment relationship. My clinical supervisor also suggested that Anthony was offering me a "test case" to see how I would respond to his rage, dysregulation, suffering, and sadism. Anthony was very likely, though not intentionally, seeing if my reaction to him would fit with his internal working model for relationships, which would have meant some version or combination of retaliatory rage, deflated helplessness, impotent pleading, or indifferent withdrawal.

It is easy to overlook the reality that clients are often conducting their own assessment of us as therapists in early sessions, seeking to test whether we have the capacity to dwell with them in the emotional and existential turbulence they are experiencing. While I by no means "passed" the test, neither did I move into the kinds of worst-case scenarios Anthony's working model anticipated. When Anthony arrived on time for his next session, I decided to myself to call it a draw.

Cognitive Neuroscience

Attachment research is connecting in ever-growing ways to cognitive neuroscience and interpersonal neurobiology research, helping psychotherapists better understand the physiological, brain, and body consequences of secure and insecure early attachment (Cozolino & Santos, 2014; Flores, 2010; Lewis, Amini, & Lannon, 2000; Schore, 2001; van der Kolk, 2014). Important examples of this include the capacities for emotion regulation, mentalization, and empathy that are so often the product of secure early-attachment relationships, as well as the corresponding struggles in these arenas when early attachment was characterized by extreme stress, parental misattunement, trauma, loss, abuse, and neglect. Schore (2012) identified the abilities to tolerate negative affect and regulate relational stress as emanating from repeated, reliable, emotionally attuned relational processes and experiences of coregulation between caretaker and child. The caretaker's capacity to consistently, though not perfectly, understand and respond to the child's affective communications, without withdrawing from, retaliating against, or shaming the child lives at the heart of these developmental achievements that impact internal templates about relational spirituality.

Alongside attunement, a caretaker's skill in reestablishing and repairing emotional and relational contact with the child after inevitable relational ruptures and misattunement is vital (Schore, 2012). This rupture and repair process, which allows the child to reexperience positive emotions after periods of distress and dysregulation, provides the neurocognitive and limbic building blocks for the kinds of emotional and relational resilience and trust that can positively impact healthy relational spirituality. It is also important to affirm the importance of diagnostic considerations in treatment planning, particularly related to Anthony's mood, and to have regular pharmacological contributions to his care.

Six months into individual treatment with Anthony, he shared the following story:

ANTHONY: My mom picked me up from school yesterday. I was waiting with some of my friends, but it had been a really bad day and just wanted to go home. Well, she, of course, rolls down the window and starts making a big deal, showing off in front of my friends, like she always does. The next thing I know, she invites three of them over to our house to do homework without asking me. Just what I fucking needed. When my friends finally left, we got into this huge fight. She's screaming at me, telling me it's good for me to have friends and that she was just trying to help. And I'm screaming back at her that she is fucking clueless about me and what's good for me. We didn't talk for the rest of the night. Fuck her.

While there are a host of different theory-informed ways Anthony's psychotherapist might respond to this account, RSM's grounding in attachment theory would place an emphasis on the attachment "soundtrack" that accompanies the content of the encounter. Instead of being a transient, repairable episode of misattunement, frustration, and anger, Anthony's description is characterized more by intense mutual dysregulation and sharp disconnection, with both Anthony and Karina feeling misunderstood, victimized, and ashamed. What stands out is not so much the rupture, which is not so unusual in the context of adolescent development and parenting. It is the absence of resilience, mindfulness, perspective-taking, and forgiveness following the rupture. It is as if neither Anthony nor Karina can picture and move toward a better outcome. Given their shared attachment history, it is worth considering the degree to which this absence of hope is, in part, an echo or dissonant chord carried forward from their early, shared attachment difficulties.

It also raises the question of how the psychotherapist might address this all-too-familiar family scenario. Family therapy provided a systemic space within which to do some of the work. Within the immediacy of this individual psychotherapy session, however, I found myself holding competing thoughts about how to respond. On the one hand, I agreed with some of Karina's perspective in wanting Anthony to stay connected with his friends and appreciated Karina's efforts in trying to facilitate that connection by making herself and the family home available for this. At the same time, I was aware that Anthony could experience Karina's extroverted style and relentless hospitality as forceful, patronizing, and invalidating of his own more introverted interpersonal style and developmental push toward autonomy. In addition, there was something about Anthony's posture and affect, wherein a deep sadness seemed to underlie his angry, expletive-laced description that felt important to acknowledge.

GSS: It sounds like it was really hard in that moment to feel so lonely and misunderstood.

Hoping to foster Anthony's capacity for self-reflection and to continue building our attachment-based alliance, I moved toward this more supportive intervention, trusting that he and I would have ongoing opportunities to explore, validate, and challenge his perceptions, feelings, and thoughts about his relational suffering and struggles. This is an in-the-moment choice to emphasize dwelling, and the relational security that early attachment injuries require from individual psychotherapy, while carefully holding Anthony's simultaneous though backgrounded need for the growth and learning that come from seeking.

Religion and Spirituality

Attachment theory is an excellent conversation partner with many religious traditions and spiritual frameworks and practices (E. B. Davis, Granqvist, & Sharp, 2018; Granqvist & Kirkpatrick, 2016). Attachment theory speaks powerfully to the human need for belonging, self-worth in relation to others and the greater world, and the relational mind's capacity for making meaning. In these ways, it becomes another lens through which the spiritual–existential–religious–theological (SERT) elements of personhood and relationship, both constructive and destructive, secure and insecure, can be explored and better understood through the healing process of psychotherapy.

The first words we hear from Anthony in this chapter are fraught with pain, self-hatred, and rage—and they are words filled with spiritual meaning and anguish. He describes himself as evil and worthless, rails profanely against his own body and sexuality, and declares judgment on himself, concluding that his demise might serve as a sacrifice benefiting humankind. The RSM's appreciation for the religious/spiritual nature of Anthony's suffering adds depth to our understanding of and empathy for him. To illustrate this, we offer the following example.

Earlier in the chapter, we began to consider some of the attachment-based developmental and relational conditions contributing to Anthony's self-hatred and emotional dysregulation. We believe that these attachment injuries converge and interact with Anthony's sexuality and spirituality in complex and powerful ways, as well. Both of Anthony's parents were raised in religious homes, Maronite Catholic and Roman Catholic, but they chose not to emphasize religion in the lives of their children, beyond occasional worship-service attendance. Later discussions with each parent about Anthony's sexual orientation revealed their feeling caught between two important aspects of their faith traditions. Namely, they lived in tension between believing in a loving, if distant, God and being raised in church communities that were not gay-affirming. When Anthony came out to them, they reported that it did not come as a surprise; nonetheless, the reality of his coming out caught each of them off guard, contributing to an unexpected collision between Anthony's sexuality and their mostly dormant, internalized religious beliefs and bias. With good intentions, Karina and Nick offered Anthony superficial support, but there was no further acknowledgment or discussion among anyone in the family about Anthony's sexual orientation until after he entered treatment.

Given the family's vulnerability for attachment-based relational ruptures, it is not surprising that Anthony experienced his parents' avoidance as another version of crushing misattunement, making his body and sexual orientation direct targets of his self-hatred and dysregulation, as if he somehow wanted to escape dwelling in his body because his sexuality did not seem to find a place of dwelling in his family. It became necessary in individual therapy to create a hospitable space (dwelling) within which Anthony could expand the vocabulary of his suffering and begin exploration (seeking) related to his sexuality, to draw off some of the accumulated toxins of parental, religious, and societal misattunement and prejudice, and consider other narratives and meanings.

CLINICAL VIGNETTE 2: DIFFERENTIATION SYSTEM FOCUS

Anthony, now 18 months into treatment—through much turmoil and many ruptures and repairs with his parents, chaotic relationships with peers, and ongoing work on his sexuality and internalized homophobia—graduates from high school and is preparing for his first semester at college. Having just turned 18, he now holds the right to consent to treatment on his own and, importantly, has legal protections around the confidentiality of his treatment and treatment records, something of which he is very aware. The general level of his self-destructive and self-defeating behaviors has decreased substantially in acuity. However, he has settled into a set of peer relationships that revolve around high levels of daily marijuana use and low levels of academic or vocational interest or direction. I find myself relieved that I do not worry about him as much as I used to. Anthony enters the office for his weekly therapy session, clearly prepared to talk about something.

ANTHONY: So, if I told you about something that happened in the past, would you still tell my parents?

GSS: I get the feeling you have something you want to tell me?

ANTHONY: Duh. But I'm not going to tell you if you're going to tell them.

GSS: I don't know, Anthony. I think by now you have a sense that you have a lot of room in here to say what you have to say and that we'll figure out together whether to involve your parents. And that hasn't changed from my perspective. Is there something making that feel more uncertain for you?

ANTHONY: This happened a long time ago. Back when I used to hang out with Linda.

GSS: Okay.

ANTHONY: It's important. I want to tell you.

Anthony goes on to share how he is currently experiencing posttraumatic stress disorder symptoms related to two episodes of trading sex in order to secure crack cocaine and heroin as a 16-year-old, at the time when he and his family had just entered treatment. I sigh, realizing how much I didn't know, and that Anthony had kept hidden, during that time. Anthony weeps—something that he rarely does—and speaks in detail about how much terror, in the form of flashbacks, intrusive memories, and nightmares, he experiences at night, especially when he is alone. He talks with me about how his current friends and their intense marijuana use provide some emotional buffering from these symptoms, though not with as much effectiveness over the past several months. After several conversations between us, Anthony decides that he wants his parents to know that he is struggling with intense fear and loneliness, especially at night, but he does not want to share the specific traumatic content associated with his dangerous sexual activity with them. I support his decision (see Table 8.2).

Differentiation of self (DoS; see Chapter 6, this volume), a concept developed by family therapist Murray Bowen (1978), refers to the process within families by which individual members learn to find relational and emotional balance within the family system and to navigate the anxieties of difference. According to Bowenian theory, in family systems where dynamics like closeness and autonomy and thinking and feeling are unbalanced, there tend to be frequent breakdowns in communication, rigidity of family roles, reactive anxiety to intimacy and separation, and difficulty managing strong emotions. In contrast, well-differentiated families and family members are characterized by spontaneity, resilience, creative problem solving, effective responses to stress, acceptance of differences, and greater comfort moving between closeness and solitude. In Chapter 6, we offered an overview of research on DoS and demonstrated empirical connections to numerous indicators of psychological, relational, spiritual, and intercultural dimensions of well-being and maturity. Although developed primarily within a family therapy clinical context, DoS has important implications for treatment planning in individual therapy, especially through the concepts of differentiated intrapersonal and interpersonal functioning (Jankowski, Sandage, & Hill, 2013), which are further discussed below. In addition, it has important connections to and resonance with

TABLE 8.2. Relational Spirituality Model (RSM) Assessment and Intervention With Differentiation System Focus in Individual Therapy

Assessment	1. Assess family capacity for relational and emotional balance.
	2. Assess capacity for intrapersonal and interpersonal differentiation.
	3. Assess capacity for navigating difference and tolerance of closeness and solitude.
	4. Assess family roles—rigid or flexible.
	5. Identify intrinsic versus extrinsic SERT beliefs, practices, and relationships.
Intervention	1. Use therapeutic crucible to move between empathic support and tolerable challenge.
	2. Help clients to balance closeness and intimacy with solitude, agency, and autonomy.
	3. Help clients move from dissociation, somatic trauma, self-hatred, and shame to self-reflection, inner connection and cohesion, and mindful awareness of competing self-aspects.
	4. Welcome and negotiate differences.
	5. Identify RSM resources that invite SERT experience integrated with emotional and relational balance.

attachment and intersubjectivity, the two other developmental systems of focus in the RSM.

In the above clinical vignette, we encounter 18-year-old Anthony after 1 and a half years of treatment, and there are several notable changes in him from a DoS perspective. First, he arrives at the session on his own and takes initiative in setting an agenda that will involve a negotiation about an uncertain outcome. He is in a developmental transition of trying to move out into the world with greater autonomy, and this activates his seeking a secure base to facilitate further differentiation. This is a very different presentation than 18 months earlier, when Anthony was laying in his mother's lap and then entering our session with dysregulated fury about the limits placed on him by his parents. Also, the severity, dangerousness, and destructiveness of Anthony's behavior and interpersonal conflicts have markedly decreased since beginning treatment. For the past 18 months, Anthony and his family appear to have been weathering an acute and potentially lethal storm, and as part of that Anthony is demonstrating some developmentally appropriate capacities for the individuation side of differentiation. As the vignette illustrates, though, the coast is far from clear, and Anthony's differentiation and growth are accompanied by his growing awareness and articulation of deep and profound suffering and trauma. As mentioned in Chapter 4, we find it is common for spiritual and existential struggles and associated searches for healing to intensify during liminal periods of individual or family transition when relational structures of dwelling and meaning become ambiguous. In addition, his reliance on heavy marijuana use as a self-medication strategy for emotion regulation has become chronic and, from his perspective, nonnegotiable, something we also take up later in the chapter.

Differentiated Intrapersonal Functioning

Differentiated intrapersonal functioning refers to a person's capacity to identify within themselves multiple "self-aspects." *Self-aspects*, a concept developed by Dimaggio (2006), is similar to the concept of self-states from the relational psychoanalytic tradition. Bromberg (2011) defined *self-states* as "highly individualized modules of being, each configured by its own organization of cognitions, beliefs, dominant affect and mood, access to memory, skills, behaviors, values, actions, and regulatory physiology" (p.73). Differentiated intrapersonal functioning consists of "opening up space . . . for emotional and behavioral self-regulation, whereby emotional states are monitored with a mindfulness of one's multiple self-aspects, enabling perspective taking and dialogue between differing self-aspects" (Jankowski, Sandage, & Hill, 2013, p. 2). Undifferentiated intrapersonal functioning is characterized by either a lack of awareness of the multiplicity of selves making up a person's inner world, or by a flooding of competing self-aspects, resulting in cognitive disorganization, emotional dysregulation, and behavioral and relational instability.

The vignette above poignantly illustrates some of the contrasts between Anthony's differentiated and undifferentiated intrapersonal functioning.

Anthony makes reference to several behavioral markers, which taken together offer a portrayal of the undifferentiated chaos of his inner world when he entered treatment: multiple suicide attempts and overdoses; dangerous, high-risk sexual activity to procure potent, addictive, mood-altering substances; a merged, poorly bounded, exclusive relationship with one peer (Linda) who was often controlling and sadistic; and extreme self-hatred targeting his own body and sexuality. With the help of distress tolerance and emotion regulation skills, psychopharmacology, and weekly psychotherapy and family therapy, Anthony worked incredibly hard in the first 18 months of treatment to "open up space" within himself and between himself and others. He was able to begin shifting his intrapersonal world from dissociation, somatic trauma, self-hatred, and shame to an internal experience that offered moments of self-reflection, hints of inner connection, and a mindful awareness of the often-competing self-aspects within him, giving him access to begin to try to mentalize his previously disowned or rejected vulnerability, agency, and hope. He then brought to the session a more intrapersonally differentiated approach to our work, and in this session, the stakes felt high in how I responded to him. He and I had not talked about the boundary between our sessions and his parents for a long time. While it seemed like he was bringing this to me as a negotiation between us, I also had the distinct sense that he was also negotiating something within himself, between self-aspects, if you will. The moment felt to me like one that required more space for Anthony to sit, accompanied by me, in the internal tension and developmental crucible of intrapersonal differentiation for a kind of integration of dwelling and seeking. This would require him to modulate his emotions and mindfully take in that he had the internal (and now legal) authority to decide whether and what to tell me. Under other circumstances, I might have been more assuring or explicit about the therapeutic container and contract, but it felt in this instance that we were already using the therapeutic container to work out and extend Anthony's DoS.

The work of intrapersonal differentiation was not only something in which Anthony had to engage. The above vignette also shows how much I [GSS], as Anthony's therapist, had to be working on my own differentiation to remain connected with Anthony in this new intense cycle of seeking. A key part of RSM is its insistence on the therapist being accountable for and engaged with their own internal processes, biases, subjective reactions, and personal developmental history in relation to the work we do with any of our psychotherapy clients. For me, this meant making room for the shame I felt at "missing" all that Anthony was experiencing when we first started treatment, and my existential discomfort with feeling out of control in relation to an "other" who is out of control. It meant making room for uncertainty about how to manage this information with Anthony's family, imagining their potential anger and blame about how much I did not know about their son, or knew and did not disclose to them. It meant dealing with my horror and shock at what Anthony had shared and the pain I felt in allowing myself to empathize with the posttraumatic impact on him now. Making this kind of room was by no means a solitary event, as I sought out regular consultation during which I could share my emotional reactions, while also having time and space to consider specific clinical choices and options. I also found myself holding more closely to some of the simple rhythms of my own life, including basic aspects of self-care (nutrition, rest, sleep, physical activity), relational connectedness with family and friends, and religious and spiritual life.

Differentiated Interpersonal Functioning

Differentiated interpersonal functioning and differentiated intrapersonal functioning have a bidirectional relationship. On the one hand, mindful awareness, openness, and hospitality toward one's own internal self-aspects or self-states, which can often be contradictory and conflicting, make it more possible and likely that a person will engage interpersonally in life-giving and relationship-enhancing ways. At the same time, the capacity for differentiated intrapersonal functioning is built through secure relational interaction and contact with close others that is characterized by the healthy balance and attributes found in differentiated interpersonal functioning. Some of these attributes include relational hospitality and openness to the other; an ability to welcome and negotiate differences between oneself and another person; a consistent ability to negotiate between needs for closeness and intimacy and solitude and autonomy; and an ability to regulate emotions in relationships, without falling into extremes of anxious merger/fusion or total disengagement/dismissal.

Anthony's movement toward improved differentiated interpersonal functioning proved to be a mixed bag. He continued to demonstrate and report a significant amount of mistrust toward his parents, most adults (including his therapist), and all but a tiny handful of friends. He struggled to spend any time alone, especially at night, when his posttraumatic symptoms typically increased. And he spent most of his peer social time with the same group of five or six friends who gathered together after school to smoke pot, rarely moving outside of his comfort zone or challenging himself or being challenged by others. At the same time, Anthony had several things working in his favor as he attempted to be more interpersonally differentiated. One of these was the power of his developmental strengths, driven by things like his keen intelligence, his growing curiosity about himself, and some of his attachment behaviors that demonstrated a warmth and openness to others, through smiles and humor, that were not as apparent when he first entered treatment. Another factor in Anthony's favor was having parents who were willing to struggle with their own intrapersonal and interpersonal differentiation. Their initial desperation to find expert help to "take over" Anthony's parenting had moved incrementally toward a more differentiated existential stance, with a mixture of interest and involvement with him and a shift toward emphasizing a relationship with their son rather than control over or abandonment of him. The vignette, in a way, mirrors this process of interpersonal differentiation, as Anthony enters a negotiation with me [GSS] that could end up being either a power struggle or a differentiated consideration of relational options. For most of his life, Anthony's attempted relational spirituality solutions for getting help for his suffering or trying to get his needs met was to choose either rage, self-protective dissociation, or avoidance. The vignette suggests that he is becoming more capable of seeking and using space within himself and with a "trusted enough" other to expand his relational options to risk the much more fraught, but potentially healing, path of interpersonally differentiated connection and negotiation.

CLINICAL VIGNETTE 3: SERT THEMES

Anthony, now 20 years old and 3 years into treatment, has continued both to struggle and to make progress. He spent 4 weeks in intensive outpatient treatment, to address substance abuse issues (alcohol, marijuana) and continuing difficulties with emotion regulation, and he benefited from this treatment. We continue in weekly psychotherapy, he is working full-time, and he has been in a stable dating relationship for 6 months. He is also now dealing with news of Karina's recent diagnosis of leukemia.

ANTHONY: Did you know that I pray?

GSS: (pause) I didn't know that. (pause)

ANTHONY: I do (quietly, softly). I pray for my mother, my family, and Mark. I thank God.

GSS: You thank God. Anthony, there are so many things I'd like to ask you about your prayer. If this doesn't sound like a question you want to answer, let me know. What do your prayers sound like?

ANTHONY: What do they sound like? I don't know. What do you mean?

GSS: Yes, sorry. I don't think I even have the question right in my own mind yet. It's just that you haven't always felt so grateful for your life. It's like seeing something new in you, starting to grow.

ANTHONY: (smiles mischievously) Don't get too excited. I don't always feel so grateful now, either. But sometimes I do, and when I do, I like to pray; to say thank you, or to ask for help.

GSS: That seems like a big deal, that you feel like it's okay for you to receive good things from God, and to receive help.

ANTHONY: Yeah, it is a pretty big deal.

We share this vignette for a couple of reasons. The first, more obvious one is that SERT themes are an important aspect of the RSM. On the surface, it seems to be a natural fit. What more could we ask for than a clear, explicit religious behavior like prayer showing up in therapy? The second reason, less obvious and more paradoxical, is that Anthony's initiating a discussion about his prayer life came as a complete surprise to me [GSS] as his therapist. Here we are, working within a therapeutic ecosystem at the Danielsen Institute that emphasizes attention to and awareness of the whole person, including religious and spiritual life, and yet I am caught off guard and at a loss for words when Anthony offers his description of praying. In our experience providing training and consultation to both new and seasoned clinicians, it is not unusual for therapists to struggle when engaging with clients around explicit SERT themes, concerns, and practices. Within our training programs at the Danielsen Institute, an important part of how we take up this struggle is through a weekly, interdisciplinary, small-group training seminar we call the SERT Group (Rupert, Moon, & Sandage, 2018; see also Chapter 11, this volume), which is composed of both senior staff clinicians and clinical and research training fellows. The task of the seminar is to help practicing and training clinicians to develop the sensibilities and skills, through didactics and shared depth-relational process, to be aware, accountable, creative, and clinically effective in the engagement of SERT issues in psychotherapeutic care. Three key strategies we use to engage this task are described next.

Therapist Accountability for SERT

First, we believe that it is vitally important for psychotherapists to be aware of their own religious and spiritual values, beliefs, worldview, practices, and commitments (or absence thereof) in order to act as a safeguard against potentially destructive bias, prejudice, and misuse of power in their work with clients (Stavros & Sandage, 2014; Strawn, Wright, & Jones, 2014). This is because a clinician's particular orientation toward SERT dynamics often has important implications for key therapeutic assumptions about things like human nature, change, healing, brokenness, psychopathology, healthy relationships, meaning in life, and many other key elements that are part of the psychotherapeutic process and relationship. Pargament (2007) made this point in writing, "Knowingly or unknowingly, the spirituality of the therapist permeates his or her understanding of people, problems, and change. Spiritually integrated psychotherapy makes explicit the importance of the therapist's own orientation to spirituality" (p.187). This kind of self-awareness is an important aspect of intercultural competence and applies to many dimensions of a clinician's identity, including race, social class, ethnicity, gender, sexuality, disability status, age, and others. In relation to religion and spirituality specifically, "countertransference" risks can include distorted extremes of pathologizing or idealizing a client's spirituality, as well as misusing the power and influence of the therapeutic alliance in ways that are either proselytizing or are coercively deconstructing of a client's spirituality based on the therapist's beliefs.

In the work with Anthony, several areas of awareness and accountability required attention. One of these was my [GSS] identification with the religious background of Anthony and his parents. Being born, raised, and still practicing as a Greek (Eastern) Orthodox Christian, I had some ideas about the more ritualistic, monastic, and hierarchical aspects of Maronite and Roman Catholic Church cultures, as well as the importance of ethnicity for Lebanese American Christians and Italian American Catholics. This general identification made me vulnerable to taking assumptive shortcuts in working with Anthony, which I believe I did. For example, I was really surprised to learn that he had a practice of personal prayer. My assumptions about the impact of his parents' distance from religious life created a blind spot in me and in the therapy about Anthony's spiritual life. As the child of inactive Catholic parents distanced from their own religious faith, I assumed there was no context within which a desire to pray, or to have any formal spiritual life, would emerge in Anthony. My unsteadiness was apparent to Anthony, and my short, sincere apology to him was part of trying to reestablish contact with him around his praying.

A related area that required greater therapist self-awareness was the tension and competing worldviews represented in the following: how the Eastern Orthodox Christian and Catholic Churches view same-sex attraction; my personal and professional orientation toward sexuality; and Anthony's struggle and growth around his own sexuality. From the perspective of deeply held values and personal and professional ethics, I was practicing from an affirming stance in relation to Anthony's sexuality and his developmental journey into meaningful adult intimacy and relationships. At the same time, I lived in and valued a liturgical, sacramental, familial, communal, contemplative religious life within the Eastern Orthodox Church, wherein there is uncertainty and tension related to expressions of human sexuality, sexual orientation, and the hospitality and openness that is in short supply for sexual minorities in the formal life of the Church. I believe I was vulnerable to reenacting the solution to this dilemma that Anthony's parents had chosen, namely superficial acceptance followed by invalidating silence. Peer relationships and consultation and regular intercultural training became necessary vehicles for keeping open space within myself and between myself and Anthony, for him to use as he confronted the fears of rejection, internalized homophobia, and toxic self-hatred that he could experience when trying to explore desires for relational security and deeper intimacy in his young adult life.

SERT for the Therapist

A second way in which we believe it can be important for psychotherapists to engage with SERT dimensions is by accessing SERT resources for the therapist's health, psychological and emotional well-being, and meaning making, all in the service of clinical competence and effectiveness. Here it is crucial for us to be clear that we are not privileging or recommending any particular, formal, denominational, structured, or organized religious belief system. We are relying on an understanding of spirituality more broadly defined as *ways of relating to that which a person considers sacred or of ultimate importance to them.* For some, this may include or be embodied within a specific religious faith tradition. For others, sacredness or ultimate importance flows primarily from other sources, including any number of life-giving experiences, relationships, activities, and value commitments. The point here is that psychotherapists, especially those whose clients experience deep suffering and trauma, require their own deep wells from which to draw sustaining connection and meaning. McWilliams (2014), Wallin (2014), Akhtar (2014), Sheppard (2014), Aron (2004), Fayek (2004), Sorenson (2004a), and Rizzuto (2004) have provided excellent religiously and ethnically diverse examples of how master clinicians' spiritual lives are inextricably tied to and in mutual influence with their clinical practice and thinking.[2]

In working with Anthony, I [GSS] found it important to access personal SERT resources to help sustain my own sense of resilience, hope, and courage. These resources tended to be a loose combination of conceptual, relational, and behavioral SERT elements, resonant with but not exclusive to my identity as an Eastern Orthodox Christian. One particularly important line of thinking and experience was an appreciation for how often I was confronted with mystery, surprise, and paradox in working with Anthony. There are two examples of this shared in our vignettes: Anthony's disclosure about his risky sexual activity to procure drugs and his disclosure about prayer. While these are very different kinds of disclosures, they share something in common—they both shed light on the depth, mystery, surprise, and paradox associated with Anthony's life, our work together in therapy, and by extension with human life and relationships more generally.

The Eastern Orthodox Christian faith tradition is steeped in ancient spiritual and liturgical practice that emphasizes the mystical, paradoxical relationships that exist between light and darkness, life and death, suffering and healing, freedom and captivity (Ware, 2002). I believe that my exposure to and participation in the tradition, both before meeting Anthony and during the time that we were working together, provided a conceptual framework for appreciating that I was not, and could not be, in control of Anthony's behavior. Instead, it provided a framework more geared toward a humble acceptance of Anthony as he was and as he presented himself, knowing there was so much more to him than I could ever truly know.

Paradoxically, this stance of humility relieved me of some of the burdens of anxiety and shame to which I was vulnerable and freed me to be more present to Anthony in his suffering, rather than trying to avoid or control it. In addition, Eastern Orthodox Christianity is characterized by its cycles of hourly, daily, weekly, yearly, and seasonal rhythms of prayer, worship, fellowship, feasts, and fasting. When practiced in relationally meaningful and

---

[2]Video presentations of many of these authors discussing the mutual influence of spiritual life and clinical practice are available for free viewing on the Danielsen Institute website (http://www.bu.edu/danielsen/video-library/the-skillful-soul-of-the-psychotherapist-2012-merle-jordan-conference/).

enlivening ways, these rhythms can offer a sense of security and spiritual dwelling in the context of life's inevitable disruptions and injuries. They also can act as a secure base, allowing for the possibility of seeking and journeying, engaging in exploration into unfamiliar territory. I benefited greatly from these rhythms, and this was an important part of what gave me trust in the process with Anthony, even in light of the shocking surprises I experienced from time to time in our work together. For me, these SERT rhythms resonate with the healthy vocational and relational rhythms of the psychotherapist: clinical practice, clinical training, peer consultation, and engagement with clinical research and scholarship. I find both sets to be sustaining and necessary elements, each feeding the other, of effective and ethical clinical work.

SERT for the Therapy

A third way that SERT considerations come into play in psychotherapy are those moments and situations when either a client or a therapist draws upon their own SERT experiences, insights, practices, and awareness and offers it explicitly within the therapy itself. When initiated by the therapist, this is a scenario that requires careful discernment, wisdom, and experience, for reasons described earlier. At the same time, psychotherapists committed to the healing and growth of their clients must regularly make clinical decisions about how and when to use different parts of themselves within the therapeutic process. We believe that there are moments in therapy when the explicit discussion of SERT issues and dynamics, including the therapist's perspectives on these issues, can be helpful and can embody a kind of attuned best practice in psychotherapy. When SERT themes and material are brought into therapy by the client, it is important that the therapist receive it with an open, welcoming, nonreactive, nonjudgmental stance. This kind of therapeutic response helps to communicate to the client that whatever is alive in them—whether they are experiencing it constructively or destructively, in a creative way or a deconstructing way—there is adequate space within themselves, the therapy, and the therapist to work with it thoughtfully.

To this point in the treatment, Anthony and I had engaged in very few conversations about his religious beliefs or practices, none of which I had considered particularly memorable or notable. Religion was something that was in the background of therapy, and I believe this had just as much do with me as it did with Anthony. When Anthony brought his prayer life into the foreground in therapy, it created opportunities and questions regarding the place of SERT issues, and more specifically Anthony's spiritual life, in treatment and in his relationship with his therapist. The first of these questions, we believe, had to do with hospitality and whether there was relationally secure space within the therapy and the therapeutic relationship for this more explicitly religious content. In the vignette, once I [GSS] metabolized my initial surprise, my response was intended to send the kind of welcoming signal described above, an opening of space for Anthony and me to explore the content and meaning of his prayer.

Another question that seems important to the exchange is what it means for Anthony to be "getting better," looking at his prayers of gratitude and petition for help as possible symbols of an underlying process of healing. Anthony, in a half-teasing way, is quick to put the brakes on any possible overinvestment on the therapist's part (e.g., "Don't get too excited . . ."), while still holding on to the importance of the experience for him.

A third question has to do with Anthony's embracing a relational prayer practice as a life-giving resource in the context of an institutional church perspective which sees him as deeply flawed with regard to his sexuality. There appears to be something spiritually important happening within Anthony: Call it secure attachment to God; or differentiation from traditional church teachings on sexuality; or an experience of intersubjective connection with the divine. In relation to each of these possibilities and questions, we believe it is important that the psychotherapist be a hospitable facilitator of the client's process for dwelling and seeking around SERT issues. Anthony is in the midst of unprecedented developmental movement (working full-time, in a committed relationship) and family crisis (Karina's cancer diagnosis), and he has brought into therapy a relational spirituality strategy to help him navigate these turbulent waters. By being attuned to Anthony's deep need at this time for relational security with God, and exploring Anthony's way of believing and praying, we believe the therapist is providing the necessary ingredients for Anthony to live his life, metabolize his traumatic development, and be resilient in the face of the inevitable sorrow and suffering that will come.

CLINICAL VIGNETTE 4: INTERSUBJECTIVITY SYSTEM FOCUS

Anthony is now 23 years old, 6 years into treatment, living with a partner, working full-time, and halfway to his bachelor's degree. His mother passed away 2 years ago, and Anthony is still grieving, at times intensely. He made the decision to be present and care for Karina in her final months of life, something about which he is glad and proud, though he continues to be haunted by images and sensations connected with her physical decline and death. In this session, he is considering getting his medical marijuana card, a subject about which I [GSS] have been maintaining a stance of curiosity and skeptical neutrality.

ANTHONY: So, I need that letter from you to get the marijuana card.

GSS: I know. Can I just ask you first, how does the marijuana help you?

ANTHONY: (quickly becomes tearful) It's the only thing that brings me relief.

GSS: Relief from what, Anthony?

ANTHONY: When those thoughts, the assaultive thoughts, are attacking, it's like . . . it keeps them from landing. It's like they're there, but I can just move on, like I don't give a shit what they're saying. Of course, the problem can be that I just don't give a shit about a lot of things at that point. But it's worth it. (He becomes tearful again.)

GSS: What is it?

ANTHONY: (crying). It's just that those thoughts, they tell me how awful I am, how disgusting and worthless, and it infects anything I'm trying to do. It's like they burrow into me and possess me.

GSS: Anthony, please let me know if this feels at all accurate or not. We've been talking and thinking a lot about your mother recently. Is there anything about your relationship with her that could be connected to what you just described?

ANTHONY: (tearfully, tentatively) Maybe.

GSS: Are you thinking something?

ANTHONY: She, well really both of my parents, they expected me to be so wonderful. When I was little, all they did was brag to people about how smart I was. They used to tell their friends I could order my own meals at restaurants when I was 3 years old (I smile. Anthony continues sadly.). But they left me alone. I was so alone. She didn't see ME. And then I was so awful. To myself. To them.

GSS: You were in a lot of pain then. And you are now, too. You know, for really important reasons, you chose to stay close to your mother when she was sick. I so admire how you were with her. Being with her, loving her as she died. (softly) You saw HER.

ANTHONY: (nodding and weeping) And now she's gone. She never got to see me turn my life around. I want her to see that I have a life, that I turned out okay, that I'm not just a fuck-up.

Anthony and I sit quietly for a few moments while he continues to weep. (See Table 8.3.)

Intersubjectivity (see Chapter 7) is a concept that emerges from contemporary relational psychoanalytic approaches to psychotherapy. The contemporary relational emphasis in psychoanalytic theory and practice draws from several theoretical tributaries, including American interpersonal psychoanalysis, British object relations theory, attachment theory, self psychology, and American psychoanalytic feminism (Mitchell & Aron, 2013). Central to this approach to individual psychotherapy is the idea that client and therapist enter into and cocreate a relational, intersubjective process whose healing potentials are realized in sometimes turbulent and often non-linear movement toward relational security, affective honesty, mutual recognition, and

TABLE 8.3. Relational Spirituality Model (RSM) Assessment and Intervention With Intersubjectivity System Focus in Individual Therapy

Assessment	1. Recognize enactments and other collapses in the intersubjective space.
	2. Assess intensity of loneliness and longing for connection.
	3. Assess intensity and meaning of self-hatred.
	4. Track emergence of contradictory self-states.
	5. Assess presence of dissociation vs. connection in SERT experience, practices, and relationships.
Intervention	1. Avoid the temptation to retaliate or withdraw.
	2. Strike a balance between staying connected to client's subjective experience and holding on to one's own subjective experience.
	3. Use reparative strategies and return to the rupture.
	4. Find a "third way" through collapses into complementarity.
	5. Assist with affect regulation through cycles of activation and regulation.
	6. Identify RSM resources that do not collapse into right/wrong, good/bad, saint/sinner dualities.

exploration. Therapy is intersubjective when space exists for the subjective experiences of both the client and the therapist in ways that lead to mutual recognition. Inevitable, transient collapses of the intersubjective space occur regularly in therapy, when client and therapist are confronted with asymmetries of power; differences based in culture, race, ethnicity, socioeconomic status, gender, sexuality, age, and other aspects of personal identity (Maroda, 2018); and, dissociative experiences in either or both parties that are evoked by relational dynamics triggering memories of relational and developmental trauma (Bromberg, 2011).

Another vital aspect of intersubjectivity is what Schore (2017) described as the psychobiology of psychotherapy, wherein limbic, right-brain, nonverbal, somatic, and affective experiences of both client and therapist combine and interact in ways that communicate and demonstrate the complex relational hopes, fears, expectations, conflicts, and pathways to healing that infuse the therapeutic relationship and container. In working with clients who have suffered significant relational trauma, interactions between the subjectivities of client and therapist can often contain high levels of conflict and mistrust, something Bromberg (2011) described as intersubjective collision or enactment.

Enactments

Enactments in psychotherapy are those times when a client and therapist become caught in a conflictual way of relating to one another that involves haunting familiarity and dissociation, frequently for both parties, often leaving each party feeling misunderstood or miscast by the other (Bromberg, 2011; Maroda, 2018). In addition, both client and therapist can experience anxiety, confusion, diminished relational security, difficulty thinking flexibly, and a sense of losing oneself in the context of the enactment. It is within enactments that psychotherapists are called upon to do some of their most important work, as the client's (and perhaps the therapist's) deepest existential anxieties about worst-case relational outcomes become limbically activated through in-therapy experiences of broken trust and misattunement between client and therapist. Within this crucible of relational tension, it is incumbent upon the therapist to accomplish some combination of the following: recognize the signs of an enactment, within herself and her client, affectively and relationally; avoid the temptation to retaliate against or withdraw from the client; strike a balance between staying in relationship with the subjective experience of the client while still holding on to her own subjective experience; use reparative strategies of humility, like "acknowledging fallibility, being accountable for doing harm, apologizing, forgiving, expressing and receiving gratitude" (Shaw, 2010, p. 56), to help the client modulate negative affect and elicit positive affect; and return with the client to the experience of the rupture with the goal of bringing greater perspective to it, as well as acknowledging the shared reparative journey.

Finding a Third Way

When Anthony brought us back to the question of a medical marijuana card, I [GSS] was aware of an initial pull in me toward a power struggle. I was ambivalent about what it would mean to "legitimize" Anthony's use of marijuana as a psychotropic strategy for emotion regulation, and I had not resolved in my own mind the question of providing a letter for him. I was also strongly inclined in this moment to steer away from Anthony's emotions, to ask a more "practical" question about other ways in which he can find relief and regulation, and in so doing to hopefully steer him away from the medical marijuana card without having to refuse his request. I knew endurance physical training had been helpful for him. I hoped that therapy was another source of relief. Fortunately, I had been receiving consultation from my SERT Group on the therapy with Anthony and had been helped by colleagues to be aware of times in our work when our intersubjective space collapsed, often around issues of power and control. In that consultation, I had shared how Anthony's parents had so often, in fear for his life, been swept away into similar power struggles with him and how that rarely ended well.

I had also been hooked by the way that Anthony himself was trying to hold open some space by taking a playful poke at his marijuana use and its demotivating side effects. There was something in his tone of voice and eye contact when he said this that contributed to my backing off from a control orientation and waiting to regain my internal balance. In slowing things down within myself and reorienting to Anthony, I felt his emotion rising and asked a simple question to follow that ("What is it?"), to which Anthony responded powerfully. His description of being infected and possessed by assaultive, self-hating thoughts invited me into a new language for his intense emotional dysregulation, and I am still jarred by its intensity. It is another surprise in our work together, though this time it is not a surprise about his behavior—it is a surprise about his power to symbolize with words, affect, and relational connection the episodic and awful insidiousness of this aspect of his inner experience of relational selfhood, rather than acting it out dissociatively or self-destructively.

Then, unbidden, I had my own intrusive thought and impulse: I wanted to tell Anthony that I found his description to be one of the most moving and poetic things I had ever heard as a therapist, to praise him and validate his unique talent and intelligence. It is hard to say just what happened next. Most simply put, I had another thought. A more nuanced description would be that another thought came to me, or even, was given to me. The thought was, "Don't make him the 3-year old who could order his own meal at the restaurant." So, for the second time, I used right-brain processing to avoid intersubjective collapse and to find another possibility, a Third, that involved recognizing Anthony's grief and love by following the trail of his tears toward his mother.

CONCLUSION

Relational spirituality and individual psychotherapy are guideposts to healing practice that tap into some of our most fundamental human needs about existence and ultimate concerns. Attachment theory highlights how vital attunement, relational security, and secure base and safe haven functions are. Differentiation of self holds up the balancing of intimacy and autonomy, thinking and feeling. Intersubjectivity reminds us of the sheer force of our relational biology and social brain, and the importance of space to accommodate the subjectivity of persons who need both deep connection and self-integrity. And attention to SERT dimensions and traditions connects us to the diverse and ancient ways in which these truths about relational humanity have been held and taught over thousands of years, allows us to work with our clients' ultimate concerns, and helps us negotiate the helpful and destructive experiences that can occur in religious contexts. Practiced with care and skill, individual psychotherapy can be an agent of growth, positive change, and healing in the face of deep suffering and trauma. And in order to live out its most promising potentials, it must be practiced, taught, and studied within the relational ecologies of self-reflective, energized, and vital communities of learning. In Chapter 9, we consider what this RSM process looks like in couple therapy.

Relational Spirituality in Couple Therapy

Who we are and who we become depends, in part, on whom we love.
—T. LEWIS, F. AMINI, AND R. LANNON, *A GENERAL THEORY OF LOVE* (2000, P. 142)

This opening quote by Thomas, Amini, and Lannon in their excellent book on attachment and interpersonal neurobiology speaks to the developmental and existential significance of our relationships with those we love. Many things influence "who we become," including social and cultural dynamics along with a multitude of other factors. But as we summarized in Chapter 5, a huge body of empirical research shows our closest relational bonds are tremendously formative contributors to who we become (Mikulincer & Shaver, 2016). This means our early life attachment with parents, family, and other caregivers influences our selections of romantic partners and friendships because of internal working models of relationship in the limbic brain. In some cases this is concerning, because insecure attachments put in place rather unhealthy templates about "love" which continue to disappoint. Yet relational models of therapeutic change, such as that advocated by Lewis et al., hold out hope for possibilities of "limbic revision" (p. 142) as individuals with insecure working models form meaningful relationships with those who have more secure attachment capacities (including therapists). This is also the hope offered by many spiritual and religious traditions that call people to grow in love and that also promote sacred love as a key source of spiritual transformation.

http://dx.doi.org/10.1037/0000174-010
Relational Spirituality in Psychotherapy: Healing Suffering and Promoting Growth,
by S. J. Sandage, D. Rupert, G. S. Stavros, and N. G. Devor

We share these assumptions about relational development, love, and transformation in our relational spirituality model (RSM). Chapter 8 applied the RSM to a case of individual therapy that also included family therapy work. In this chapter, we apply the RSM to a case of couple therapy. Prior publications have applied conceptual and practical aspects of our relational spirituality approach to couple therapy cases focused on challenges of forgiveness (Shults & Sandage, 2006; Worthington & Sandage, 2016), spiritual and religious problems in couples (Sandage, Bell, Moon, & Ruffing, 2019), and the possibilities of theological integration within couple therapy (Sandage & Brown, 2018). Since we have laid out the theoretical contours of our RSM in Chapters 1 through 7 of this book, we focus here on case description and dialogue, along with key assessment and intervention strategies drawing on the three relational development systems of focus in the RSM—attachment, differentiation, and intersubjectivity.

COUPLE THERAPY CASE STUDY

This case study will be used to illustrate ways of applying the RSM in couple therapy. We will lay out some initial information and then a series of vignettes over the course of therapy with some considerations at each phase of the process, which parallels the work of therapy with clinical impressions always based on partial information and dynamics that are unfolding. Alexis (age 34; African American; heterosexual cisgender woman) and Nick (age 36; Dutch and Anglo-American; heterosexual cisgender man) had been married for 10 years and had a 4-year-old daughter (Amelia). They pursued therapy with Michelle (age 48; Irish American; lesbian cisgender woman) during a period of transition after Alexis accepted a significant promotion into a leadership position in a large nonprofit social service organization. Conflicts had emerged for them about whether to try to have more children and differences on work–family balance as Alexis's obligations at work had expanded. But beneath these situational conflicts, both Nick and Alexis realized neither had felt really connected or intimate with each other for several years. Nick explained, "It's like she's always on the move, and I can't get access to her anymore. But if she does slow down, she's disappointed in me, or about to be disappointed, so why even try to relate to her?" Alexis responded, "He says he wants me to pursue my goals, but then he pouts and withdraws when I do. It feels like he's trying to suck my dreams out of me. He used to be supportive and fun to be around. I don't understand what happened to *that* guy."

Many important dynamics are already emerging in this brief description, and we will summarize some key dynamics that would be areas of focus in our RSM-based approach.

Transition and Existential Concerns

Like many couples seeking therapy, Alexis and Nick sought help during a major transition in their couple and family life as their relational system was changing and they were having difficulties collaborating amid those changes. They were both intelligent and had solid communication skills (when not dysregulated), in addition to other strengths we note below. In couple therapy based on the RSM, we focus particular attention to the interlocking conflicts that typically emerge as a couple system starts to change. It is dangerous to form strong interpretations from limited data, but some clinical hypotheses can be generated from their differing struggles voiced in relation to this transition. Nick seems to feel left behind, or that he has lost access to Alexis (possible abandonment anxiety), and Alexis seems to feel she is in a double bind of being encouraged to seek after her goals but then punished with Nick's pouting, which registers with her as trying to "suck her dreams out of her" (possible engulfment anxiety). These are powerful existential themes for each of them, and from an RSM perspective we would note that both seem to feel that Alexis's movement toward seeking new opportunities has somehow resulted in difficulties connecting or dwelling together.

Therapist Countertransference

We consider it crucial that we remain attuned to our personal affective and embodied responses to cases and value contemporary perspectives on countertransference that call for self-awareness of ways our responses can provide both helpful information or potential distortion (based on projection) in understanding clients. Michelle, a highly experienced couple therapist, was struck by an unusual feeling of intimidation during the intake session, which had her doing some emotional backpedaling. In debriefing later with her consultation group, she realized she observed a high level of resentment between Nick and Alexis, but she also got in touch with her own sense of a much more profound feeling of sadness in both. This is another impression that needs to be held loosely until more information is available, although this depth of profound sadness was later confirmed.

Interracial and Intercultural Dynamics

Alexis and Nick obviously differed in race and ethnicity. These are issues we would want to further explore in terms of what those differences might mean to each of them, how they have experienced and navigated those differences, and any ways they have tried to support and learn from one another (Waldman & Rubalcava, 2005). Couples can also differ tremendously in their interest in and openness to these kinds of questions, and neither Alexis nor Nick offered much when asked about this in the intake. This was less about the two of them having nothing to say and more about their shared reticence to venture into those vulnerable areas until they knew Michelle better. Boyd-Franklin (2010) noted that African Americans can have a "healthy cultural suspicion" about therapy in general, but this particularly makes sense in working with a White therapist (p. 986). White males like Nick have often learned to minimize their race and ethnicity, which limits their self-awareness about how those factors may influence their approach to relationships. Michelle needed to be patient in assessing this area and came back to it several times in their work together.

For her part, Michelle also needed to factor her own intersectional dynamics (e.g., gender orientation, race, ethnicity, sexual orientation, religiosity) into her awareness as she entered into dialogue with this couple on diversity issues. She was triangulated in opposing directions on gender and race, which added to some of the undercurrents of anxiety she felt at the outset. In her consultation group, Michelle processed ways her painful background growing up in an evangelical Christian church as a lesbian caused her to have reactions of sympathy for Alexis and frustration that Nick did not respond to her social justice concerns sooner (described below). But as a Unitarian Universalist, she was also aware of some anxiety that her religious affiliation, if "outed," may be problematic for both (i.e., too liberal for Nick and too White for Alexis). This processing helped Michelle get regrounded in a differentiated stance of relational spirituality.

Disappointment Dynamics

Disappointment is another key theme we seek to assess in the RSM and a particularly powerful dynamic in couple and family relationships (Sandage, Bell, Moon, & Ruffing, 2019; Schnarch, 1997; Worthington & Sandage, 2016). It can feel difficult to disappoint someone we are close to, but feeling one is a disappointment to a spouse or family member is often highly shaming. This can represent an example of what Bromberg (2011) described as the disconfirmation of one's existence in developmental and relational trauma (see Chapter 4, this volume). It can also be challenging to manage and regulate feelings of disappointment toward a spouse without conveying shame and unforgiveness, and over time this can turn into the contempt that is particularly toxic in relationships (Gottman, 2011).

Nick and Alexis were in an interlocking disappointment dynamic that is part of their disconnection, and our RSM approach would lead us to further assess ways in which these disappointment dynamics might parallel and unconsciously reactivate: (a) earlier family of origin disappointment dynamics, and (b) relational spirituality disappointment dynamics (i.e., disappointment with the sacred, or feeling spiritually or existentially like a disappointment in the core of selfhood). Disappointment dynamics involving interlocking shame and unforgiveness in couples like this often represent grief that is being avoided or defended against in some way. In fact, chronic disappointment in a partner can provide a powerful displacement that distracts from the pain and anxiety of deeper spiritual and existential grief. And for this couple the relationship is not sufficiently safe and differentiated to allow for them to connect in grief at the outset of therapy (Worthington & Sandage, 2016).

Relational Dynamics of Wanting

Our RSM also places great emphasis on the relational dynamics of *wanting*, or how each partner's dreams, desires, and goals play out in the balance of conflict and collaboration in the couple relationship. Schnarch (1991, 1997, 2009) has provided innovative and clinically useful insights about the role of wanting and desire in couples, as expressing one's wants can be quite vulnerable and revealing of subjective aspects of selfhood that could be shamed and rejected. Yet not revealing one's authentic desires will shut down intimacy and growth. Personal dreams, fantasies, desires, and goals all tap into vital existential parts of the self and the seeking system. Potential movement toward growth can involve actualizing one's potential and deeply personal meanings about living a generative life, and this can be challenging to coordinate with the wants, desires, and goals of an adult partner.

But wanting can be incredibly anxiety-provoking for some persons, particularly in the context of relationships, like that of Nick and Alexis, that are fraught with power and control struggles and anxieties about the potential consequences if one or both persons seek after their goals. This can lead one or both partners to focus on communicating what they do not want rather than what they do want in their relationship as a control strategy that limits vulnerability and the existential or spiritual pain of deeper disappointment. In couple therapy, it is important to try to assess what each partner actually wants in and for their relationship, and in the case of Nick and Alexis this was ambiguous at the outset. It did become clear both were committed to working on their marriage, which was a necessity if couple therapy was to eventually prove effective.

CLINICAL VIGNETTE 1: RELATIONAL SPIRITUALITY DYNAMICS

Relational spirituality differences had also developed between Nick and Alexis in ways that were alienating in their marriage. In an early session, they started to unpack some key episodes in their relational spirituality estrangement. They had both belonged to a large, predominantly White Evangelical Christian nondenominational church when they met and remained active there for several years. However, about five years ago Alexis became disenchanted with the church's seemingly passive or "conservative" stand on several social issues, particularly racism and environmental concerns. She initially voiced those concerns to her church leaders (all White men), whom she experienced as dismissive and even condescending in some cases. Nick did not disagree with her views, but he did not actively join her in that advocacy and argued they needed to be patient with the church and the leaders. He had been attending that church for over half his life and drew a lot of support from long-time relationships, which started when he joined the high school youth group during an emotionally turbulent adolescence.

Alexis explained to Michelle that she and Nick had "gone in different directions with our spirituality." When asked to explain, she recounted a particularly painful episode of years earlier during a large strategic planning meeting at the church where she asked pointed questions of the leaders about whether they intended to try to become more diverse as a church to better reflect their surrounding community. After the meeting, James (an associate pastor and Nick's former youth ministry leader) walked past the two of them and said to Nick, "You better rein her in before she spews more of that venom here," and then walked off.

ALEXIS: (shaking her head and raising her voice in anger) Nick said nothing. That was the moment I knew that church was full of shit and I was done with it. It also confirmed once and for all that Nick would not have my back. He just let it go. (long pause)

NICK: (looking away from Alexis and out the office window) At the time, I didn't really get it . . . and I thought she was pushing the leaders too hard. Like she often pushed me too hard. But over the years, I have come to see they were wrong on these issues and she was right. I'm sure their response to her was racist and I basically stopped going to church there a couple years ago. She dropped her faith but I can't really do that.

ALEXIS: (forcefully and looking at Michelle) I didn't drop all faith. I pursued Afrocentric spirituality once I realized White religions would always be disempowering and oppressive.

NICK: Okay, I meant that you dropped Christianity . . . and that is no longer something we share. Though actually I'm not really sure where I am at spiritually at this point. I tried going to another church for a while, but I didn't know anyone there and it felt empty. (starting to sound agitated) And this is all stuff we can't even talk about. I worry about what this means for Amelia and how we will raise her. It feels like you are just doing your own thing spiritually and won't communicate about these issues.

ALEXIS: (turning to look at Nick) There you go, trying to guilt me about taking care of myself and doing what I find meaningful. That guilt and control is stuff you learned at that church and it doesn't work on me anymore. That's why I don't like talking about this with you!

This interaction starts to reveal some of the dynamics in their relational spiritualities as individuals and as a couple. This painful and possibly traumatic experience narrated by Alexis leads to information about Nick's own spiritual and family history. From an RSM perspective, we would pay attention to the ways this episode may have represented a developmental collision of their relational spiritualities at a level that should be further assessed for relational trauma. At the culmination of this conflict, Alexis appears to have been individuating as an African American female in a pre-dominantly White church led by men who enacted racism and sexism (the latter in telling Nick to "rein her in," using an emotionally abusive and dehumanizing analogy expressing hostility toward her social justice advocacy). This unfolded in a relational spirituality context of the church "home" (i.e., place of dwelling) that Nick had turned to and depended upon for stability during a multifaceted family crisis. Nick's relational spirituality had seemed to remain tilted more toward dwelling than seeking until the time of that conflict with Alexis, although we could wonder if his initial move toward developing an interracial relationship with Alexis, a woman who would eventually differ from his church home, was an unconscious move toward seeking. It is unfortunate that his own racial identity and social justice awareness at that time did not help him negotiate his racial and gender privilege to be more supportive of Alexis and attached to her in her relational trauma and suffering (see Liu, 2017). Eventually, this conflict contributed to his deidealization of the church and some growth in awareness of racism, but he had not found a way to repair this rupture and attachment injury with Alexis or deal with his own spiritual struggles that ensued.

After hearing their respective narratives and further assessing the impact of this chapter in their relationship over several sessions, Michelle was able to offer this framing to Alexis and Nick:

> Clearly, this was a very painful chapter in your relationship for each of you, and you each lost something very important, and I sense you have not healed from it. Alexis, you took significant risks in speaking out for your spiritual beliefs and values in the hope your church leaders would take steps with you toward justice, but instead you met with the racism, sexism, and exclusion in the church that you had already experienced in our society. It sounds like you had longed for Nick to be with you in this suffering and to show he was willing to be excluded with you even if it meant losing his spiritual home. But that is not how he responded at that time, so you found a way to move on spiritually without him and develop new sources of strength. And although you've stayed married, you lost trust Nick would be with you in the most important times . . . which is a huge thing to lose. Am I understanding this right?" (Alexis, tearing up and looking down, nods affirmatively.)

Michelle continues,

> And Nick, it sounds like this period was complicated for you given your long history at that church and the important role that community had played for you at the beginning of your spiritual journey. It sounds like you have tried to confront yourself about some of the realities of racism and the unfairness of how Alexis was treated there. And I have to believe that, in addition to losing her trust, you also lost your own spiritual grounding, is that right? (He nods.) And I'm not clear about what all you have tried to communicate about all this to Alexis, but I get the sense it has been hard for you to find a way to try to repair this with her and show her you are committed to fighting injustice with her."

This intervention by Michelle carries risks of one or both clients feeling misunderstood and disconfirming her conceptualization, but that scenario would likely offer assessment information. Michelle has offered a plausible empathic and systemic framing that (a) unpacks their respective injuries with attunement to the developmental significance, (b) connects relational and spiritual themes for each, and (c) evokes the idea they have both suffered losses without flattening the difference in racial and gender privilege. In this case, Alexis and Nick each felt understood and this served to strengthen their working alliance with Michelle, although they each had enough insecurity in their working models of attachment to be anxious and guarded about feeling hopeful about someone who was supposed to be helpful.

CLINICAL VIGNETTE 2: ATTACHMENT SYSTEM FOCUS

The attachment system is one of three primary developmental systems we seek to assess and engage in the RSM (see Chapter 5) and was prioritized in the treatment planning in this case. Further assessment of Nick's and Alexis's relational development histories identified several important dynamics. Nick grew up the youngest of three children in a rather emotionally disengaged upper-middle-class family that was rocked by his parents' divorce when he was 15. His mom had discovered his father having a second affair, and "all hell broke loose for about six months with tons of yelling and crying and finally he moved out." Nick had never been very close with his father, who seemed to Nick to prefer his more athletic older brother and sister. Nick's mom started drinking at that time, and with both siblings in college the burden fell on Nick to try to manage her depression and drinking. That was the year he started attending the youth group at that church with a friend, and he had a conversion experience on a retreat which he described by saying, "God became my rock. I knew I would be okay whatever happened to my family." Nick's mom eventually went to counseling and got sober, although she continued to try to rely on him for support. Nick and his dad (now remarried) had developed a more friendly, though superficial, relationship in recent years since the birth of Amelia. Nick had been in individual therapy for the past 2 years, which had helped relieve some significant symptoms of depression and activated him to be more assertive at work. But he continued to feel a nagging sense of guilt interspersed with anxiety about where his life was going.

Alexis was the oldest of five children. Her father died in a car accident when she was 14, which required her mom to drop out of a graduate program in education and take on two jobs to provide for the family—as a teacher at a state prison and a counselor at a group home. Alexis admired her mother's resilience, her work ethic, and her commitment to social change and empowering others. But after becoming a mother herself, she started to reflect on what she had lost in drawing a parentified role in her family, giving so much of her adolescence and early adulthood to caring for her siblings and their complicated struggles while missing out on parental guidance during such formative years in her own development. While she loved and respected her mother, she had also started to realize she did not really know her at a deep level. Her mom was now dealing with some serious health problems, perhaps from years of chronic stress and overwork in tough settings. Whenever Alexis would slow down long enough to really feel deeper than the surface anxieties and frustrations, she experienced a painful dread of impending losses. Some of her only solace and hopefulness had come in exploring her racial and cultural heritage through personal reading, a discussion group with other African American women from her social justice involvements, and the use of ritual practices and prayers to ancestral spirits.

Assessment of Attachment Systems

Nick and Alexis showed contrasting attachment styles, which is common among couples in therapy. Nick showed signs of a preoccupied attachment style with a tendency under stress to doubt his own internal resources and to solicit lots of help from others, whom he would tend to idealize as stronger and wiser than himself. But this idealization of others could quickly turn to anxious frustration and desperation if they were not responsive to his solicitations. This internal working model of relationships was shaped by enmeshment with his mom, who had intense problems he could never completely resolve (resulting in guilt), and a father whom he experienced as mostly disapproving or rejecting. Nick's emotional turbulence and lack of cohesive selfhood made it hard for him to consistently pursue goals or even clarify his own beliefs and values. He believed in a personal God, but struggled with inconsistency in spiritual practice and often felt like a disappointment to God (note the parallel to projections about Alexis). (See Table 9.1.)

Alexis showed a mixed attachment picture of some dismissive attachment behaviors combined with some capacities for secure attachment developed through healthy relational experiences. Consistent with dismissive attachment, she tended to cope with stress through tenacious self-sufficiency and repressing emotional vulnerability. She mostly preferred to think of herself as independent and strong, and felt shame about seeking help from others. Like many with a dismissive attachment style, she could be courageous and exhibit a high pain tolerance but struggled with empathy, forgiveness, and admitting wrong. Alexis showed some positive signs of attachment security in her spirituality practices and in building community with other African American women. But she preferred to stay focused on relational spirituality dynamics that were positive, intellectual, or activist in emotional tone and tended to avoid situations that involved relying on others (human, divine, or ancestral) for help. This pattern had been shaped by the ways her family of origin avoided processing the grief of her father's tragic death, as well as the demands this placed on her mother as a single parent who had limited emotional availability for Alexis in the context of holding multiple stressful jobs and having younger children with more obvious struggles.

TABLE 9.1. Relational Spirituality Model (RSM) Assessment and Intervention With Attachment System Focus in Couple Therapy

Assessment	1. Note specific treatment goals of each member of couple system and how they may reflect attachment and relational spirituality dynamics (e.g., dwelling, seeking, struggles).
	2. Assess attachment styles and track their impact on relational patterns.
	3. Assess family-of-origin dynamics related to attachment with attention to key losses, disruptions, and transitions.
	4. Assess relational spirituality dynamics, strengths, and resources reflective of the attachment system (safe haven, secure base).
	5. Note ways individual clients and the couple system attach with therapist, and how therapist's attachment style interacts with this process.
Intervention	1. Cultivate securely attached working alliance in light of attachment styles within the couple system.
	2. Therapist metabolizes countertransference about mistrust and attachment insecurity and idealization within the working relationships with clients, drawing on consultation and other relational resources.
	3. Coconstruct a developmental crucible framing of treatment while conveying a stance of complex hope.
	4. Normalize anxiety and invite reflection on its role in relational, existential, and spiritual dynamics (the relational spirituality triangle).
	5. Foster corrective attachment experiences.

These attachment system differences between Nick and Alexis had led to a common distance–pursuer cycle in their marriage (S. M. Johnson, 2019), with Alexis often emotionally distancing and Nick pursuing during stressful or conflictual times. Alexis had been socialized to seek distance during stress and to try to self-regulate, and this style felt abandoning to Nick and confusing for his internal working model of pursuing relational support when anxious. In contrast, Nick's anxious pursuit and need to "talk things out" following a conflict felt engulfing to Alexis. He did not seem physically dangerous to her, but his desire for relational regulation distracted her from her learned methods of coping. When this pattern was in play, they would both end up frustrated, overwhelmed, and then worn out. Nick would go away feeling lonely and Alexis would be angry.

Attachment-Based Intervention Strategies

There is not space to consider all the attachment-based intervention strategies Michelle might have used, but we will highlight some key ones. First, our RSM focuses on seeking to establish a relationally secure attachment and working alliance with the couple, since we consider relational sources of gain to provide key mechanisms of change. This can be complicated since Alexis and Nick have different attachment styles, so Michelle needed to pace them somewhat differently (e.g., giving Alexis some emotional space and being consistently responsive to Nick's concerns in nonanxious ways without reinforcing his sense of neediness or inadequacy). Cultivating a good alliance with a couple is tricky because the therapist is in a triangulated position, and it requires flexibility in positioning to not convey a stance of being aligned with one partner over the other.

In the early going, Nick sometimes seemed to probe for more disclosure from Michelle or lingered at the office door before leaving a session. Alexis conveyed suspicion about the need for some of Michelle's questions related to her internal process and started one session with a series of questions of her own about Michelle's credentials and training. For both Nick and Alexis, this represented their attachment systems seeking to adapt to the therapy relationship. Michelle drew upon her consultation group to metabolize her own affective responses to these moves and to reflect on her positioning and the ways her countertransference sometimes had her leaning toward one partner. In this way, Michelle used her own professional attachment relationships to keep herself in a position to cultivate healthier attachment dynamics in this couple system (a key RSM strategy).

By session eight, this couple was experiencing what systems theorists describe as first-order change or some initial behavioral improvements resulting from reduced anxiety levels in their relationship, and they were each developing a positive transference with Michelle. She had conveyed a "hopeful but no quick fix" therapeutic frame and cultivated the understanding that they needed to work together to reflect on the patterns in their relationship and explore the different feelings and meanings for each of them (thus normalizing difference). Michelle probed for their respective anxieties and offered some brief psychoeducation on the role of anxiety based on the RSM framework of normalizing realities of anxiety without minimizing the distress involved (see Chapter 4). She was able to start to help both Nick and Alexis become aware that their immediate or surface anxieties were connected to deeper existential and spiritual concerns that became activated in their marital conflicts. Initially, they were both unconvinced there was this much "meaning" to their conflicts and they simply wanted to feel better about things. But Michelle's relational capacities to stay emotionally present and nonreactive (mindful dwelling), combined with her confidence about the value of exploring both underlying meanings and practical strategies for better collaboration (mentalized seeking), eventually began to facilitate their own curiosity and reflective capacities. It started to feel empowering for them to consider connections within the relational spirituality triangle (i.e., their relational dynamics, their family of origin relationships, and their relational spiritualities).

Over the next several months, Michelle was also able to pace in some corrective relational lead moves to begin to shift the attachment templates of both Alexis and Nick. This involved small doses of Michelle kind of "moving toward" Alexis during sessions in ways that challenged her dismissive style to invite more relational warmth, proximity, and vulnerability while respecting her need for boundaries of autonomy (or softening; see S. M. Johnson, 2019). For example, Michelle started one session saying, "Thanks for the call about running late tonight. I was thinking how, Nick, you are the one who calls about rescheduling and these kinds of things, which is fine. I was just trying to remember, Alexis, if I had given you both one of my cards with my number to get in touch with me if you need to." This type of move can actually feel quite confrontive to a client with a dismissive attachment style, but when offered with warmth it can communicate an availability and concern that counters their internal narrative.

With Nick, Michelle's corrective lead moves were less about moving toward him and more about not getting "boxed in" or reactive to his pursuer moves with her while scaffolding his efforts at self-regulation (Holmes, 2001). One enactment during a heated regressive moment went like this:

NICK: (to Michelle and with anxious intensity and frustration) You say I am supposed to manage my own anxiety, but I still don't understand how I am supposed to do that.

MICHELLE: (noticing the "supposed to" language was a different relational message than what she intended to communicate but choosing to stick with the present moment) I'm not sure either . . . (pause) . . . but I am willing to explore options with you to see what will work for you . . . (pause). What have you tried . . . ?

NICK: (still looking frustrated and "pouty" in the way Alexis complained about) I don't know. . . . I thought you could tell me what will work (with a slight smile and now sounding more anxious than angry).

MICHELLE: (softening her tone a bit but still speaking to the adult part of Nick) Well, let's think together about it for minute. I want to be helpful to you, but since we are all different, I can't presume to know exactly what will necessarily help you with your anxiety at these kinds of moments in your marriage. . . . I think it may help you if we consider some options and then you kind of experiment with some ways to try to calm yourself between sessions and then report back so we can see if we can develop some options.

NICK: (sounding a bit more regulated but still tentative and somewhat sad) Well . . . a couple weeks ago I was feeling alone one night, and Alexis was wiped out from work and didn't seem interested in connecting, which was frustrating. So I went out for a walk and tried to pray about our marriage, but couldn't get into it. . . . And I just started looking at the stars, and it felt good to be outside. Nothing felt better in our marriage, but I guess I kind of settled down.

MICHELLE: That's an interesting example. What happened for you after your walk?

NICK: Alexis and Amelia were both already asleep. So I read a little bit from this book of prayers I like and turned in, myself.

MICHELLE: (careful to not overstate the positive effects) So, yeah, that is the kind of option or experiment I was wondering about. I sense that it didn't have some magical effect on your feelings about your marriage at that moment, but you did find a way to soothe some of the painful feelings you were having, a little bit. And, in the midst of feeling anxious and alone, you found a way to be with yourself, and with nature, and eventually even with your spirituality—I would be interested to understand that part better—in a way that brought some grounding. Am I right?

This intervention strategy offered Nick enough relational connection to scaffold his own reflection and exploration of possible self-regulation strategies. In attachment terms, Michelle was attaching to provide a secure base experience, which fits with our RSM integration of dwelling and seeking. Clients with a preoccupied style, and particularly those with relational trauma around abandonment themes, may become more anxious if their efforts at self-regulation are framed too optimistically, as they may fear the therapist will start to pull back too much. Michelle allowed Nick to struggle a bit with himself and his anxiety, but he eventually generated some ideas. This was a form of self-regulation in session even as they considered self-regulation strategies outside of sessions. If Nick had become more dysregulated and unable to generate any ideas, Michelle may have needed to provide more structure and scaffolding. But it was helpful that Michelle stayed grounded herself and did not become anxious to please or satisfy Nick when he pressured, nor judgmental about his struggles.

Alexis also benefited from being out of the "hot seat" of Nick's anxious demand for help and able to watch how Michelle responded to him, which is an advantage of a relational treatment modality such as couple therapy. In some cases, a spouse in Alexis's position might feel jealous or defensive that the therapist can seem more effective with their partner than they are. Of course, the attachment dynamics and emotional history are so much less intense between a therapist and client than within a couple relationship, which is a useful point of discussion in therapy if those kinds of jealous feelings surface.

We have also drawn on theorists like Kohut (1977) and Jones (2002) to suggest idealization is a normal dynamic within both psychological and spiritual development, and it is common for a certain idealization of the therapist to develop in the limbic transference when therapy is starting to feel helpful. This can represent a kind of hopefulness about the attachment and the therapy experience. In this case, neither Nick nor Alexis felt deep jealousy about Michelle's relationship with their spouse, but rather they each began to playfully invoke her in their minds; for example, self-mentalizing the question "I wonder how Michelle would respond to this?" This indicated Michelle was becoming a useful attachment figure for each of them outside of sessions.

We are struck by parallels to relational spirituality dynamics of healing in so many traditions, where spiritual growth is mediated through a relationship (or "working alliance") with a guide, teacher, priest, rabbi, imam, spiritual director, shaman, saint, ancestor, or other sacred figure who leads the person toward healing and growth. This parallel is a major point in Jerome Frank's classic work *Persuasion and Healing: A Comparative Study of Psychotherapy* (Frank & Frank, 1993), and this comparison also factors into Wampold and Imel's (2015) contextual model of psychotherapy and their emphasis on relational sources of change.

CLINICAL VIGNETTE 3: DIFFERENTIATION SYSTEM FOCUS

The differentiation system is the second of the three primary developmental systems we seek to assess and engage in the RSM and focuses on self-identity development, self-regulation capacities, interpersonal flexibility, and diversity competence, or the ability to relate across differences (see Chapter 6). The differentiation system functions to negotiate tensions between preserving the integrity of self-identity and core values, on the one hand, while also responding to social and relational pulls for the flexibility to cooperate and collaborate amidst differences. This is obviously a crucial developmental system for couples, particularly in diverse and egalitarian social contexts that provide increasingly high levels of both freedom and ambiguity about differing ways of structuring intimate relationships. In the RSM, we assume couples need robust capacities for differentiation to collaborate over time across these numerous and complex areas of relational functioning. Yet growth in differentiation is often existentially difficult and necessitates the development of values, meaning systems, and forms of relational spirituality that can motivate and sustain the quest to integrate dwelling and seeking. In this case, the differentiation system came into treatment planning focus in the second phase of therapy.

Assessment of Differentiation Systems

There are numerous areas of potential interdependence that can be assessed in couple relationships to get a sense of dynamics of differentiation and capacities for collaboration. Some key areas (if relevant to a given case) include parenting, sexuality, finances, in-laws, and sociocultural or relational spirituality differences, since these are areas where dilemmas about collaboration frequently emerge over time (Schnarch, 1997; Worthington & Sandage, 2016).

Alexis and Nick tended to agree on parenting practices and shared an intense love for Amelia, which was a strength and one of their few unifying dynamics. It is important to notice the patterns in areas where collaboration is working. Michelle helped them realize they both had abilities in caring for others as an area of common ground. Up to this point, Amelia (at this age) had not presented significant reasons for Alexis and Nick to experience power struggles as parents (although parenting Amelia around spirituality and religion was brewing as a potential conflict). However, caring for one another as a couple amidst their differences was more challenging.

When they started couple therapy, they found themselves at a point in their marital journey where they were struggling with many of their differences, and the breaches seemed to be widening while the connections were fading. Now, about six months into therapy, Alexis and Nick had each made some progress on self-awareness and skills for managing their own anxieties, which are two important dimensions of differentiation of self. They felt kinder and more comfortable with one another, but rather than resolving all tension, this created the safety to open the door to deeper differences between them. This fit the existential dynamic where relaxing of surface level anxieties can allow for facing depth dimensions of ultimate anxieties and concerns in the suffering–trauma matrix (described in Chapter 4). (See Table 9.2.)

Differentiation-Based Intervention Strategies

A key to growth in differentiation is helping a couple learn to manage the anxiety of exploring areas of difference, so Michelle began to help them press into differences. Nick and Alexis each wanted a better sexual relationship and

TABLE 9.2. Relational Spirituality Model (RSM) Assessment and Intervention With Differentiation System Focus in Couple Therapy

Assessment	1. Assess dynamics of differentiation (fusion, cutoff, reactivity) and capacities for collaboration in the couple system (including areas collaboration works and breaks down).
	2. Track specific patterns in breakdowns in collaboration.
	3. Assess family-of-origin and sociocultural dynamics related to differentiation and the diversity competence of the couple system.
	4. Note ways the differentiation system interacts with relational spirituality dynamics (including existential) and ways the couple system may be struggling to balance pulls toward dwelling and seeking.
	5. Watch for pulls toward homeostasis and/or change in the couple system as they make initial progress in treatment.
Intervention	1. Normalize differences and intentionally explore differences in the couple system.
	2. Cultivate capacities for self-regulation of anxiety, disappointment, and other difficult emotions related to the relationship.
	3. Help clients in their self-identity work and relational spirituality development and to consider ways to bring those parts of self into the couple relationship.
	4. Normalize intimacy anxiety while also helping clients consider ways they can self-regulate and respond compassionately and nonreactively to one another to explore greater intimacy.
	5. Promote well-planned experiments or risks in collaboration for learning and self-awareness rather than immediate "success."

were confused about why they were struggling in that area. They had found it difficult to talk about sex with each other, but were now better able to tolerate exploring these issues. Both also knew they had trouble connecting and collaborating around certain episodes of suffering, like the conflict with the church and Alexis's concerns about her mother's health. It had seemed to Nick like he had tried to connect with Alexis around his own emotional struggles, but now with greater self-awareness he could see that he really didn't trust Alexis, or anyone for that matter, to care for him at those times. Previously, Michelle had worked on self-regulation with Nick so she decided to further probe the connection side of differentiation:

MICHELLE: (to Nick) What makes it difficult to trust that Alexis will care for you at those times?

NICK: I don't know . . . (starting to sound like he was passively withdrawing into the shame vortex of dissociation; Bromberg, 2011).

MICHELLE: (feeling both anxious and frustrated but taking a deep breath to stay grounded and leaning forward slightly) Take a minute to think about it. . . . This can be hard to access, but, regardless of what you are showing on the outside in these situations, something keeps you from really trusting she cares for you.

NICK: (after a couple moments) I can't stand the risk of losing it . . .

Nick was surprised by his own insight, which rose to his conscious mind from a deeper place. Michelle could have drawn out this existentially provocative insight with Nick, and she did make a quick note on the pad by her chair ("risk of loss") to track the theme. But she wanted to wrap the themes of trust and risk back toward Alexis to further assess the relational dynamics and see how this landed with her.

MICHELLE: Nick, that sounds like an important insight . . . that a part of you wants to be cared for while another part may calculate that the risk of losing love and care is too great. I can imagine ways that makes sense from what you've described in your experience with your parents, and I'd like to understand that better. . . . But, Alexis, I am also wondering what is happening in you when Nick is in that place of wanting support from you but, at the same time, being afraid of losing you?

ALEXIS: (sounding confused and somewhat defensive) Ah . . . I'm not sure. I mean, at those times I see him asking for help but I think I have known there is some other message beneath that that leads me to feel I can't win. . . . But I don't get the part about losing me.

MICHELLE: (deciding the issues are important enough to press a lead move) His fear of losing you is confusing?

ALEXIS: Yeah . . . well, no . . . I guess we could lose people at any time.

MICHELLE: (allowing a pause as Alexis looks away) What are you thinking about?

ALEXIS: (starting to cry) My dad.

Nick reached over at this point to take her hand, and this offered a valuable experience of softening (Johnson, 2019) and connection around insight about existential vulnerabilities. The interaction revealed the relational impact of anxiety and traumatic loss. Alexis and Nick both knew the pain of unexpected loss in their families of origin. The losses were different, but each had been shocked and injured during a formative time of adolescent development. In the present, Nick would seem to demand support from Alexis, but internally he was "playing not to lose again," as he had in his family of origin. Alexis knew how to give tangible support based on her parentified youth, but now she came to realize Nick's fear of loss triggered her own unprocessed feelings about losing her dad. Initially, she resented Nick for this, but with Michelle's help she started to move into her own grief process. Loss is a powerful psychological, existential, and spiritual theme that can activate each of the relational development systems in differing ways (Paine et al., 2017) and include themes of relational intimacy (Cernero, Strawn, & Abernethy, 2017).

After laying further groundwork of connecting with them around their respective loss dynamics, Michelle made the paradoxical move of trying to help them find some grounding for differentiation by "putting them in the same boat": "It seems to me you both lost your fathers way too soon, at a time when you should have been moving out into the world and forming your identity. But instead, you were each left to care for others."

As they finished what had been an emotionally intense but relationally balanced session, Nick and Alexis both looked tired but more open and present to each other. Alexis laughed and commented,

> I just thought of how, after my dad died, my uncle Rodney [his brother] would sometimes come around to play cards with all of us kids, which was so fun. And he would always tease us and say he was giving us 'life lessons on how to lose.' I guess that is kind of what therapy is about, learning how to deal with loss, huh?

The expression of humor and allusion to an important relational figure in her life (Uncle Rodney) were positive signs. But this was also an example of how clients can sometimes give the best articulation of the specific developmental crucible, which makes sense in the light of the meaning they help coconstruct (Worthington & Sandage, 2016; see also Chapter 3, this volume). Michelle reflected later that she would have framed their developmental crucible as a couple around the theme of learning how to process loss together, but Alexis was the first one to express this crucible theme.

Consistent with many depth-oriented and systemic theories, we believe couples are often attracted to one another and pair up due to some unconscious developmental processes that beckon each of them toward growth.

This RSM way of thinking is consistent with many spiritual and religious traditions that suggest, in a myriad of different ways, that the process of spiritual transformation starts with an invitation to a quest or a journey that is a liminal passageway into a forest, a wilderness, a desert, an ordeal, a belly of a whale, or some other archetypal dark space (Shults & Sandage, 2006; see also Chapter 3, this volume). We must be careful not to idealize or minimize the suffering (sometimes traumatic) that follows, and obviously many relationships end with far more tragedy than transformation. Yet what is striking in many couple therapy cases, such as Alexis and Nick, is a plausible narrative hypothesis that the neurobiology of their limbic attractors (Lewis, Amini, & Lannon, 2000) may have caused them to implicitly recognize some common relational and existential wounds and familiarity. Unfortunately, they subsequently found themselves in a spiritual holding environment that was not sufficiently differentiated to help support them with the specific healing and growth they needed, and the pain of this rupture had pulled them in opposing and estranging directions as a couple.

Whatever happened to draw them together, they did some constructive work of attachment and differentiation together over the next few months around processing their earlier losses and other family of origin dynamics. They still had disappointments in each other, but it helped to better understand and gain some mutual empathy for the relational lessons each had learned about emotions, conflicts, differences, and other issues. As is often the case, the work on loss raised existential and spiritual dynamics for each of them related to their views of suffering (Chapter 4). Michelle invited each of them to reflect on what they had come to believe about suffering: Why we suffer? What it means to suffer? How one should try to cope with suffering? This could seem like a risky move because it opened up another area of significant difference in this couple, that of relational spirituality. But growing the differentiation system in a couple requires working on differences, and they had already showed some movement toward greater openness and acceptance of differences.

Alexis was actually eager to share more about her spiritual beliefs and practices in the space of therapy, where it was feeling safer to express differences. She described some of her Afrocentric and Yoruban understanding of suffering as a "normal part of human existence where there is both good and evil." This dialectical perspective was combined with the belief that malevolent spirits can cause various kinds of suffering, destructiveness, and misfortune; and she had learned prayers and other ritual practices to call on her ancestral spirits and *orishas* (lower messenger deities or personified natural forces) for spiritual empowerment. She was particularly drawn to orisha spirits that dwell in water. Her views included elements of animistic causation and a kind of soul-building orientation with her belief that one needed to relate to the good spirits to grow in the ability to contend with the evil spirits. Michelle noted her countertransference pulled her toward interest in Alexis's spirituality and even some idealization, since it was so new to her. She tried to remain curious but systemically balanced in her stance toward the couple and their contrasting spiritual orientations and struggles.

Elaborating these particular elements of Alexis's relational spirituality helped thicken the therapy dialogue beyond the typical clinical emphases that can reduce the process down to biopsychosocial realms of experience (Dueck & Reimer, 2009). Michelle eventually asked a key RSM question: "Are there ways we can integrate your spiritual practices and help from the ancestral spirits and orishas into our work here in therapy, to help you with your healing both individually and as a couple?" Alexis's Afrocentric spirituality had served her individuation, and she had not previously found it safe, or even plausible, to integrate it into her marriage. As a minority spiritual orientation in the United States, this also presented certain challenges in spiritual practice for Alexis and experiences of negation and exclusion (Sandage, Bell, et al., 2019; Tummala-Narra, 2016). Nick claimed he had asked about her beliefs and practices out of genuine openness in recent years, but it had felt loaded to Alexis. Even now, part of her was afraid to bring her relational spirituality into her marriage, not so much because of fear of judgement, but out of fear of losing something sacred that was hers. Yet she also knew that she could not be herself in her marriage without doing so, and this integrity dilemma (Chapter 6) moved her toward the path of differentiation and willingness to share more of her spirituality with Nick.

Nick was less clear about his current beliefs related to suffering. Previously, he had adopted a common "Providence-oriented" theological view from his church that God was in control of everything that happened. He explained, "I think that my family was in so much chaos in those early years that it felt good to believe that someone was in control, and that someone was God. He was my rock." This god image seemed to offer Nick stability and grounding for spiritual dwelling that insulated him, to some extent, from the turbulence in this family. But his marital conflicts with Alexis started to crack "the rock" of stabilization, which was tied up with his church family and the leaders. We could say his relational spirituality became destabilized over this marital–church conflict and the loss of existential control over his life, and he had not really been able to reconstruct a new form of relational spirituality in its place.

He still considered himself a Christian, and he had attended a new church a few times that seemed to emphasize an image of God as more compassionate than controlling of all things. Michelle tuned into some countertransference on this matter; as both a therapist and a Unitarian she valued this more relationally warm and "process-oriented" view of spirituality and thought it would serve Nick better in his healing and development than the prior control-oriented spirituality. But she also knew he was moving toward differentiation and did not need another figure in his life trying to direct him toward what he should believe. She tried to stay focused on remaining curious and mentalizing with him on these matters and asking similar seeking questions about whether there were ways they could integrate his spirituality into their couple therapy work. And she put an internal check on her own desire to validate some of the relational content in his emerging beliefs.

CLINICAL VIGNETTE 4: INTERSUBJECTIVITY SYSTEM FOCUS

The intersubjectivity system is the third of the primary developmental systems we seek to assess and engage in the RSM and focuses on patterns of relational interactions, developmental capacities for intimacy and mutual recognition, and processes of seeking to repair inevitable ruptures that can hinder relationships (see Chapter 7). The intersubjectivity system came into treatment focus during the third and final phase of therapy.

Assessment of Intersubjectivity

Just over a year into couple therapy, Nick and Alexis had made progress in changing relational patterns of disconnection, accepting some of their differences, and collaborating on work–family coordination. Additionally, processing some of their grief about family-of-origin dynamics had set the stage for them to seek greater intimacy with each other, and this is actually a very vulnerable phase of the couple change process. Although the attachment, differentiation, and intersubjectivity systems are somewhat overlapping in their functions, the quest for greater emotional, sexual, and spiritual intimacy is a unique developmental challenge of intersubjectivity for couples and is not synonymous with reducing conflict, gaining greater emotional trust and safety, or being more open to differences. Each of those relational achievements can help pave the way to desiring more authentic intimacy, but existential anxiety can often run underneath powerful experiences of intimacy particularly among couples who have drifted away from that level of knowing and being known. (See Table 9.3.)

Alexis and Nick had gone away for a weekend, with Amelia staying with Nick's sister. They had not had a full weekend as just a couple since before Amelia was born. The first night they had intense sex, which they both greatly enjoyed. Alexis had opened up in therapy about her desire for Nick to be more sexually confident and assertive, and she explained that in recent years it sometimes felt like she needed to shore up his self-esteem while trying to enjoy the encounter. She was usually so tired from work and parenting that it was challenging enough to tune in to her own body, much less try to take care of his insecurity. On this first night, Nick had brought himself forward with a mix of passion and tenderness she found to be wonderful. Afterward, they held each other as they fell asleep.

The next morning at breakfast Alexis was more withdrawn, and after some probing by Nick she said there had been a story about a racial hate crime in the news, and she found herself thinking about the harassment by Pastor James back at the church years before. She was angry and said, "You just left me alone in that! I still can't believe you wouldn't take my side."

TABLE 9.3. Relational Spirituality Model (RSM) Assessment and Intervention With Intersubjectivity System Focus in Couple Therapy

Assessment	1. Assess strengths and barriers related to different forms of intimacy in the couple system (emotional, sexual, spiritual, recreational).
	2. Explore clients' understandings of their suffering and ways those may express important worldview and diversity dynamics (suffering–trauma matrix).
	3. Assess couple's capacity for intersubjective solidarity in suffering and growth.
	4. Assess capacities for rupture, repair, and forgiveness.
	5. Note spiritual and existential strengths in couple system that might be engaged for growth in intersubjectivity.
Intervention	1. Explore risks in greater intimacy in various domains.
	2. Foster corrective experiences in intersubjectivity building on growth in attachment security and differentiation.
	3. Scaffold possibilities for relational repair and forgiveness in couple system.
	4. Therapist models relational repair of ruptures and seeks to understand the meaning of enactments.
	5. Therapist stewards relational spirituality process in therapy with humility and openness to allow third space for creative growth.

Nick was thrown by what felt like emotional whiplash going from the connection the night before to this conflict. He defended back, "I thought we talked about that in therapy. Where is this coming from?"

Alexis replied, "We did talk about it, but that doesn't mean it's not triggering when I remember how you just stood there and let me get treated that way. How am I supposed to trust you?"

They were alienated and emotionally cut off the rest of the weekend and called that Monday to move up their next session with Michelle (a sign of attachment). Several areas of their relationship were converging—sexuality and the desire for intimacy, attachment templates that were changing but still fragile, anxiety about trust and lingering unforgiveness, and diversity and justice differences between them that needed more work. It seemed noteworthy that Nick had made a positive intimacy move that Alexis had requested, followed by her struggle with awareness of deeper injuries and trust dilemmas in their relationship about solidarity in suffering. The old Nick would have been devastated by this response from Alexis, but he now had more tools for differentiation. And he also sensed that although Alexis was hurt and upset, she was being fair about the reality that they had not really dealt with this past rupture. In our experience, this kind of nonlinear pattern and iterative process of change is relatively common in therapy with certain kinds of progress being followed by (a) certain "after tremors" of destabilization as the overall relational system reorganizes (Gelo & Salvatore, 2016) and (b) possibilities of working on other developmental challenges given the prior gains (Worthington & Sandage, 2016).

Intersubjectivity-Based Intervention Strategies

Michelle helped them settle into about six months of work, not exclusively on this rupture event, but largely focused on the wider suffering–trauma matrix involving intersectional dynamics of racism, sexism, religious communities, social justice, and authentic forgiveness and repair (as opposed to denial). The episode at the church was an experience of relational trauma for Alexis; that is, a violation or betrayal of connection (Herman, 2015). As an African American woman she had suffered chronic exposure to racialized and gendered trauma with numerous incidents in her history (Helms, Nicolas, & Green, 2012), and she benefited from some culturally sensitive individual trauma therapy with one of Michelle's close colleagues to keep the treatments well-integrated. Alexis was able to state that her desire was not to punish Nick out of bitterness for the episode with James, but she wanted to see him work harder at his awareness of diversity and privilege and to take a more active, self-directed stance on social justice issues so they "could be on the same page" (a kind of well-differentiated intersubjectivity). Nick felt a growing desire to do this work, and he was able to gain awareness that he was being invited to similar kinds of growth in both sexuality and social activism—showing courage and commitment to authentically connect in spite of the existential risks. Michelle was able to help Nick check in with his own integrity to make sure he was not just trying to please Alexis out of anxiety about losing her, but seeking to develop himself out of his own core values. Nick was also able to voice his own desire for Alexis to pull back from some of her work preoccupation for the sake of their couple and family connection, while being clear he was not asking her to forfeit her career goals. This was a significant challenge for Alexis, not so much because she wanted to be so focused on work but because she had spent so much of her life working and seeking after new goals that more mindfully dwelling in close attachments took a different kind of internal work of affect regulation. Michelle worked to help them each keep their communication in session in relational postures that were more mindful and intersubjective and to recover from lapses into complementary one-up/one-down stances of power and control (Benjamin, 2018; Maddock & Larson, 2004).

Like many relational theories of change in therapy, our RSM places a strong emphasis on corrective relational experiences that shift a recurring and problematic pattern in new directions of growth. Nick came to the clearer awareness that he had not learned to stand up to people, particularly men, because he would rather lose himself than their support and approval. This was true of Pastor James, but also of his father. He had never communicated how his father's distance and affairs had impacted him or what he had missed in their lack of relationship until recent years. This became a kind of growth crucible for Nick that was spiritual, psychological, and existential, and Alexis joined him in this growth crucible as she realized she needed to try to trust his commitment to growth without seeking to manage it for him. This represented a kind of well-differentiated collaboration between the two of them in working toward growth in relational spirituality, which is a key part of positive change in couple therapy (Sandage, Bell, et al., 2019; Worthington & Sandage, 2016).

Nick decided he would start with James and made an appointment with him to communicate that his actions toward Alexis years earlier were wrong. He was well prepared to offer a clear and simple message of how James's actions were problematic and that he hoped he would reflect on that reality. Not surprisingly, James became defensive and tried to argue; however, Nick refused to debate, reiterated his point, and said good-bye as he left. There was nothing clearly transformative about this single confrontation. But Nick had found the courage and differentiation to go back to a place that was once sacred for him before it became a desecrated scene of rupture and relational trauma in his marriage and his relational spirituality. And he put his own integrity and his marriage over old loyalties. Nick and Alexis went on to get involved in a social activism organization together, their first collaboration in that kind of effort to work against systemic suffering and to promote social well-being and justice. They had more work to do in couple therapy over the next year or so, but the remaining growth was much easier as they constructed a new way of being in life together.

CONCLUSION

This chapter opened with a reflection on the role of relational love in forming who we are, and this couple case study depicted the ways Alexis and Nick needed transformed templates about taking the risks involved in love. A long-term couple therapy case like this one (48 sessions over about two and a half years) involves more complex dynamics and interventions than can be described in a single chapter, but we have tried to highlight key therapeutic moves and developments based on our RSM emphases on attachment, differentiation, and intersubjectivity. In Chapter 10, we turn our attention to applying the RSM to another relational modality of treatment—group therapy.

10

Relational Spirituality in Group Therapy

It is the affective sharing of one's inner world and then the acceptance by others that seem of paramount importance. To be accepted by others challenges the client's belief that he or she [sic] is basically repugnant, unacceptable, or unlovable.

—I. YALOM AND M. LESZCZ, *THE THEORY AND PRACTICE OF GROUP THERAPY* (2005, P. 56)

The previous two chapters considered clinical applications of the relational spirituality model (RSM) to cases of individual therapy (which included family therapy) and couple therapy. In this chapter, we apply the RSM to group therapy and consider the three relational development systems that provide areas of clinical focus in the RSM—attachment, differentiation, and intersubjectivity—and how those systems operate in relation to spiritual–existential–religious–theological (SERT) dynamics in group therapy. Through our use of literature, research, and group therapy vignettes, it should become clear over the course of the chapter that RSM is a model grounded in clinical theory while simultaneously being responsive to the particular personhood and journey of each client. This opening quote by Yalom and Leszcz speaks to the power of relational dynamics in group therapy to heal core parts of the person that can easily be considered existential and even spiritual within many traditions.

Group psychotherapy is an efficient, well-established, evidence-based mental health treatment modality (Burlingame et al., 2013). At the same time, it tends

http://dx.doi.org/10.1037/0000174-011
Relational Spirituality in Psychotherapy: Healing Suffering and Promoting Growth,
by S. J. Sandage, D. Rupert, G. S. Stavros, and N. G. Devor

to be underappreciated and underused by many mental health practitioners and institutions (Marmarosh, Markin, & Spiegel, 2013). This may have to do with a number of factors, including a bias toward individual therapy among behavioral health clinicians, a paucity of training in group psychotherapy, and a preference for individual therapy among patients seeking psychotherapy (Shechtman & Kiezel, 2016). Despite these factors, there is continuing interest in the effectiveness and efficacy of group psychotherapy as a vehicle for addressing and healing the psychopathology, loneliness, and suffering that emanate from relational trauma, loss, neglect, and abuse. In addition, there is a body of literature and research related to SERT themes and approaches in group psychotherapy. Cornish and Wade (2010) provided a literature review, as well as practice guidelines for addressing SERT issues within different group structures, including homogenous groups (specific populations, diagnoses, demographics), heterogeneous groups, and structured and unstructured groups.

There are many possible configurations, structures, and approaches to group psychotherapy. This chapter focuses on theory, practice, and research associated with interpersonal process group therapy, whose relational emphasis makes it particularly resonant with RSM as a healing vehicle that invites relational experiences of both dwelling and seeking. The poignant elegance of interpersonal group psychotherapy is that it gathers together a group of previously unrelated people, typically between eight and 10 participants, including group leaders. Together the group members take on the task of relating to one another while also creating space, a developmental crucible, within which each group member can reflect on the experience of being in relationship with others. Inevitably, both the relationships themselves and the reflections on those relationships are windows into the complex relational expectations and histories of each person in the group. Group members, through their own courageous efforts and the facilitation of group leaders, have opportunities to challenge and expand upon the often distorted and limiting relational expectations they hold for themselves and others, toward more life-giving, life-affirming experiences of security, interdependence, exploration, spontaneity, aliveness, and meaning-making. This continuous and often tumultuous process of relating and reflecting lies at the heart of the healing power of group therapy.

CLINICAL VIGNETTE 1: ATTACHMENT SYSTEM FOCUS

A long-term interpersonal psychotherapy group meets weekly at a local community mental health clinic. The group has been active for 3 years, and its membership is made up of both longer term members and more recent additions, four women and three men (Note: client demographics will be progressively revealed throughout the chapter as the group process unfolds). The group is currently being co-led by two postdoctoral psychology trainees: Rebecca, a female clinician trained in a clinical psychology program, and John, a male clinician trained in a counseling psychology program. Rebecca was raised in a practicing, conservative Jewish home and is not currently practicing or directly connected to her faith tradition. She attends yoga classes regularly, in addition to participating in yoga retreats several times each year. John, in addition to his doctoral degree in psychology, has a master's degree from a Protestant Christian seminary and is active in his local United Methodist church community.

Rebecca has been leading the group by herself for the past year, and John joined the group as coleader 2 weeks ago. In his introduction to the group, John provided some of his training background, including the school from which he had earned his PhD and some of his previous training experiences. He did not, however, disclose his seminary background in either of his first two sessions with the group, and in general did not share this information when he introduced himself in professional settings. The first vignette takes place in John's third week as coleader of the group.

Leo, a 27-year-old man who has been in the group for just over a year, begins the session by saying there is something he needs to tell the group. He proceeds to disclose that he Googled the new coleader John and discovered that John attended a Christian seminary prior to getting his degree in psychology. Leo continues by stating that, while he does not necessarily have a problem with this, he wonders whether it means that John will be practicing some kind of "Christian counseling" in the group, stating, "I'm not sure I would be up for that." John's multiple forms of social privilege as a White, Christian, cisgender man seem to contribute to questions about how he will handle power dynamics.

Vanessa, who has also been in the group for over a year and is sitting next to Leo, reacts strongly to Leo's news, stating, "Are you kidding me? We should have been told that ahead of time." Vanessa is a 24-year-old woman who was adopted at 2 years of age from a household in which she experienced notable neglect and physical abuse. Her adoptive parents, who provided a stable and secure home for her, were and are practicing members of the United Methodist Church, and Vanessa has not yet told them that she is gay and currently in a relationship with a woman. The group has been the one place where Vanessa has begun to open up about her sexuality and the fear, hurt, and loneliness she feels about keeping it hidden from her adoptive parents.

All group members sit in tense silence for a moment, while coleaders John and Rebecca look at each other across the circle, each of them feeling temporarily stuck and unable to think clearly about how to respond to Leo and Vanessa. (See Table 10.1.)

Taking an Attachment-Informed Approach to Group Therapy

Attachment theory offers an invaluable lens with which to observe, understand, stabilize, and heal the relational expectations, experiences, and capacities of group therapy clients beset by emotional suffering and trauma. *Attachment* is the biological, evolution-based imperative for humans to manage distress and threats to survival through maintaining relational proximity to and security with other humans, with relational experiences during infancy and early

TABLE 10.1. Relational Spirituality Model (RSM) Assessment and Intervention With Attachment System Focus in Group Therapy

Assessment	1. Identify group members' early relational traumas, losses, neglect, and abuse.
	2. Stay alert to the array of attachment styles, needs, and behaviors that emerge within the group members and group process.
	3. Assess group members' capacities for emotion regulation, mentalization, mutual perspective-taking, and empathy.
	4. Identify threats posed by SERT differences in the group and how they intersect with group members' struggles outside of therapy.
	5. Assess attachment style connected with SERT experience and behavior.
Intervention	1. Recognize enactments of family attachment dynamics and seek nondestructive, corrective relational experiences.
	2. Appreciate the confusing, contradictory, and paradoxical content, behavior, and group process that accompany anxiety in group members.
	3. Maintain a group climate and culture that invites, contains, and creates space for each group member's perspective and subjective experience.
	4. Name and normalize potential sources of anxiety and threat for group members.
	5. Identify RSM and group resources that provide experiences of dwelling and seeking, support and challenge in group process.

Note. SERT = spiritual–existential–religious–theological.

childhood being particularly influential in establishing patterned expectations for relational security and insecurity. Attachment theorists and researchers (Ainsworth & Eichberg, 1991; Bowlby, 1988b; Main, 1995) have used the term *internal working models* for these patterned expectations and have developed a taxonomy of attachment styles to describe them. Applying these attachment styles to group psychotherapy, Marmarosh et al. (2013) offered guidance in relation to clinical presentations and treatment goals for group psychotherapy clients.

Secure Attachment

Secure attachment is characterized by a combination of relational security and a capacity for exploration through the accessing of both *secure base* and *safe haven* relational functions within the group. Securely attached persons in a group psychotherapy context are typically more able to balance needs for connection and autonomy, security and exploration, and dwelling and seeking within the group, and typically have reliable and resilient capacities for emotion regulation and anxiety tolerance (Marmarosh et al., 2013).

Dismissive Attachment

Clients with a dismissive attachment style are more likely to deemphasize the value of being part of the group, minimize the importance or impact other group members have on them personally, and put a greater emphasis on their own personal strengths and goals. Not surprisingly, these clients are often seen as aloof, unaffected by feedback and attempts at connection by other group members. They can have a difficult time weathering the inevitable ruptures and conflicts of the group process, putting them at risk for leaving the group prematurely. Group therapy goals for clients with a dismissive attachment style include eliciting core affect through empathy, developing insight into underlying feelings and defenses, increasing mentalization, verbalizing and tolerating feelings, and encouraging personal feedback (Marmarosh et al., 2013).

Preoccupied Attachment

Clients with preoccupied attachment often present in group psychotherapy as being initially adept at winning acceptance by and protection from the group, by skillfully reading and responding to the needs and preferences of other group members and by displaying a kind of fragile vulnerability that inhibits challenges and confrontation by others. Eventually, however, the group process results in relational injuries, perceived slights, and increasing anxiety around belonging for the preoccupied client, setting the stage for the hard work of relational growth and change. Group therapy goals for clients with a preoccupied attachment style include increasing mentalization, facilitating insight into underlying feelings, encouraging interpersonal feedback, and regulating affect (Marmarosh et al., 2013).

Fearful-Avoidant Attachment

Group therapy clients with a fearful-avoidant attachment style often present themselves and interact with other group members in ways that are self-protective but can be off-putting, hard to understand, paradoxical, and evocative. Because these group members can act out their relational struggles in such inconsistent and extreme ways, it can often be difficult for other group members to empathize, stay connected, and demonstrate vulnerability with them in group, making the role of group leaders that much more important in working with them. Group therapy goals for fearful-avoidant members include facilitating emotion regulation through empathy, increasing mentalization, putting emotions into words, identifying relational templates, expectations, and distortions, encouraging interpersonal feedback, and developing insight into the impact of trauma on the client (Marmarosh et al., 2013).

Empirical Evidence for Attachment in Group Therapy

Empirical evidence supports the importance of attachment, both theoretically and as an outcome variable, in group psychotherapy research (Marmarosh et al., 2013). Maxwell, Tasca, Ritchie, Balfour, and Bissada (2014) utilized group psychodynamic interpersonal psychotherapy (GPIP) to treat patients with binge-eating disorder and found that attachment anxiety and attachment avoidance decreased at 12 months posttreatment, with decreases in attachment anxiety and avoidance being significantly related to decreases in interpersonal problems, and reduced attachment anxiety being significantly related to decreases in depressive symptoms. Keating and colleagues (2014) found that group attachment insecurity and overall attachment insecurity decreased in GPIP participants one-year post treatment. Lawson, Barnes, Madkins, and Francois-Lamonte (2006) reported that 13 of 33 men being treated for partner violence with integrated cognitive behavior therapy/ psychodynamic group psychotherapy changed from insecure to secure attachment style, experienced less depression and anxiety than men with unchanged attachment style, and reported increased comfort in closeness and depending on others. So there is some evidence group therapy can improve attachment system functioning. Yet Wade et al. (2018) noted that clients high in attachment avoidance (or dismissive attachment) may tend to do better in structured psychoeducational groups than process-oriented group therapy, at least in the short term. This raises important treatment planning considerations about the type of groups that might fit best for particular clients at certain phase of treatment.

Cognitive Neuroscience and Attachment

The biological and neurological foundations for the human capacity and need for attachment security and emotional attunement are becoming more frequently considered and discussed in relation to psychotherapy (Cozolino & Santos, 2014; Flores, 2010; Lewis et al., 2000; Schore, 2001; van der Kolk, 2014). Psychotherapists and cognitive neuroscientists have now begun to consider, more specifically, group psychotherapy's potential as vehicle for this kind of healing process. Flores and Porges (2017) noted this clinical potential:

> Because the relational models of group therapy inherently provide a social environment that requires its members to emotionally engage each other interpersonally in recurring face-to-face social interactions, it naturally promotes many of the most crucial elements necessary for the promotion of the neural substrates required for attachment and affect regulation. (p. 206)

They continued:

> The active engagement of one person's social engagement system with another person's social engagement system lies at the heart of all psychotherapy, interpersonal learning, exploration, discovery, change, emotional regulation, and the maintenance of mutually gratifying relationships. (p. 213)

Given the conceptual resonance and empirical support that connect attachment theory with group psychotherapy, attending to attachment style and dynamics in groups whose focus is on interpersonal learning, growth, and change is vital. Each communication made by a group member, either explicit or implicit, has potential significance for every other group member and for the group as a whole. Group leaders have the considerable task of trying to maintain a group climate and culture that invites, contains, and creates space for each group member's perspective and subjective experience, while staying awake to and aware of the array of attachment styles, needs, and behaviors that emerge within the group therapy context.

Trust and Existential Concerns in Group Therapy

In the vignette, Leo's disclosure that he Googled the new coleader raises important questions regarding his own clinical status, progress, and healing, as well as for what his behavior represents for other group members, group leaders, and the group as a whole. A closer look at Leo reveals a 27-year-old, single, white, Irish American, heterosexual man with a history of early physical and emotional abuse, often sadistically carried out, by his stepfather. The entry into the group of a new male coleader proves to be an emotionally evocative and dysregulating event for Leo, engaging his attachment behavioral system to deal with the anxiety and threat associated with the new coleader. His seeking to establish some existential control over an unknown male authority figure can be understood as a means of self-protection, a kind of aggressive expression of insecure attachment intended to restore a sense of relational control and safety within the group. Leo's behavior also suggests that he is playing a protective role for other group members who are less likely to openly articulate or demonstrate their fear and suspiciousness. The entry into the group of any new member, let alone a new leader, is often fraught with the expectations, hopes, and especially the attachment-related anxieties of each group member, strongly informed by their individual developmental relational histories and attachment styles. Both consciously and unconsciously, profoundly influenced by internal working models, each group member prepares for the new leader's arrival. And Leo rolls out the group's welcome mat in a very distinctive and understandable way, characterized by caution and suspicion.

The news of John's religious background and training also comes as an unwanted surprise to Vanessa, a surprise that she experiences more like a threatening and intrusive shock, activating Vanessa's attachment behavioral system and fight–flight response. Bromberg (2011) described relationally oriented approaches to psychotherapy as being full of surprises, with an important therapeutic goal being an increased capacity to distinguish between what is relationally novel and what is dangerous. Vanessa's early developmental experiences of abuse and neglect, as well as the relative security provided by her adoptive parents, contribute to her finding herself in a confusing and frightening existential moment. The real but fragile trust she has built within the group is now threatened by the arrival of a stranger, someone whom Vanessa's internal working model suggests has the power to reject or displace her and her budding courage to explore more intimate ways of relating.

It is also important to note that for both Leo and Vanessa, John's religious training seems to activate anxiety about the threat of sacred power and control that surpasses the normal anxiety that comes with the addition of a new group coleader. This is an example of relational spirituality dynamics that are complicated by deep existential anxieties and, potentially, mutual projection processes. At least in Vanessa's case, this vignette also suggests powerful ways SERT dynamics in the clinical setting may intersect with clients' SERT struggles outside of therapy. Wade and colleagues (2014) provided a helpful clinical case application addressing issues in working with SERT themes in a process-oriented psychotherapy group. Among the questions they addressed is when group leaders might move toward or away from explicitly spiritual and religious content in the group. Given the intensity and powerful convergence of SERT issues with the overall group process at this point in time, we would support the group leaders' efforts to hold open as much space as is possible and tolerable for the group to continue this discussion.

CLINICAL VIGNETTE 2: DIFFERENTIATION SYSTEM FOCUS

MARYBETH: I don't see what the big deal is. So he went to seminary.

ERICA: C'mon Marybeth, you know why it's a big deal to Vanessa.

MARYBETH: (looking slightly irritated at Erica) Do I?

(Erica rolls her eyes and breathes hard through her nose.)

REBECCA: (gently, stretching her hands toward Erica and Marybeth) Hold on for just one second. Marybeth, is it possible for you to give a thought as to why Vanessa might be upset to hear about John's religious background?

MARYBETH: (takes a breath and pauses) Well, maybe she's afraid that she'll be rejected or that John will be judging her, because of her relationship with Megan, you know. Her parents don't even know about that.

REBECCA: Vanessa, does that sound at all accurate.

VANESSA: (in tears with her head down) Yes.

REBECCA: (pausing a moment) Is there more that you want to say?

VANESSA: (tearful but breathing more easily) Not right now.

REBECCA: It can be so hard to trust someone you don't know, especially when the stakes feel so high. It probably doesn't make sense to let your guard down too quickly. My guess is that Vanessa isn't the only one feeling anxious about having a new coleader.

(John nods his head and meets the eyes of the group members who are looking at him.)

REBECCA: Would others be willing to share what it is like to have John joining the group?

(John breathes a quiet sigh as he and Rebecca exchange a brief look of mutual reassurance.)

(See Table 10.2.)

TABLE 10.2. Relational Spirituality Model (RSM) Assessment and Intervention With Differentiation System Focus in Group Therapy

Assessment	1. Assess group members' capacity for intrapersonal and interpersonal differentiation.
	2. Assess group members' capacity for navigating difference and tolerating closeness and solitude.
	3. Identify subgroups within the overall group.
	4. Identify intrinsic versus extrinsic SERT beliefs, practices, and relationships.
Intervention	1. Use therapeutic crucible to move between empathic support and tolerable challenge.
	2. Help group members to balance belonging and intimacy with agency and autonomy.
	3. Group leaders avoid identifying completely with any one subgroup.
	4. Welcome and negotiate differences between group members.
	5. Invite SERT experience of group members without idealizing or devaluing any one system of belief, practice, or experience.

Note. SERT = spiritual–existential–religious–theological.

The Therapist's Differentiation of Self

Differentiation of self is a term first developed by family therapist Murray Bowen (1978) to describe the therapeutic process that family members undergo in becoming "unstuck" from one another, when their "stuckness" contributes to poor communication, rigid family roles, reactive anxiety to both intimacy and separateness, and poor emotional regulation capacities. Bowen advocated for family members to develop "person to person" relationships with one another, allowing each member to both experience interpersonal intimacy and maintain autonomy within the family system. Skowron, Kozlowski, and Pincus (2010) further developed the concept of differentiation of self beyond the family context:

> Differentiation of self is defined as the capacity of a system and its members to manage emotional reactivity, allow for both intimacy and autonomy in relationships, and engage in adaptive problem solving. It involves the capacity to think clearly in the midst of strong emotions and to modulate one's emotional reactions and self-soothe emotions such as anxiety, anger, or fear. (p. 305)

While there is little available research on the relationship between differentiation of self and group psychotherapy process or outcomes, the conceptual implications seem clear. Differentiation is a particularly important relational dynamic for making space for diversity in a group process, including SERT diversity (see Chapter 6). Differentiation of self is a concept that is strongly resonant with attachment theory. Both theories attend to a person's need for closeness and autonomy in relationships, the capacity for emotion regulation as a developmental achievement, and a harmonious balance of emotional and cognitive functioning (Worthington & Sandage, 2016), all of which are valuable considerations in group psychotherapy.

Establishing Relational Security and Safety to Explore

Returning to the clinical vignette, a good example of differentiation of self is when the coleader, Rebecca, opens the group discussion to the possibility that having a new coleader join the group may be understandably anxiety-provoking for group members. Rebecca is in the unique position of being part of two subgroups within the larger psychotherapy group. She is an "old" member of the group, someone who was part of the group prior to John's arrival as coleader. She is also part of the "new" coleadership subgroup with John. A less differentiated intervention option at this tender and anxious moment would be for Rebecca to deflect her own discomfort and anxiety onto her new coleader by closing the circle around the subgroup of "old" members, including herself, keeping John on the outside as an unwelcomed "other." She could do this by remaining silent in the face of group members' comments or by validating and intensifying group members' suspicion of John. For example, Rebecca might say, "I think the group feels justifiably shaken by John not sharing this part of his background sooner. Perhaps John could explain his reasons for not disclosing this to the group when he first entered." In technical terms, this "throwing John under the bus" could be seen as a retreat by Rebecca into the temporary and tenuous comfort and emotional safety of belonging (to the old group) and away from a more differentiated intervention that balances both belonging and autonomy, as well as cognitive and emotional functioning, amid this relational transition in the group.

Another less than ideal option would be to close the circle around a different subgroup, the new coleadership subgroup, by explicitly allying with John and using the power and authority of leadership to "other" the patient subgroup. For example, Rebecca might say, "I wonder if focusing on John is a way of avoiding how much mistrust already exists among the other members of this group." In similar fashion, this intervention would draw sharp distinctions between subgroups and attribute unwanted, uncomfortable affect and motivations to the "othered" group, in this case, the patient subgroup. By attributing mistrust exclusively to group members, Rebecca may be able to temporarily preserve a sense of relational security and reduced anxiety for herself and perhaps for her coleader, John. However, this would be at the expense of the group members observing a more differentiated response by the group therapist(s), and it would invite the rigidity, fear, and conflict that inevitably infect a system when relational stuckness overrides differentiated, person-to-person relating. Additionally, this would run the risk of the group therapist re-producing negative relational spirituality dynamics in the group in a manner that is isomorphic (or consistent with) Leo's and Vanessa's relational spirituality concerns that seem to transcend the group.

With 1 year of experience and relationship-building with the group, however, Rebecca senses that she might be in a better position than John to initially open up more space for the group's anxiety about a new coleader, without identifying herself exclusively with either subgroup. In doing so, she demonstrates and embodies the important work of differentiation by balancing belonging and autonomy, thinking and feeling, and maintaining her ability to make clinical decisions in the midst of the escalating emotional climate in the group and among the group members. Instead of locating the source of tension solely in a person (John), a subgroup (the group members), or a single issue (John's religious background), Rebecca creates more emotional and relational space for each group member to consider their own experience of the transition of having a new co-leader join the group. "It can be so hard to trust someone you don't know. My guess is that Vanessa isn't the only one feeling anxious about having a new coleader." She helps to create the conditions for each group member to respond to the anxiety in the group in a more differentiated way, closer to the particularities of their own personal developmental histories, values, affective states, religious and spiritual lives, and cultural backgrounds. Thus, she also helps to reestablish some much-needed relational security and affect regulation for her coleader and moves the group toward less reactive forms of seeking meaning as they shift the dwelling dynamics of the group.

CLINICAL VIGNETTE 3: INTERSUBJECTIVITY SYSTEM FOCUS

LEO: Why don't we ask him? Dude, do you, like, have something against same-sex relationships because of your religion?

(All eyes turn to John.)

JOHN: I'm actually relieved that you asked, Leo. None of you really know me yet, and I'm only beginning to get to know each of you. But, as I understand it, my role here is, together with Rebecca, to help create a space within this group for each of you to learn about yourselves and one another, and what it's like to be in relationship with each other. (This is language from the group contract, which was reviewed when John entered the group 2 weeks earlier.)

ERICA: (with an edge to her voice) I appreciate you saying that, but that wasn't really the question. What about Vanessa's relationship with Megan?

JOHN: If you're asking whether my religious beliefs or values keep me from affirming a same-sex relationship, they certainly do not. At the same time, I don't think I know enough about their relationship to say a lot more about it. But my hope would be that our work in the group can help you, Vanessa, to have a better relationship with Megan, and with your parents, if that's what you want.

(See Table 10.3.)

TABLE 10.3. Relational Spirituality Model (RSM) Assessment and Intervention With Intersubjectivity System Focus in Group Therapy

Assessment	1. Recognize enactments, complementarity, and collapses in the group's intersubjective space.
	2. Assess flexibility versus rigidity of group roles enacted by group members.
	3. Assess group members' capacities for recognizing and naming complementarity and enactments.
	4. Track emergence of contradictory self-states in group members, triggered by anxiety and shame.
	5. Assess presence of dissociation/avoidance/conflict versus connection/acceptance/exploration in group members' SERT experiences, practices, and relationships.
Intervention	1. Avoid the temptation to retaliate against or withdraw from group members and their subjective experience.
	2. Model and facilitate a balance between staying connected to group members' subjective experiences and holding onto one's own subjective experience.
	3. Use and facilitate reparative strategies to restore relational security and group cohesion—apologizing, forgiving, appropriate self-disclosure.
	4. Return to interpersonal ruptures through contained exploration and sharing of group members' subjective experiences.
	5. Identify RSM resources that do not collapse into right/wrong, good/bad, saint/sinner dualities.

Note. SERT = spiritual–existential–religious–theological.

Promoting Hospitality Amid Conflict

Contemporary relational psychoanalytic theory is a third relational-development system of focus within the RSM, and the intersubjectivity system is also very important for group psychotherapy. With attachment theory providing the RSM with a developmental and diagnostic lens, and differentiation of self providing a systemic lens, relational psychoanalytic theory contributes a depth psychology lens for understanding the processes and outcomes of group psychotherapy. Within contemporary psychoanalytic literature, the concept of intersubjectivity provides a particularly useful and poignant way of appreciating how group members' histories of loss, neglect, abuse, coercion, seduction, exploitation, or abandonment continue to play out in their lives and relationships, including within the group psychotherapy environment itself (Aviv, 2010; A. Berman, 2014; B. D. Cohen, 2000; Paine et al., 2017). From an intersubjective point of view, group members and coleaders become partners in a complex and tenuous project. Members of the group attempt to bring themselves into the developmental crucible of relationship with one another, risking the rejection, abandonment, and mistreatment that many group members are anticipating based upon their troubled relational histories. At the same time, members of the group commit themselves to cocreating intersubjective space, through acceptance and understanding, for one another's subjective reality and experience while trying not to diminish, shame, retaliate against, masochistically surrender to, or idealize one another.

Two key concepts related to intersubjectivity that have particular relevance for group psychotherapy are *complementarity* and *intersubjective space*. Complementarity is the tendency for relational interactions to be reduced to a confrontation of polar opposites, whether that be in the form of ideas (right vs. wrong), loyalty (with vs. against), power (strong vs. weak), morality (good vs. evil), trauma (perpetrator vs. victim), and many others (Benjamin, 2004, 2018). Complementarity in group psychotherapy is often the product of anxiety within the group that group members attempt to manage by reducing ambiguity, avoiding complexity, and calling for clear lines that demarcate emotional safety from emotional danger. Such episodes of complementarity, or complementary relating, can put intense pressure on group members and group leaders to declare themselves on one side of an issue about which their feelings may be more complicated and unclear, even to themselves.

In a sense, complementarity is the opposite of intersubjectivity, to the extent that intersubjectivity is characterized by a hospitable invitation to the more unpredictable, spontaneous, paradoxical, conflicted, and dissociated parts of the self. In order to provide and maintain this hospitable stance, the members and coleaders of the group must strive toward the creation of intersubjective space. The intersubjective space in group psychotherapy can be thought of as the psychological field formed by the different subjective realities of each of the group members and group leaders (Stolorow & Atwood, 1992). To the extent that the group process leaves adequate room for the holding and validation of each person's complex subjectivity, the conditions for growth and healing remain in place. Conversely, when the group process is driven more by fear, mistrust, and a sense of relational danger, the intersubjective space is at risk of collapsing, and there is less room for creativity, intimacy, problem-solving, and exploration.

An important and somewhat paradoxical consideration, however, is that the restoration of intersubjective space following a collapse into complementarity can be among the most healing aspects of group psychotherapy. Relational psychoanalytic theorists have referred to this process as "rupture and repair," and they consider it to be both developmentally ubiquitous (Beebe & Lachmann, 1994) and unavoidable and necessary as a vehicle for healing, growth and change in psychotherapy (Muran et al., 2009). Therapeutic repairs of these inevitable ruptures can take many forms, but they are often characterized in one of two ways. The first is through an opportunity to explore, maybe for the first time, the kinds of deep fears and feelings that tend to inhibit the authentic expression of feelings, wishes, desires, and protests on the part of the group members. The second is through the containment, acceptance, and eventual diminishment of intense, self-protective emotions and conflicts that group members often assume will result in the loss of relationship and connection (Safran & Kraus, 2014).

While there is little available literature on the relationship between intersubjectivity, SERT themes, and group therapy, there are connections between intersubjectivity and SERT themes that have important implications for group therapy (Paine et al., 2017). Tummala-Narra (2009) affirmed the specific importance of an intersubjective approach to treatment in inviting and exploring the subjective SERT experiences, questions, practices, and conflicts in both clients and therapists. Lord (2010) described a kind of "sacred" intersubjective space as "a disciplined and carefully tended crucible that we (clients and therapist) develop together as a source of spiritual energy and healing" (p. 270). Our experience as group therapists resonates with both the importance and difficulty of promoting intersubjective hospitality and resisting the forces of complementarity, especially in the context of SERT themes, which tend to be highly loaded with potential for disconnection, on the one hand, and relational growth and healing, on the other.

Holding Intersubjective Space for the Group

This vignette demonstrates the competing forces of complementarity and intersubjectivity as the group continues to wrestle with its anxiety and mistrust. Leo once again plays a powerful role in questioning new coleader John's religious beliefs in an attempt to expose the potential threat they may pose to his own sense of relational security, as well as to the safety of the group. Leo's question is important in several ways. From a content perspective, it is an important question about religious or theological beliefs and diversity in the group therapy clinical setting. From a process perspective, it is important in its structure, as it represents an example of complementarity being used to collapse the intersubjective space as a means of reducing an incredibly complex issue into a yes-or-no question. In the heat of the moment, the group is implicitly calling upon Leo to settle this issue quickly and cleanly, and in so doing, to banish the threat of traumatically reexperienced rejection and shame that John's (unarticulated) beliefs may represent in that moment. This clinical vignette also reveals potential intersections between theological belief systems and religious institutions outside the clinical setting with psychological and relational dynamics emerging within the therapy space.

John finds himself in a very difficult situation, with the powerful forces of therapeutic rupture and complementarity bearing down on his subjectivity, likely raising his anxiety and making it more difficult for him to access his capacities for a flexible, space-creating response. Nonetheless, he musters a solid attempt at repair by nonreactively opening the interaction up to more than a binary question, drawing upon the structure of the group contract as a vehicle for doing this. Not surprisingly, another member of the group, Erica, continues to push for a more definitive response from John. Here, John must make an in-the-moment technical decision about how to proceed. One option is for him to maintain his approach of trying to open up more discussion by validating group members' anxiety, without moving towards self-disclosure, which might risk "taking the bait" of complementarity. This kind of intervention would tend to emphasize John's leadership role, something that makes him different from the group members and gives him the authority to avoid the direct question.

Another option, which John chooses, is to go ahead and offer some important self-disclosure related to Leo's and Erica's questions. Some of the most powerful and important moments in group psychotherapy begin with group leaders and members temporarily entering a space of emotional, cognitive, and relational dysregulation. One of the risks in these moments is that the intersubjective space within which the group is working collapses. As a way of counteracting such collapse, an intersubjective approach to group psychotherapy understands the roles of the group leaders to include a mutual, two-way influence between leader and member. In other words, the leaders are not simply facilitators of a process, but they are also engaged in direct ways of relating with each of the group members, affecting and being affected by those relationships. John's sharing with the group that his religious beliefs do not prevent him from affirming same-sex relationships is an important, culturally sensitive intervention that helps to create more space rather than collapse further into complementarity. It brings him into his role and relationships within the group in a transparent way that helps create more relational safety, while at the same time does not assert more than he is authentically able to say about Vanessa's relationship with Megan and with her parents.

CLINICAL VIGNETTE 4: DIVERSITY, CULTURE, AND POWER

This vignette takes place 1 week later, 45 minutes into the 75-minute group, and comes on the heels of some cohesive and connected discussion among group members related to the previous week's group. The group seems to have moved away, at least temporarily, from the complementarity of the previous week's group and its focus on John.

Erica is a single, African American, Protestant (African Methodist Episcopal), female group member in her late 20s, a practicing social worker, and a recovering alcoholic with a history of sexual abuse by a middle school teacher. Marybeth is a single, white, Catholic, female group member in her mid-20s, studying for her master's in counseling. She has a developmental history notable for growing up with a severely depressed and withdrawn mother and absent father. Bo is a single, Chinese American, Protestant (Presbyterian), male group member, son of Chinese immigrants, 30 years old, working as a software programmer, with a developmental history of physical and emotional abuse by his father throughout his adolescence.

MARYBETH: Erica, I want to say something to you, but I'm afraid you'll get angry with me if I bring it up.

ERICA: It's up to you, Marybeth.

MARYBETH: (sighs anxiously) Oh, man. Okay. I didn't like it last week when you called me out about the thing with John going to seminary.

ERICA: Well, I thought you were wrong for not seeing why it was a problem.

MARYBETH: Why does it have to be that way? You know, a part of me doesn't see it as a problem. How do we know if he's homophobic just because he's a Christian? I get it, how it was painful for Vanessa. But you didn't have to come down on me like that, like I'm some sort of bad person.

ERICA: Maybe you got it eventually, but that's not how you started. You left Vanessa hanging.

MARYBETH: There you go again. Coming down on me again. What makes you so perfect?

REBECCA: Can I jump in? Marybeth, is it okay with you if I change your question to Erica a little bit?

MARYBETH: Fine.

REBECCA: Erica, can you say anything about why it was so important to you, personally, that Marybeth protect Vanessa, to get it right in that way?

ERICA: Because it's the right thing to do.

REBECCA: Yes, but can you share anything with us about why it's so important to YOU that Marybeth get it right?

ERICA: (her eyes open wide and she lowers her head) Do I have to?

REBECCA: Of course not. But I have a feeling that whatever you're going to say is really important. For you AND for the group.

ERICA: (pauses) Because if Marybeth doesn't see it, maybe nobody sees it.

JOHN: Sees what, Erica?

ERICA: Sees that Vanessa was in trouble. That she needed help.

BO: Maybe you're afraid that nobody will help YOU when you're in trouble.

ERICA: Well. Nobody ever has.

BO: I feel that way a lot, too. Most people just think I'm obnoxious. I liked it when you stuck up for Vanessa, Erica. But maybe you want somebody to stick up for you. You're always so strong. Like you don't need anybody.

ERICA: (quietly) I can't need anybody.

Diversity, Culture, and Power in Relational Dynamics

Interactions within a process-oriented psychotherapy group have important implications when considered from the perspectives of diversity, culture, and power. By taking intersecting dynamics of diversity, sociocultural identity, and social justice and power factors into consideration, a deeper level of nuanced understanding of the clinical process becomes possible, positively affecting clinical outcomes. Tummala-Narra (2016) explained:

> The recognition of traumatic loss, backdrop of social change, political struggles, and privilege is further important for theorizing that is authentic and not presumptive of universal truths, but rather is one that seeks a more complex truth concerning mental life in a pluralistic society. This is perhaps more important than ever before in a highly technological American society, as we continue to struggle with social and political issues such as racism, immigration policy, and same-sex marriage that have an important impact on both a collective psyche and individual psychological well-being. (p. 28)

In this spirit, care must be taken by the leaders of process-oriented psychotherapy groups to minimize the potential negative impacts of the group process when it inevitably enacts dominant group–minority group dynamics that result in experiences of oppression, exclusion, microaggression, and shame (Eason, 2009). These diversity and power dynamics, inasmuch as they affect the inner lives, relationships, identities, and self-understanding of group members are influencing the group process and, therefore, the clinical outcomes of the group. Because these dynamics are often subtle and unconscious, group leaders require substantial training in multicultural awareness, intercultural development, and the ways in which a process-oriented group can mirror the dynamics within the larger culture and society. Without this training, there is a risk that dominant group norms will hold sway in the group, potentially marginalizing and silencing the unique experiences, suffering, and resources of minority-group members. And from a social justice perspective, it is important for group leaders to have the training and personal awareness to recognize the impact of socially oppressive realities such as racism, sexism, and heterosexism on group members, as well as the skill to work with these issues clinically in the moment.

Supporting Difficult Conversations in Group Therapy

In the opening vignette, the group was challenged with metabolizing the threat that the new coleader John's Christian identity held for Vanessa, particularly around her sexuality and her fear that John's beliefs would marginalize and condemn her for her intimate relationship with her partner. While the process was complicated and understandably messy, members of the group were able to mobilize around this issue and help create space to both support Vanessa and allow for John to free himself from the projections of fear and judgment that he represented for several group members. John's coleader, Rebecca, played an important role in helping to contain group members' reactivity by regulating her own emotions, facilitating group members' regulation of their emotions, and providing intersubjective space and relational security for the group, thus allowing for further exploration of group members' anxiety about John joining the group as the new coleader.

In this current vignette, it is important for the coleaders to be finely attuned to the presence and impact of racial dynamics as Marybeth and Bo interact with Erica. The vignette begins with Marybeth wanting to address her feelings about Erica's criticism of her during the previous group. There are several things to which the coleaders might attend in the context of this vignette. The first is the group's history in dealing with issues of race. If the group in general, and these group members specifically, have a solid and stable history discussing race openly with one another, Rebecca and John might choose to point towards the group members' different racial backgrounds early in the process, as way of inviting the overt recognition of this difference and the complexity it contributes to the discussion. Rebecca or John might offer something like, "This is such an important conversation. I wonder if thinking about racial differences might be useful in understanding one another's feelings and viewpoints."

If the group's discussions of race have not gone well in the past, and Rebecca and John become aware of growing anxiety among group members, they might consider a more active intervention. For example, they might ask more direct questions and reframe interactions between members in a way that both acknowledges and contains the discussion, including race. For example, "Erica, there have been times when you have felt that others in the group, including Marybeth, have been especially hard on you because you are African American. How are you feeling about how this discussion is going?" Or, "Bo, you shared that you think that people think of you as obnoxious. Has it ever seemed to you that those assessments of you might be based on racism?"

Finally, if the group does not have much experience talking together about race, it may make sense to emphasize and foster the development of alliances among group members and with group coleaders that will provide a secure foundation from which race can be explored more explicitly at another time. For example, "This is such a candid and tender conversation you are having with one another. What is making it possible for each of you to let your guards down in this way?" Or, "Bo, you and Erica have been able to share something important. How were you able to reach out to her in the way you just did?" It is also important for clinicians, especially those of racial privilege, to remain aware that wading into these kinds of traumatic justice-related topics can activate powerful waves of fear, pain and spiritual and existential dysregulation but may also be necessary to cultivate deeper group solidarity in the multiple forms of suffering group members are holding.

CLINICAL SUPERVISION VIGNETTE: SELF OF THE THERAPIST

The setting for this vignette is a supervision session that includes the two group coleaders, Rebecca and John, and their clinical supervisor, Marie, a seasoned group clinician and supervisor who is a Peruvian immigrant and a practicing Roman Catholic. The session takes place the week after the previous vignette. Rebecca and John just finished giving Marie a summary of the previous two group therapy sessions.

MARIE: Well, it sounds like the group is really alive and that the two of you are doing a good job staying with them. Where were you feeling the most heat?

(Rebecca and John look at each other and smile, each inviting the other to begin.)

REBECCA: Well, I don't know if you agree with this, John. But I thought the most intensity, and my highest anxiety, was when Leo and Vanessa brought up your religious beliefs.

JOHN: Oh, yes. I agree.

MARIE: Tell me.

JOHN: Well, it felt like two worlds colliding. I was anxious enough getting started with the group, and I was just starting to feel a little more comfortable. Like knowing each group member's name and Rebecca giving me a sense of each of them. Then, wham! Leo brings in this news about me going to seminary, and Vanessa is triggered and so upset. It happened so fast. I never saw it coming.

MARIE: Ah, welcome to working with a group that is dealing with trauma. They've already taught you something about what if feels like to be in their skin.

(Rebecca smiles and John sighs.)

MARIE: So, John. Can I ask you how the content of the group's concern affected you, as something of a challenge to your religious faith and beliefs?

JOHN: Sure. I actually think that added to how off-balance I felt.

MARIE: So, the collision was not just between you and the group? There was also an inner collision?

JOHN: Maybe not a collision, but there was something.

MARIE: Say more, if you like.

JOHN: You know, when I was in seminary, we never really had to think very broadly about sexuality. There was this quiet agreement that the Scriptures laid out an easy, healthy path for heterosexual attraction, marriage, and parenthood. There we all were, with gay friends, classmates, and family members, and yet we did our best, or worst, to keep their sexuality outside that easy space by not talking about it. Or by talking around it.

REBECCA: So, what happened?

JOHN: I'd like to say I had some dramatic revelation about justice and inclusivity, but it wasn't really like that. It was more like some of us voted with our feet. We finished seminary and instead of getting ordained, we became social workers and psychologists.

MARIE: And when Vanessa and Leo and Erica challenged your beliefs, what happened inside you?

JOHN: I think I realized that a part of me had never really articulated with my mouth what my feet were trying to say.

REBECCA: What is that?

JOHN: Maybe something like, sexuality and sexual orientation are at the heart of who we are as persons, and they connect us to a lot of our hopes and dreams. I think we all need wise and loving and nurturing spaces to be healthy sexually. That feels holy to me. And our culture and society and churches can make that a lot harder, even fight against it, if you're gay.

Self-Awareness and Use of the Self in Therapy

A key element of the RSM is the importance of therapist reflection on and awareness of the impact of their own personal development, vulnerabilities, strengths, traumas, beliefs, values, assumptions, and worldview on their work and roles as clinicians and clinical supervisors. Under the concept of countertransference, many psychodynamically trained psychotherapists have been cautioned to bracket out the influence of their own subjectivity on the therapeutic process. However, more recent relational psychoanalytic approaches to psychotherapy have suggested that therapist subjectivity, or self-of-the-therapist influence, can just as readily have a beneficial impact on the therapeutic process (Bromberg, 2011; Wallin, 2007). In addition, Cornish, Wade, and Knight (2013) found that therapist spirituality, therapist training in religion and spirituality, and therapist comfort with spiritual discussions were associated with more frequent use of spiritual interventions in group therapy, as well as lower perceived barriers to incorporating spirituality into group psychotherapy. Psychotherapists can approach self of the therapist awareness through self-reflection, peer consultation, personal therapy, and continuing education, resulting in a greater accountability for the impact of their unique selfhood on clients and the therapy process (see Chapter 11). By extension, it is not only ethically necessary but clinically vital for psychotherapists to explore and be aware of their own religious and spiritual sensibilities, histories, practices, and beliefs and to consider carefully how religion and spirituality inform and influence their clinical work (Stavros & Sandage, 2014). In our experience, there are three primary reasons for this. One reason is to protect clients from the potentially negative impacts of the therapist's religious and spiritual values, biases, and assumptions. Pargament (2007) explained:

> For better or worse, the therapist's own attitudes and approaches to the sacred, and to religion more generally, will have an impact on their work with clients. Spiritual awareness is the most effective antidote to the dangers of spiritual imposition on clients. (p. 335)

A second reason for clinicians to be aware of their spiritual and religious assumptions and values is that the work of the psychotherapist, particularly if one is dealing with the intense suffering and emotional dysregulation of traumatized clients, can be extremely difficult and stressful. The deep wisdom embedded within many religious and spiritual traditions and practices can often serve as an important resource for therapists as they seek to stay grounded, balanced, present, and regulated in the face of their clients' suffering, as well as to find meaning in the challenging work of the psychotherapist.

A third reason for self-awareness of our spiritual and religious perspectives is that, when carefully considered, it might be important to authentically share some version of the therapist's religious or spiritual perspective or experience with a particular client. For example, there may be times when a Buddhist perspective on mindfulness and anger, or a Talmudic approach to simultaneously competing truths, or an Eastern Orthodox Christian approach to paradox might be well-suited to the particular therapeutic moment with a particular client. While emphasizing and adhering to vital ethical principles for avoiding proselytizing or coercive influence with clients, the metaphors, meanings, and relational ethics of many religious and spiritual traditions can be life-giving and useful vehicles for change and healing within psychotherapeutic practice.

Secure Relating and Deepening Exploration in Clinical Supervision

The preceding vignette helps to demonstrate how both group members and group coleaders require a relationally secure and structured space to do their work. Several notable things happen within the context of this supervision session. Some of the supervisor's interventions are oriented toward the creation of a robust relational container for the supervision. Other interventions make use of that container to hold the necessary challenges by the group supervisor, enabling coleaders to explore both the group's process and their own contributions, responses, and reactions to that process.

After getting a sense of the group process, the supervisor, Marie, uses a very efficient intervention with her supervisees, Rebecca and John. Marie chooses not to emphasize only one side of the relational security–exploration dialectic. Rather, she validates the coleaders experience of the group as particularly intense, provides genuinely positive feedback to them in how they are working with the intensity, and then nudges the coleaders to deepen their exploration and understanding of the group's process. Thus, she effectively balances dwelling and seeking in her supervisory relational style. Another important part of the supervision vignette is when Marie suggests that John's reaction to "two worlds colliding" can be used as a self-of-the-therapist strategy for experientially understanding and empathizing with the hypervigilance, emotional reactivity, and catastrophizing that clients with trauma histories can experience.

Marie then models for Rebecca and John a combination of secure relating and deepening exploration that invites the two of them into a process of meaning-making and growth. Had Marie sensed that John was shaken, emotionally dysregulated, or flooded with shame at this point in the supervision, she would likely have not moved as quickly into asking him about the more personal meaning of his "collision with the group." In that situation, it would have likely been more appropriate to affirm the group leaders' roles, to validate the group's and the group leaders' resilience, and to appreciate and contextualize the conflict in the light of anxiety about a new coleader joining the group. However, Marie likely sensed some sturdiness and readiness in John and decided to directly and hospitably invite the discussion of John's religious background into the supervision. Had there not been such a direct connection between John's religious history, his role as coleader, and the group process, it may not have been appropriate to move in this direction. Marie also needed to make sure she was sufficiently grounded and differentiated in relation to these particular religious issues to be able to handle the discussion. However, given the convergence of personal history, leadership role, and group process, the intervention was clinically and developmentally relevant and fruitful.

CONCLUSION

As this chapter demonstrates, the RSM is a multifaceted, complex model that simultaneously brings multiple considerations to bear in relation to group psychotherapy: it emphasizes three interlocking developmental systems—attachment theory, differentiation, and intersubjectivity—which illuminate multidimensional relational depth approaches to working with groups; it calls for close attention to power, diversity, and multicultural awareness, sensitivity, and skill; it insists on therapist self-awareness; and it takes seriously and draws on the ancient, healing wisdom of diverse religious traditions and practices, while attending to clients' ultimate concerns and the possible damage done in the name of religious belief and faith. The RSM steers group therapists toward stewardship of group relationships, group processes, and group structures that are hospitable, open, sturdy, and life-giving across a diverse mosaic of clients and group leaders. It attempts to impart the skills and sensibilities necessary to contain and metabolize the more destructive and self-destructive ways in which people can interact. Finally, the model attempts to make it more possible for complex and fundamental human needs—belonging and exploring, dwelling and seeking, loving and learning—to take root and flourish, within and between persons.

11

Relational Spirituality and Therapist Formation

Being a therapist means understanding first and foremost who you are, and where you are relative to other people.

—B. GREENE (AS CITED IN LEVITT & PIAZZA-BONIN, 2017, P. 135)

Becoming relationally adept as well as spiritually and culturally aware and sensitive psychotherapists is a lifelong endeavor. In a similar fashion, artisans master a craft, paradoxically, by remaining open to learning—perhaps especially so as they reach the most skilled level of their craft. Through mentoring, longstanding collegial relationships, and reflection on experience they continually learn and transform their skills. The same lifelong learning process is true for psychotherapist expertise as well. In this chapter, we examine the implications of our relational spirituality model (RSM) for the training, continuing education, and well-being of the psychotherapist. Our conviction, which we explain below, is that relationships and communities of practice are essential to our growth as psychotherapists. We explore the development of psychotherapists in two ways: (a) what it takes to become a relationally adept and spiritually/culturally attuned therapist in general, and (b) how therapists can learn to be more effective in attending to spiritual–existential–religious–theological (SERT; Rupert, Moon, & Sandage, 2018) dimensions in their own lives as well as their practice.

One approach to these questions is through the story with which we began this book in Chapter 1—the account of a young woman, Sofia, suffering with

http://dx.doi.org/10.1037/0000174-012
Relational Spirituality in Psychotherapy: Healing Suffering and Promoting Growth,
by S. J. Sandage, D. Rupert, G. S. Stavros, and N. G. Devor

cystic fibrosis. Sofia's medical team seemed misattuned to the depth of her existential struggles, questions of meaning, and need for relational engagement. In contrast, she found an outpatient psychotherapist who listened to her spiritual lament and intense relational conflict with God, and who related to her with warmth and irreverent humor. How do we understand such different responses to Sofia? Is it possible that training and collegial contexts that value relational engagement and relational spirituality attention to SERT questions and concerns might make a significant difference in how we respond to patients like Sofia and accompany them in their suffering? If so, how might our collegial relationships enable us to be more capable, personally and professionally, of being present and able to listen to Sofia and other clients who challenge our core beliefs about human existence? These questions concern how therapists develop across their lives in a process of ongoing formation.

DEFINING THERAPIST FORMATION

We propose the concept of *therapist formation* as a primary metaphor for the development of clinicians in and through relationships. The concept of therapist formation acknowledges the impact of relating with clients like Sofia, whose traumatic experiences can erode our capacities for hope and resilience. It also focuses our attention on the ways training communities and collegial consultations may guide and guard us, and our clients, in this sometimes dangerous, sometimes promising work. The concept of therapist formation additionally suggests that professional growth for relational therapists includes cultivating attitudes and personal/professional capacities as well as increasing knowledge and skills, and thus requires relational and experiential learning as well as more traditional methods of training.

We choose the metaphor of formation with its roots in spiritual traditions because it is resonant with a relational, developmental approach. The wisdom and practice of many ancient religious traditions offer some vital lessons about formation that are especially relevant to the development and growth of psychotherapists. For example, in many spiritual traditions formation is practiced in relationship with mentors and communities of practice; attends especially to right-brain affective and relational processes, not only left-brain training focused on content (Schore, 2018); acknowledges the necessity of a crucible for growth to occur; requires the cultivation of particular characteristics such as self-awareness, differentiation of self, and cultural humility; attends to holistic self-care; and is facilitated through the engagement of one's own spiritual and existential journey.

On the theme of practicing in relationship, religious approaches to formation tend to emphasize a relational dialectic of mutual seeking between guides and seekers. Typically, formation requires an apprenticeship with a guide (e.g., Hinduism's guru, the Murshid in Sufism, the Zaddik in Hasidic Jewish communities, the Anam Cara or Soul Friend of Celtic Christianity). Both Eastern and

Western traditions stress the danger of formation without guides and/or companions. In her tour de force, *A History of God*, Karen Armstrong (1993) noted that "all religions have insisted that the mystical journey can only be undertaken under the guidance of an expert, who can monitor the experience, guide the novice past the perilous places, and make sure that he [sic] is not exceeding his strength" like some novice mystics who died or went mad (p. 213).

Formation is an uncommon term in literature on psychotherapy and clinical training, although there is discussion of spiritual formation in the training of doctoral-level psychologists at some Christian-affiliated, American Psychological Association–approved programs (Flanagan et al., 2013). Since our clinical and training context is diverse and pluralistic, we do not focus on a singular religious tradition, but rather draw from multiple sources, including the mental health training literature and various religious and spiritual traditions. Moreover, our emphasis is on formation of therapists rather than spiritual formation, while acknowledging that these processes may be interrelated. While spiritual formation pertains to spiritual growth as defined by relevant communities, therapist formation in the RSM involves well-being and growth in the core relational systems of attachment, differentiation, and intersubjectivity, and the cultivation of essential attitudes, skills, and practices for effective clinical care. These attitudes, skills, and practices have been described in prior chapters, and include factors like cultural humility, dwelling and seeking, accompaniment, meaning-making, self-awareness, presence, affect regulation, crucible experiences, rupture and repair, mutual recognition, and consultation. Our view of therapist formation has resonance with ideas and practices from several psychotherapy traditions, such as the self of the therapist emphasis in family therapy, the psychoanalytic emphasis on personal therapy and growth in self-awareness, and the accent in humanistic and other relational therapies on the personal qualities of therapists. Each of these perspectives holds up the idea that the personhood of the therapist is a crucial factor in the healing effects of psychotherapy, equally or even more influential than a set of particular skills or techniques.

Skills and capacities for addressing spiritual, religious, and existential concerns in clinical practice are an important aspect of the RSM. Yet research indicates that graduate students and practicing psychotherapists alike report limited to nonexistent clinical training in spirituality and religion (Bartoli, 2007; Saunders, Petrik, & Miller, 2014; Vieten et al., 2013). We have already described problems that can arise from a lack of attention to SERT dynamics in clinical practice, as well as the risk of clinical bias. Saunders et al. (2014) provided a simple but sobering illustration of the potential impact of insufficient training as they noted that therapists without training in assessing and intervening in spiritual and religious concerns are more likely to ask if religion is a resource and fail to ask if it is a problem. Examples like these inform the growing ethical stance and clinical imperative that psychotherapists learn to routinely include spiritual and religious matters in assessment and intervention and also grow in self-awareness about their own values and perspectives in this area (Vieten et al., 2016).

However, the concerns about psychotherapist effectiveness and growth over time are not restricted to competence with SERT issues. Researchers remind us that we routinely overestimate our effectiveness and increasingly advocate deliberate practice as an inoculation against our false optimism (Chow et al., 2015). A further professional embarrassment is documented in Stirman, Gutner, Langdon, and Graham (2016), who reported that most clinicians do not rely on research to inform their practice. Obviously, professional knowledge changes over time, and research suggests practitioners vary significantly in their openness to new information and innovations in practice (Aarons, Hurlburt, & Horwitz, 2011). If our overestimation of our abilities and our lack of integration of research into practice were not enough to cause concern, consider that competence can degrade over time. Estimates of the half-life of psychological knowledge range from 9 down to 7 years (W. B. Johnson et al., 2014). Perhaps most concerning, research has indicated that therapist effectiveness tends to diminish (rather than improve) over time (Goldberg et al., 2016). Clinical practice is highly stressful with chronic exposure to human suffering. Altogether these findings raise complicated questions about the formation and well-being of therapists and emphasize the importance of practicing in relationship as a means of accountability for personal and professional competence and well-being.

In clinical training in general, and more specifically in training for SERT competencies, there is a growing literature, with numerous books, courses, and continuing education resources now available. Examples include Russell and Yarhouse (2006) and Vieten et al. (2013). Vieten and colleagues (2013) proposed three attitudes (respect for religious and spiritual diversity, along with awareness of how therapist backgrounds in spirituality and religion influence our practice), seven areas of knowledge (increasing knowledge about the diversity of spirituality and religion and how those can impact positively and negatively impact well-being, as well as knowledge about ethical issues related to spirituality and religion), and six specific skills (integrating awareness of spirituality and religion in assessment and intervention, staying current with research). These competencies, with which we would agree, were identified through a review of professional literature and an online survey with expert scholars and clinicians. In a follow-up study, Vieten et al. (2016) surveyed a general sample of psychologists and found additional support for these 16 competencies. Interestingly, two of the competencies that received the highest endorsement were in the attitude domain: "Psychologists demonstrate empathy, respect, and appreciation for clients from diverse spiritual, religious or secular backgrounds and affiliations" and "Psychologists are aware of how their own spiritual and/or religious background and beliefs may influence their clinical practice, and their attitudes, perceptions, and assumptions about the nature of psychological processes" (p. 99).

In addition to these attitudes, knowledge, and skills identified by Vieten et al. (2016), this volume emphasizes specific competencies found in the RSM. The RSM explores how dialectics of spiritual dwelling and seeking impact client well-being and developmental growth, particularly within experiences of trauma and suffering. Building on attitudes of "empathy, respect and appreciation for diversity" (Vieten et al., 2013, p.135), the RSM emphasizes commitment to thick understandings of spiritual, religious, and existential processes within diverse contexts and traditions. In the area of knowledge, the RSM integrates knowledge of three relational development systems of attachment, differentiation, and intersubjectivity, particularly as they intersect with client SERT factors and cultural contexts. In the attachment system, we look for ways that safe haven and secure base patterns map onto patterns of spiritual and religious dwelling and seeking, and their implications for healing and growth. The differentiation system involves knowledge of, and skilled assessment and intervention in, the dialectics of connection and autonomy and ways of relating to difference. Knowledge and skills in the intersubjective system enables us to assess and intervene in relational enactments, ruptures and repairs, and pathways toward finding the third space. We have pointed to the need for knowledge of diverse perspectives on the meaning of suffering across various worldviews and traditions. We also describe in this chapter the foundation of therapist formation in relationship in training and in ongoing consultation throughout our professional lives. Awareness of our own SERT backgrounds and the ways we process the changing spiritual, religious, and existential backdrop of existence, and how this impacts our clinical work, is essential to the RSM. Accessing what is sacred to the clinician and accessing our SERT resources enables us to be more fully present in the witness of client suffering. We are mindful as well of the need for the RSM to be practiced within a relational ecology of a clinic and research program to continue to renew ourselves and our field.

While training in content areas and skills is essential both to spiritually and culturally sensitive practice, attitudes are considered the foundation that enables skill and knowledge development. Perhaps many clinicians know intuitively that workshops and online training are not enough. C. E. Hill, Spiegel, Hoffman, Kivlighan, and Gelso (2017) found that in learning to provide psychotherapy, "therapists perceived that hands-on experiences with clients, personal therapy, and supervision were the most helpful factors in their growth" (p. 185). Stirman et al. (2016) pointed out that when performance based on workshop or online training is measured, proficiency typically falls short of benchmarks required for clinical-trial clinicians and requires ongoing support and consultation to achieve adequate skills and improve clinical outcomes. It is in candid relational dialogue with others where our attitudes about spiritual and religious diversity and our "blind spots" may surface in ways that allow corrective feedback and new learning.

In addition to concern about clinical competence and client outcome, the concept of therapist formation considers how collegial relationships guide us through territory that challenges us as persons as well as clinicians. Below, we consider the potential for burnout and vicarious traumatization that comes when psychotherapists witness the trauma suffered by many psychotherapy clients. Based on our core RSM themes, we believe clinicians need relational containers of professional and personal support to sustain us in the difficult and stressful terrain of clinical practice (*dwelling*), as well as relationships that challenge us to explore and integrate fresh understandings of how we can provide the best possible care for our clients (*seeking*). In the next section, we consider the types of relationships that foster psychotherapist competence and well-being over our lifetimes.

FORMATION IN RELATIONSHIP

Our primary thesis in this chapter on therapist formation builds on a central idea of the RSM: Healthy relational processes and containers shape developmental crucibles that integrate both dwelling and seeking. Over our professional lifetimes, psychotherapists are impacted in their development through multiple relationships, including classroom interaction with professors, individual and group supervision, peer supervision, and personal psychotherapy. Consistent with our relational development focus in the RSM, it is important to note that these relational impacts on clinicians can range from salutary to harmful, with many variations of relational influence on the attachment, differentiation, and intersubjectivity systems as they shape therapist formation in clinical practice.

Relational Ecologies of Clinical Practice

We see significance in reflecting on the multidimensional *relational ecologies* of clinical practice and training settings, which involve numerous levels and kinds of relationships between professional colleagues, clinicians and administrative staff, trainees and supervisors, and administrative staff and clients (Kehoe, Hassen, & Sandage, 2016). In some settings, the relational ecology is supportive and stimulating of growth, while in other settings there can be chronic power struggles, wounds, and conflicts that impact the overall ethos, at least for certain clinicians. We have also seen clinical settings that lacked deep conflict but also seemed to lack much relational support or fresh, "growth-oriented" engagement among clinicians and other staff even if they meet regularly for case consultation, supervision, or clinic coordination. Still other clinicians are working in relative isolation without much interaction with colleagues, which is another kind of relational challenge. We consider these relational ecology dynamics, particularly dynamics of attachment, differentiation, and intersubjectivity, an important part of what we mean by relational spirituality in clinical practice. And, as discussed in Chapter 2, we also believe these kinds of systemic and ecological dynamics can impact the quality of clinical care (Sandage, Moon, et al., 2017). These differing kinds of relational ecology problems will require differing interventions from leaders to cultivate healthier, growth-generating dynamics. In the absence of such leadership, individual clinicians will likely need to do their best to differentiate from their surrounding system and seek training and consultation resources outside their system (which can also be constructive even in healthy clinical contexts).

Training and Consultation

Relational processes and containers of training and consultation are critical for therapist formation. These resources may include formal supervision/mentoring, collegial relationships, consultation groups, peer support groups, and training groups. From our perspective, the structure is less important than establishing ongoing professional relationships that include enough depth, vulnerability, and expertise to allow for meaningful support, accountability, and growth. Our understanding of psychotherapist formation in relationship resonates with a call by W. B. Johnson et al. (2014) for a "communitarian training culture." Johnson et al. contrasted the individualistic ethic of psychology, which emphasizes "individual responsibility for assessment and maintenance of competence," with the communitarian ethic expressed in the African proverb "it takes a village" to maintain professional competence and ethical accountability (p. 212). They argued that "a flourishing community of psychologists is one in which both individuals and groups of colleagues forge interconnections to address competence concerns honestly and collaboratively and bolster each other's competence" (p. 212).

Embedded in peer groups from early in training, therapists might better learn to share a collective responsibility for our community's competence. W. B. Johnson and colleagues (2014) center their competence constellation model (CCM) on a small group of five to eight primary relational mentors/colleagues who practice "high levels of mutuality, reciprocity, intimacy, self-disclosure, and engagement" (p. 214). Mentors and supervisors model communitarian values—including care and compassion, collegiality and civility, and self-care—from the beginning of training. Collegial relationships emphasize reciprocity, transparency and vulnerability, focus on professional and personal development, and seek to decrease defensiveness and increase humility.

Similar relational themes emerged in a study by Beidas and colleagues (2013) on what *experienced* clinicians found important or helpful in consultation. The identified factors were connection with other therapists, authentic interaction around actual cases, and consultant responsiveness to the particular concerns/needs of individual therapists. These findings and the CCM model focus on relational dynamics that align with and engage the attachment, differentiation, and intersubjectivity systems.

With regard to SERT competencies, relational training and consultation may help therapists to be more aware of the power we carry in the therapeutic relationship regarding SERT dynamics, including the potential for pathologizing or idealizing client spirituality, advancing our religious and/or spiritual beliefs in a proselytizing way, or constructively utilizing resources in service of our client's needs (Stavros & Sandage, 2014). Tillman, Dinsmore, Hof, and Chasek (2013) explored how therapists develop confidence in their capacity to address spiritual and religious issues in psychotherapy. One of the themes that emerged in their study concerned a learning environment that fostered interaction with others and helped trainees fill in their gaps in knowledge, awareness, and skills. Overall, their research points to an understanding of

SERT competence as constructed in multiple kinds of relationship—with clients, peers, and supervisors.

As mentioned in Chapter 2, Rupert, Moon, and Sandage (2018) described clinical training groups—SERT Groups—that seek to promote formation in relational spirituality and competence in assessing and addressing spiritual and religious issues in treatment. SERT training groups have four goals: (a) developing therapist self-awareness about one's own SERT location and background and facilitative attitudes (openness, curiosity, differentiation) toward SERT dynamics in others, (b) deepening overall knowledge and perspective about SERT factors as expressed in clinical settings, (c) facilitating skills in conducting SERT conversations and interventions, and (d) cultivating personal and professional support and accountability. At our clinic, SERT Groups include staff and trainees, are structured with an intention for diversity, and meet weekly for 75 minutes to facilitate the goals above. Key process elements include talking about our own values, perspectives, and questions, and not simply focusing on theories, ideas, or client/case material; sharing aspects of one's own background and current identifications/communities; using clinical and personal examples and stories to create specificity and avoid intellectualizing; attending to power by asking leaders to go first in being vulnerable and to make room for differences and points of tension within the group; practicing the process (and learning tacit skills) by discussing thick topics including emotions and struggles; and having enough regularity and continuity to the meetings to get to know and really engage each other. Examples of SERT Group topics include: (a) What was the religious or spiritual context in your family/community growing up, and how have you continued that and/or changed over time? (b) What are some of your strongest values and beliefs, and how do they inform your clinical work? (c) What case is troubling you the most right now, and what is it touching in you? and (d) Identify one client who seems quite different from you in some important way and reflect on how those differences are playing out in the therapy.

There are many ways clinicians could borrow from or adapt SERT group structure and processes to fit their context and still achieve the goal of fostering healthy attachment, differentiation, and intersubjectivity in the formation of their capacities for competence in addressing spiritual, existential/philosophical, religious, and theological concerns (Sandage & Brown, 2018). For example, it might be possible to invite colleagues in a consultation group to deepen and broaden conversation by sharing about each other's background and inviting explicit discussion of SERT issues, including one's personal reactions, questions, and struggles. A clinic or consultation group might also bring in a consultant with expertise in spiritual and religious competence to provide some training and self-reflection related to SERT dynamics in practice. A unique example of this is on the Danielsen Institute website.[1] It contains detailed presentations by prominent relational psychoanalytic clinicians,

---

[1]Available for free viewing online (http://www.bu.edu/danielsen/video-library/the-skillful-soul-of-the-psychotherapist-2012-merle-jordan-conference/).

including Nancy McWilliams, David Wallin, and Salman Akhtar, demonstrating how master clinicians' spiritual lives can be inextricably tied to and in mutual influence with their clinical practice and thinking. Whatever strategies are used, we believe it is vital to engage the personal/professional interface and to make oneself known to others for support and accountability.

Perhaps if more training sites created SERT-like groups, therapists would be less likely as a group overall to avoid spiritual and religious topics in the clinical domain. Like other aspects of cultural competence and cultural humility, SERT training is developmental and lifelong. But even without widespread adoption of SERT groups or other specific training models, clinicians can use peer groups to help them develop as psychotherapists skilled in addressing relational spirituality. Peer groups may have more formative impact when their membership is stable over time, enabling colleagues to develop the mutual trust necessary to foster therapist vulnerability and the openness to support and challenge. Bartoli (2007) proposed using peer supervision groups structured to create interpersonal safety to explore SERT concerns. She emphasized the psychotherapist's conscious and unconscious capacity to convey respect and openness for client spirituality and religious concerns, as well as the clinician's self-awareness of what may help or hinder such a welcoming stance. Bartoli offered specific suggestions for peer groups, such as proposing that members share their three-generational spiritual genograms with one another to promote reflection on some of the spiritual and religious narratives and legacies that shape their attitudes and work, and we have found this to be very useful in clinical training.

Supervision

Supervisors have an especially influential role in supporting the formation of beginning psychotherapists. The supervisory process is complex and must address multiple perspectives and contexts to promote optimal client care and trainee growth while also serving an evaluative, gatekeeping function. From our perspective, supervision occurs in a relationship that will engage the developmental systems of attachment, differentiation, and intersubjectivity, and the relational spiritual themes of dwelling, seeking, existential challenges, and meaning-making. Once again, the quality of the relationship is critical. For example, how does the supervisor (a) provide a safe haven and secure base to facilitate well-being and growth? (b) promote dwelling and seeking, with different emphasis depending on the needs of the clients and the supervisee? (c) assist the supervisee to identify and negotiate crucibles that feel disruptive and disorienting but may ultimately lead to growth? (d) attend to individual and cultural differences and power dynamics? (e) provide experiences of attunement without compromising differentiation? (f) tolerate tensions and repair ruptures? and (g) regulate his or her own affect and assist the trainee with affect regulation?

For example, in one supervision an older trainee in her second career was given feedback that she sometimes came across as "knowing better" and being somewhat closed-minded. A week later she shared that she had started to trust the system but now saw that false compliance was necessary, as it had been in prior training. This led to several discussions about the trainee's experience of the feedback, associations to prior training experiences, and experiences of sexism and ageism. The supervisor offered recognition and support for her autonomy and voice, and they talked about ways she might communicate her ideas without compliance or seeming arrogance. In these same discussions, the supervisee gave feedback to the supervisor and training program about a tendency to "be nice" and mostly avoid conflict but then come down hard in unexpected ways. The supervisor also became more aware of gender and age dynamics in the supervisory relationship. Both parties left with something to ponder for personal/professional growth, both felt (mostly) heard, and both continued to process the interaction with other peers and colleagues.

The literature on diversity and cultural humility also offers helpful perspective on how students learn in supervision. Watkins and Hook (2016) remarked, "It is incumbent on supervisors to make culture a welcome part of the supervisory process" (p. 10). In a similar way, how supervisors model an openness and comfort with spiritual or existential themes will enable trainees to venture into new territory. Stirman et al. (2016) suggested that modeling may have a greater impact than behavioral rehearsal in mental health care training, causing us to consider the importance of authentic engagement in supervision. Without the invitation of supervisors, students may be less likely to reflect openly on their experiences with spirituality and religious content in their clinical work. Lee and colleagues (reviewed in M. M. Miller, Korinek, & Ivey, 2006) asked first-year students to journal daily about their clinical experience and development. Their writing revealed that they were facing difficult dilemmas in ethical and spiritual terrains and were keeping silent. Having a supervisory relationship where cultural and SERT topics are initiated as part of the conversation and reflection, instead of waiting for the student's initiation, is a crucial part of the early learning process.

M. M. Miller et al. (2006) offered guidance to supervisors hoping to provide modeling for their trainees. Comprehensive questions were suggested for opening conversations in four different dimensions in which spirituality/religion and self-of-therapist concerns may arise in supervision: the client system, the supervisory system, the diversity lens, and the lens of meaning and value. An example is the following: "Is there anything in our relationship that runs counter to your spirituality?" (p. 367). A critical aspect of this approach is that it moves beyond a view of spirituality and religion as consistently positive, enabling a more complex way to relate to spiritual and religious material across interpersonal differences.

THERAPIST FORMATION IN DEVELOPMENTAL CRUCIBLES

While much training and continuing education focuses on content and didactics learned in classes, workshops, and online presentations, many clinical practice capacities must be "caught" as well as "taught," especially if they involve relational awareness and skill. More than a classroom or professional continuing education experience, research shows that clinical skills, knowledge, and attitudes are shaped through relationships that provide a certain level of support while at the same time challenging us to grow. We have been alluding throughout this chapter to a need to focus on the self of the therapist, including awareness of our own SERT and cultural backgrounds and values and convictions. In her discussion of how to "teach" the therapeutic alliance, Chazan (2015) addressed a different kind of learning, a learning that is caught:

> The centrality of the therapeutic alliance in all psychiatry practice; the prevalence of developmental trauma and the evidence base for psychotherapy in its treatment; neurobiological research supporting the importance of affect in all mental processing; psychologically sophisticated community expectations, together with the psychic hazards of working empathically with mentally disturbed patients—all point to the importance of developing psychological skills in our trainees and our obligation as educators to explicitly facilitate 'right brain' professional development with a focus on affective and relational skills. (p. 581)

Right-brain training, according to Chazan (2015), occurs in a relational context. It is not synonymous with work/life balance, mentorship, and perhaps not even psychotherapy. It is hands-on assistance with thinking about and reflecting on the emotional content of clinical work in experiential ways. Right-brain training offers a chance to identify and verbalize limbically based psychological experience before our defenses have a chance to obscure our capacity to learn. Chazan suggested several vehicles for right-brain training: a supervised "long case," supervision based on audiovisual recordings, autobiographical reflection, case discussion groups focused on uncomfortable clinical material, attending to emotional and interpersonal process, and giving trainees permission to be on a steep learning curve. Chazan's suggestions are similar to the kinds of processes encouraged in the SERT groups referenced earlier (see also the POTT training described later in this chapter; Kissil & Niño, 2017).

The deliberate practice literature offers several helpful perspectives on therapist formation. First, deliberate practice encourages attention to areas of struggle (Rousmaniere, 2016). In the RSM, we see a dialectic between affirming strengths and working on areas for growth. However, in alignment with the findings in deliberate practice, we find that encouraging ongoing consultation around *struggles and questions* is essential. Strategies include reviewing research and theory on the potential benefits of such vulnerability, asking leaders and power holders to set an example and go first, creating structures for and shared expectations around sharing difficulties, and building relational trust over time. Second, deliberate practice theory recommends consulting and training in "long-term" collegial relationships (Rousmaniere, 2016, p. 7) that invite feedback from persons who have gotten to know our tendencies and vulnerabilities. Third, the literature on deliberate practice encourages intentional effort and working through experience of strain, confusion, and "disequilibrium" (Rousmaniere, 2016, p. 7). This echoes our perspective on the necessity of persevering through developmental crucibles that challenge our current capacities. Fourth and finally, deliberate practice recognizes that all therapists, not just trainees and early career practitioners, need resources for support, accountability, and growth. As discussed above, typical forms of continuing education and many peer group conversations lack the kind of sustained and in-depth interaction that promotes increased competence. Deliberate practice adds an emphasis on getting feedback and participating in active practice in targeted areas (Rousmaniere, 2016). We encourage individual clinicians to seek out colleagues who might collaborate in more intentional and creative colearning experiences. Larger systems may benefit from redesigning in-service training to incorporate more meaningful relationships, personalized feedback, and active practice.

What part of clinical practice is better "caught" in relationship than "taught"? Punzi (2015) suggested the term *practical wisdom* to describe the reflective capacity that supports our ability to work with varying and complex clinical situations, to "understand what the problem is all about" (p. 348, referencing Schon, 1983). The development of practical wisdom, similarly to Chazan's (2015) right-brain learning, tends to be an emotionally and cognitively demanding process. Punzi doubted that practical wisdom can be taught in a classroom, as it is not about accumulating pieces of knowledge but instead requires learning through interactive processes characterized by support, permission, and an expectation of engagement by each learner. Punzi's study of psychology trainees concluded that practical wisdom was learned through iterative processes of active experience (e.g., role-playing therapy), reflection, observation of others including senior role models, and discussion. Through this sort of reflective engagement, students gained professional and personal insights, and linked theory with practice. Students also expressed that they would not have developed practical wisdom if they had to make these connections independently, on their own.

Both Chazan (2015) and Punzi (2015) moved us in the explicit direction of considering how training may impact the self of the therapist and self-awareness. Teyber and Teyber (2014) drew our attention to therapist use of self in the here-and-now process, including making process comments (comments or questions about the therapeutic relationship). Such learning can produce significant anxiety as psychotherapists discuss matters that conflict with familial prescriptions and cultural rules. Yet making process comments and having a capacity for engagement are variables that separate effective and ineffective psychotherapists, and as such are critical for psychotherapist training and client outcome. Helping psychotherapists contain their anxiety while learning to use themselves to intervene (e.g., using the psychotherapist's filtered experience to wonder out loud about the clinical relationship and interaction) is an essential aspect of training. Consider a therapist who recognizes her own growing anxiety as a client with a trauma history calmly tells her about hitchhiking home from a friend's at 3 a.m. the previous night. The therapist comments to the patient, "Maybe sometimes it can be hard to know how scared you really are, or should be."

Sandage and Jensen proposed a model of reflective practice defined by Barnett and O'Mahony in 2006 as "a learning process examining current or past practices, behaviors, or thoughts in order to make conscious choices about future action" (as cited in Sandage & Jensen, 2013, p. 96). Their reflective practice model includes *double-loop learning*, by which they mean learning that results in changes in values, strategies, and assumptions. Double-loop learning, they wrote, "is psychologically unsettling [because it asks] human beings to question the foundation of their sense of competence and self-confidence related to effective practice" (p. 96). Three criteria for double-loop learning are: openness to examining personal responsibility; willingness to play with ideas that seem wrong; and the capacity to deal with the bewilderment and frustration often inherent in learning. This involves a transformational or crucible-like approach to education and training in which anxiety and ambiguity will increase during a liminal middle phase of the process. The importance and quality of relationships or relational containers "is critical for moving through the process" (Sandage & Jensen, 2013, p. 96). What does this mean in practice? It often involves asking hard questions (without offering answers) while pacing the work and providing accompaniment.

The crucible or transformative space opened up by double-loop learning may bear some similarities to the *cultural third* described by Watkins and Hook (2016): "a unique space where cultural meanings and experiences are welcomed, respected, and privileged and can be openly explored and examined for their treatment/supervision perspective" (p. 2). What may be missing from their description, although likely implicit, is the dangerous quality implied in the metaphor of a crucible. In a crucible, in transformation, something has to die or be lost in order for something new to occur. For a cultural third to be an authentic space offering the possibility of nondefensive change, something must be let go. To encounter difference deeply enough to learn or be changed, we must relinquish certainty and familiarity (to some degree), tolerate internal and interpersonal tensions, and actively work at revising our understandings and stances.

All of these various types of learning—right-brain learning, practical wisdom, process and reflective capacities, use of the therapist's self, clinical capacities that need to be "caught" and not just "taught," and double-loop learning— are best facilitated in the kind of relationship that is both safe haven as well as secure base, empathic responsiveness to vulnerability and distress as well as support for individuation and differentiation. It is also crucial to consider systemic dynamics within a clinical organization and wider social systems that can make it particularly stressful for clinicians from nondominant groups to exercise cultural humility and enter into developmental crucibles, particularly if the surrounding systems are ethnocentric and lacking in resources to support diversity (Moon & Sandage, 2019).

FORMATION AND THERAPIST SELF-CARE

Formation in relational spirituality attends to dialectics in human existence: safe haven and secure base; connection and separateness; embeddedness and exploration. These dialectics inform our relationships with self, other, and the transcendent horizons of human experience. We encounter and negotiate these dialectics in relational webs—professional networks of mentors, supervisors, personal therapists, colleagues, and clients; and personal communities and relationships of various kinds. These relationships are the containers within which we are formed, where we bear and negotiate the heat of developmental crucibles, where we are challenged to be more transparent, more engaged, more awake, and more alive. In considering therapist self-care, we look to relational formation as a way to increase self-awareness and seek relationships of support, accountability, and growth.

To consider therapist self-care is to explore how we can become professionally lost, and how being lost can become a road to finding relationships that can hold us when we are without our moorings and challenge us when we need to become more engaged and alive in our work. We find that discussions of self-care often fall short of being truly helpful and transformative because our mental health fields often frame self-care in the same way they frame training—focusing on observable phenomena and left-brain knowledge rather than focusing on relationships, developmental systems, and personal and communal resources that ground and inspire us.

There are a number of terms used in the professional literature to describe the impact of psychotherapy on the person of the therapist, and these terms tend to focus on negative effects. Harrison and Westwood (2009) and Newell and MacNeil (2010) reviewed several prominent descriptors. The first term is *burnout*, which may be the oldest, most researched, and most comprehensive term. Burnout has three distinct domains: "overwhelming exhaustion, cynicism and detachment, and a sense of ineffectiveness and lack of accomplishment" (Clay, 2018, quoting the *Maslach Burnout Inventory Manual*, 4th ed., 2016). Burnout can result from factors within the psychotherapist, the clients served, and the organizational context of the work. The second term is *vicarious traumatization*, which focuses on changes in cognitive schemas such as safety, trust, control, and changes in spiritual and existential beliefs resulting from chronic empathic engagement with traumatized clients. Other impacts include *secondary traumatic stress*, which points towards traumatic symptoms and behaviors, and *compassion fatigue*, which seems to include elements of burnout and secondary traumatic stress.

While many authors focus on negative impacts, some have noted that even these seemingly negative effects of psychotherapy can also have a positive, life-giving aspect. For example, Harrison and Westwood (2009) found that psychotherapists who were able to embrace rather than avoid or resist the traumatic accounts of their clients were better protected from vicarious traumatization. Their study "yielded the novel finding that empathic engagement can be a protective practice for clinicians who work with traumatized clients" and that clinicians who displayed what they termed "'exquisite empathy' (a discerning, highly present, sensitively attuned, well-boundaried, heartfelt form of empathic engagement)" considered themselves "invigorated rather than depleted by their professional connections with traumatized clients" (p. 213).

What kinds of relational containers and processes are key in turning us from clinicians suffering from vicarious traumatization to clinicians engaged and more alive in and through this difficult work? We know that clinicians are resistant to using colleague-assistance programs and are not accurate when it comes to assessing their own competence (W. B. Johnson et al., 2014). Given this, how will psychotherapists know when they need help and, in turn, get the help they need without building networks of support and accountability? Bearse, McMinn, Seegobin, and Free (2013) found that a greater percentage of psychologists seek psychotherapy than the general population, but they also reported a number of barriers, such as finding an acceptable psychotherapist. Women in their study reported more struggle than men with the effects of vicarious traumatization and compassion fatigue. At the same time, female psychologists struggled with more barriers to psychotherapy than their male counterparts. Lack of time and money were a factor for both females and males, but time and money were more problematic for female psychologists. We have been struck that some clinicians continue to feel stigma about seeking therapy for themselves, yet we consider personal therapy to be not only a crucial self-care resource but also one of the best opportunities for experiential training in psychotherapy.

Several promising studies have indicated ways that clinicians can engage in relational self-care to increase self-awareness and accuracy in self-assessment and develop a relational ethic for accountability and support. One example is person-of-the-therapist training (POTT), developed by Harry Aponte. The goal of POTT is to help trainees identify their core ongoing struggles, known as *signature themes*, and the impact these struggles have on their therapeutic relationships (Aponte & Kissil, 2014). Signature themes are perceived to be obstacles; common examples are fear of rejection, need to control, and fear of being vulnerable. Rather than promoting resolution of signature themes, POTT emphasizes acceptance and learning to use them "purposefully and intentionally" in clinical work (Kissil & Niño, 2017, p. 527). POTT includes structured reflection and discussion exercises in supervision groups that explore how signature themes are present in specific cases. A thematic study of Marriage and Family Therapist students engaged in POTT (Kissil & Niño, 2017) found better self-understanding, including awareness of vulnerabilities and flaws, increased self-compassion and acceptance, and relational changes such as increased capacities to be vulnerable, seek help, and set boundaries. Kissil and Niño (2017) noted that POTT promotes clinical skills as well as attitudes and skills of self-care.

Patsiopoulos and Buchanan (2011) studied the practice of self-compassion among experienced clinicians. They found six different ways psychotherapists incorporated self-compassion in their clinical work: (a) an accepting attitude, (b) an attitude of not-knowing, (c) being less critical and more compassionate toward their inner dialogue, (d) being more present and mindful, (e) making time for themselves, and (f) acknowledging their mistakes more openly. Clinicians used self-compassion to manage the stress and impact of clinical work and reported that it positively affected their stance as psychotherapists. They reported having more realistic expectations, better balance between client and psychotherapist needs, self-correction and proactively engaging in self-care.

Barsness and Sorenson (2018) noted that in the shift to relational theory, psychotherapist neutrality has been replaced with a focus on authenticity and empathic engagement, which places high emotional and cognitive demands on the psychotherapist. Moreover, McWilliams commented that the type of persons drawn to relational psychotherapy are those who "like closeness, dislike separation, fear rejection, suffer guilt readily . . . tend to be self-critical, to be overly responsible and to put people's needs before their own" (as cited in Barsness & Sorenson, 2018, p. 105). We are wounded healers, and our wounds can be reactivated, leaving us with shame, anger and loss that can, in turn, "collapse into restricted affect, restricted relationships, restricted imagination, restricted self-love" (Barsness & Strawn, 2018, p. 311). As an antidote, they suggested resources for resilience, such as cultivating a mind-set of growth, applying our clinical theories to ourselves, and lying fallow (taking small and large breaks from clinical work). Perhaps most relevant for our RSM, these authors pointed to relational resources such as "an internal chorus" (p. 312) of those who have given us direction and support in difficult times (a frame that assumes ongoing networks of support), and allowing ourselves to learn and heal along with our clients through an encounter of genuine dialogue in which we both are transformed. As part of our RSM, we also suggest attention to spiritual and religious resources—communities, values, commitments, preferences, practices—that can offer meaning, support, or even inspiration to beleaguered therapists who have had significant exposure to human suffering and trauma through their work and perhaps also in their lives.

CONCLUSION

Formation of the therapist is a crucial component of the RSM. It refers to a wide-ranging developmental process that goes beyond the accumulation of knowledge and honing of skills to encompass paths for growth and sustenance throughout one's career. Formation involves relational processes that transcend psychotherapy and are deeply intertwined with our identities, values, personal histories, and experiences of growth, woundedness, and healing. To be formed in this way requires relationships with trusted others who help to provide both relational security and challenge. It requires the courage and humility to move beyond self-protective assumptions about ourselves and others into crucibles characterized by robust feedback, self-evaluation, and investment in growth. It also requires relational experiences that access and affect us at deep, limbic levels, expanding our capacities for encountering and tolerating the suffering of our clients, as well as our own. Finally, formation of the therapist invites us to become part of a larger legacy of formation, to find our place in the intergenerational, multicultural community of mental health providers where we can and must learn from one another.

12

Summary and Future Research Directions

In this concluding chapter, we summarize core themes and ideas of the relational spirituality model (RSM) as it applies to psychotherapy based on the previous chapters in this book, with some of these ideas also considered in other publications (Sandage, Bell, Moon, & Ruffing, 2019; Sandage & Brown, 2018; Sandage, Jensen, & Jass, 2008; Sandage & Shults, 2007; Shults & Sandage, 2006; Stavros & Sandage, 2014; Worthington & Sandage, 2016). We then outline some future research directions for this approach to spiritually integrative psychotherapy and training.

10 KEY IDEAS WITHIN THE RELATIONAL SPIRITUAL MODEL

1. *Spirituality is relational.* Spirituality is relational and involves diverse ways of relating with the sacred—whomever or whatever a person considers ultimate or of utmost importance. Individual differences in relational spirituality are influenced by implicit and unconscious neurobiological processes, interpersonal dynamics, and cultural and systemic factors. Particular forms of relational spirituality might be adaptive or maladaptive depending on the context. We view spirituality in psychotherapy as a dynamic relational process, and our understanding of relational spirituality is most readily integrated with relational models of psychotherapy like the RSM that highlight the key role of the therapeutic alliance in change. At the same time, we

http://dx.doi.org/10.1037/0000174-013
Relational Spirituality in Psychotherapy: Healing Suffering and Promoting Growth,
by S. J. Sandage, D. Rupert, G. S. Stavros, and N. G. Devor

recognize that clinicians working from other treatment approaches have found aspects of the RSM helpful for engaging spirituality in psychotherapy (Boettscher, Sandage, Latin, & Barlow, 2019; Correa & Sandage, 2018).

2. *Theories of relational development.* The RSM frames spirituality through a relational development lens focused on three developmental systems— attachment, differentiation, and intersubjectivity—which we consider central to psychological and spiritual healing and growth. These developmental systems partially overlap in influence, yet also are unique in their developmental emphases and evolutionary functions. The attachment system focuses on trust, security, and exploration through relational regulation. The differentiation system focuses on the identity aspects of self and other and the self-regulation of emotions. Particular attention is paid to how people balance their interpersonal stances in different relational contexts and manage anxiety related to difference to pursue cooperation. The intersubjectivity system focuses on patterns of interaction and their developmental effects, including capacities for intimacy, affect regulation, mutual recognition (in contrast to oppressive power dynamics), and repair of relational ruptures. RSM treatment planning involves textured assessment and intervention strategies across these three developmental systems.

3. *Diversity competence and social justice.* Diversity competence and deep commitments to social justice are core values and capacities within the RSM. As clinicians, clinical supervisors, teachers, and researchers, we need to continue to grow in diversity competence and social justice commitments, which involves an integration of dwelling and seeking. While recognizing the need to respect clients' diverse perspectives on these issues, we also assume growth in these capacities is beneficial for clients, who must also negotiate differences with others in more or less constructive ways. We believe this requires sensitive and humble consideration of clients' spiritual, existential, religious, and theological backgrounds and traditions in intersection with other diversity factors, as well as clients' preferences about how and whether those dynamics might be addressed in treatment. Clinician self-awareness is critical.

4. *Spiritual and existential dynamics as clinically relevant.* Spiritual and existential struggles are common and can negatively affect clients' psychosocial functioning over and above the impact of specific symptoms of mental health distress. Initial empirical evidence suggests spiritual well-being also may be somewhat distinct from psychological well-being, with both forms of well-being positively predicting the psychosocial functioning of clients beyond the influence of symptoms. These findings support the RSM thesis that it is typically necessary to clinically assess and engage with clients relational spirituality dynamics, including the existential, to gain a holistic understanding of their functioning that includes symptoms but also responsibly transcends reductionistic versions of the medical model of mental healthcare.

5. *Suffering–Trauma Matrix.* Suffering and trauma are always existential and necessitate clinical attention to clients' diverse views of both suffering and ultimate meaning within the suffering–trauma matrix (Rambo, 2010; Yansen, 2016). This requires ongoing learning about differing views of suffering, illness causation, and pathways for healing across sociocultural, spiritual, religious, and philosophical traditions, as well as reflection on assumptions embedded within our own perspectives and clinical approaches. Existential themes within suffering and trauma are also diverse, and we offered a heuristic taxonomy of existential themes (see Chapter 4) that may emerge in psychotherapy. Engaging these themes with sensitivity to relational spirituality dynamics can promote meaning-making and developmental growth. In the RSM, we value depth engagement with existential and spiritual dynamics; however, we also highlight the importance of helping clients develop emotion-regulation practices to manage symptoms and what we have called surface-level anxieties as a precursor to deeper developmental work around ontological anxieties.

6. *Dialectic balancing.* Human development and therapeutic change each involve ongoing, dialectical balancing of dwelling and seeking, stability and change. Therefore, spiritual dwelling and seeking are core dialectical themes within the RSM. We like to say relational spirituality is "limbic and liminal" because it involves both our pulls toward familiar relational patterns (limbic dwelling) and periodic activation of movement into unfamiliar territory (liminal seeking) for the sake of potential healing and growth. This shapes our view of therapeutic change as a multifaceted, crucible-like process involving tensions between dwelling and seeking during periods of systemic reorganization or transformation.

7. *Crucible metaphor.* The crucible is a metaphor used within numerous spiritual and religious traditions and psychotherapy theories to depict the intensification of a stressful, anxiety-provoking, and ambiguous process of change. Relational dynamics in and around psychotherapy, including the therapeutic alliance, are key factors in shaping crucibles of change. Crucible themes involve key aspects of necessary developmental growth and differ across clients, thus requiring therapists to adjust their relational style and treatment focus for a given client or client system (see Chapter 3). For crucible work, there must be enough heat and enough containment.

8. *Ongoing therapist formation.* The RSM also outlines a framework for integrating a relational approach to psychotherapy, training/consultation, research, and ongoing therapist formation. Our approach to formation emphasizes (a) therapist self-development and use of self, and (b) relational dynamics and experiential learning in training and consultation. We describe various practices and processes for formation including SERT (spiritual–existential–religious–theological) Groups (Rupert, Moon, & Sandage, 2018). Many clinicians obviously have limited time and resources for ongoing training and consultation, yet we believe the deliberate practice of relational

psychotherapy necessitates relational resources of support and fresh input for clinician well-being, effectiveness, and growth.

9. *Relational ecologies.* Psychotherapeutic practice unfolds in multilevel and multidimensional relational ecologies that impact relational spirituality dynamics (Kehoe, Hassen, & Sandage, 2016). These relational ecologies often include interactions between clients and multiple providers, administrative staff in clinical contexts, third-party payers, referring organizations, and other relational figures with a stake in the therapy process. We described initial empirical evidence that clients' working alliance with administrative staff at our clinic predicted their ratings of treatment progress over and above their working alliance with their primary therapist (Sandage, Moon, et al., 2017). Our RSM suggests it is important to consider the various relational dynamics within the liminal process of therapy that can either provide an effective holding environment or possibly have a negative impact on treatment. Relational ecology awareness also highlights the underrated role of intentional collaboration among (a) clinicians and administrative staff and (b) multiple clinical providers working with the same client system, which requires healthy clinician humility to avoid problematic triangulations and power struggles (Paine, Sandage, Rupert, Devor, & Bronstein, 2015).

10. *Research as relational.* We have argued for the value of both existential and empirical approaches to knowledge and offered a relational understanding of the research process within the RSM. The ongoing use of research is an ethical mandate for clinicians, and we have suggested that research is also part of clinicians' engaging the human seeking system in what we have depicted as open system functioning (at individual and clinic/organization levels) that represents a humble commitment to learning, accountability, and innovation in practice. Clinical research can also represent well-boundaried communication to allow client voices to provide feedback about clinical services to counter clinician tendencies to overrate progress and to provide understanding of other vital therapeutic processes. Disaggregated data analyses can offer attention to diversity dynamics and varying levels of effectiveness with differing client problems and populations. While research could be exploitive of clients, it can also be a form of power-sharing with clients, which further highlights the importance of the relational dynamics within research. Clinical research also typically involves high levels of collaboration at various levels and has the potential to create valuable relational feedback loops between clinicians, scholars, and administrators at multiple systemic levels.

FUTURE RESEARCH DIRECTIONS

Throughout this book, we have built upon bodies of research across numerous fields and have referenced studies from our own lab that have informed the RSM. There are also significant empirical literatures on spirituality and religion in psychotherapy that go well beyond the scope of this book but can be informative for clinicians and researchers interested in this broad and growing area (e.g., Captari et al., 2018; Harris, Randolph, & Gordon, 2016; Hook, Worthington, & Davis, 2012; Pargament, Mahoney, & Shafranske, 2013; Post & Wade, 2009: Shafranske, 2013; Worthington, Hook, Davis, & McDaniel, 2011). We have also noted that there are many approaches to (a) spiritually integrative psychotherapy (see the Introduction to this volume) and (b) relational spirituality (Chapter 2), and we are excited about the plurality of models and thoughtful approaches to spirituality and religion that can be studied in clinical contexts. In this final section, we briefly highlight some directions for future research on the RSM and clinical practice and training. We outline some future research possibilities in the areas of psychotherapy processes and outcomes, client preferences and therapist orientations, clinical training and consultation, and relational ecologies of psychotherapy.

PSYCHOTHERAPY PROCESSES AND OUTCOMES

We need more research, in general, on spirituality and religion in psychotherapy that links therapeutic processes and outcomes in a variety of clinical contexts and with wider sets of presenting problems. This should include both randomized clinical trials (RCTs) and practice-based research. RCTs represent a more widely known methodological approach and have certain advantages for replication and internal validity. However, we are enthusiastic about the growing movement of practice-based research through routine monitoring of clinical practice in naturalistic settings, which can enhance the ecological validity of research in many clinical settings where RCTs and tightly controlled adherence would not be feasible (Castonguay & Muran, 2016). We have also found that implementing practice-based research in our own clinical context has pulled for greater collaboration and bidirectional input from clinicians, researchers, and administrators, and this fits with our relational view of research and practice in the RSM.

As mentioned above (and in Chapter 3), our prior incremental validity research on the RSM has suggested relational spirituality dynamics can predict client psychosocial functioning over and above mental health symptoms. We are currently investigating these RSM-predicted effects over time, and it would be helpful to see various approaches to relational spirituality in clinical practice tested in this way. There are several key research questions that we consider priorities amidst the myriad of potential research directions:

1. *Based on our relational approach to psychotherapy, do positive changes in various dimensions of the therapeutic alliance account for (i.e., mediate) the impact of relational spirituality changes on clinical outcomes?* The majority of clinical studies of spiritually integrative psychotherapy have focused on cognitive behavior approaches, and there is a need to also investigate spiritual dynamics in other kinds of therapeutic approaches and with greater attention to the

therapeutic alliance. We have also suggested movements of dwelling and seeking may be common developmental processes that could occur in a variety of psychotherapeutic approaches; however, this common-factors hypothesis requires empirical testing.

2. *Do changes in various aspects of relational spirituality impact differing kinds of clinical outcomes, such as (a) reductions in mental health symptoms and (b) growth in various forms of well-being?* We consider both symptom reduction and growth in meaning-oriented well-being (Wong, 2011) important goals in psychotherapy, yet we know much less empirically about the latter. It might also be the case that developmental growth and increases in well-being could serve additional relapse prevention functions for clients (Boettscher et al., 2019). Spiritual and religious outcomes can also be particularly important to clients who are strongly committed in those areas, and outcomes have been better for such clients when spirituality and religion are thoughtfully and sensitivity engaged in treatment (Captari et al., 2018; Hook, Worthington, & Davis, 2012). Most specifically to the RSM, we are interested in the impact of positive changes in spiritual dwelling and seeking and the integration of these dimensions over time on the full range of clinical outcomes.

3. *Do positive changes in the three relational development systems (attachment, differentiation, and intersubjectivity) of focus in the RSM also account for (mediate) the impact of relational spirituality changes on clinical outcomes?* These relational development systems can be operationalized in a variety of ways and considered in relation to other prominent constructs we have considered in this book, such as mindfulness, mentalization, and affect regulation.

4. *Do clinical changes in relational spirituality follow different trajectories of change for differing clients?* Prior research at our clinic found evidence of differing trajectories of change over time using person-centered analyses and growth-mixture modeling to identify both linear and curvilinear patters of change for differing subgroups of clients on anxiety, depression, interpersonal conflict, and life satisfaction (Jankowski et al., 2019). This fits the RSM thesis that therapeutic change is often, though not always, nonlinear (Chapter 3). This same study also tested parallel growth models and found that improvements in affect regulation mediated the impact of improved relational functioning on clients' life satisfaction, which highlights the connections between relational functioning and affect regulation on client well-being. We are now testing these different trajectories of change and parallel growth models with relational spirituality factors.

5. *In addition to testing mediators and causal mechanisms of change, what might we learn by testing moderator effects to nuance, diversify, and contextualize our clinical understandings of "what works for whom and under what conditions"?* We need to disaggregate our findings to explore potential moderator effects for different spiritual and religious orientations and traditions and levels of commitment, as well as a wide range of other diversity factors (e.g., race, gender, ethnicity, sexual orientation, gender orientation, socioeconomic factors). Therapeutic

processes over time might also vary for clients with differing relational spirituality profiles; for example, comparing clients that are primarily spiritual seekers versus those scoring high on dwelling and seeking versus those low on both dimensions. Clients scoring high on spiritual struggles or with certain views of suffering may also show unique patterns of change in relational spirituality and clinical and outcomes. Much of the prior research on spirituality and religion in psychotherapy has also focused on the treatment of depression and anxiety, and there is a need for further research on a broader range of clinical problems, including complex and relational forms of trauma and relational problems in couples and families.

6. Finally, numerous virtues (e.g., forgiveness, hope, gratitude, compassion, humility) have been studied within the field of positive psychology. *What might an investigation of virtues (as either mediators or moderators of therapeutic change) add to spiritually integrative psychotherapy research* (see, e.g., Worthington & Sandage, 2016, for a review of research on relational spirituality and forgiveness in application to psychotherapy)? Virtues such as gratitude, forgiveness, and hope (among others) might represent specific forms of positive affect regulation for certain interpersonal situations that rest upon (a) broader affect regulation capacities and (b) relational development capacities. In Chapter 2, we mentioned cross-sectional evidence from our clinic that humility moderated the relationship between religious salience (or commitment) and psychosocial functioning of clients, suggesting humility may be a key virtue necessary to help keep the dynamics of relational spirituality conducive rather than deleterious to positive mental health (Paine, Sandage, Ruffing, & Hill, 2018). We also found reductions in narcissistic symptoms among clients at our clinic during the course of treatment were associated with improvements in social and sexual functioning (Bell, Jankowski, & Sandage, 2018). Forms of relational spirituality that promote narcissism, mania, chronic hostility, or shame would seem to interfere with healthy psychosocial functioning for clients, however these dynamics necessitate further research in a range of clinical contexts and populations.

CLIENT PREFERENCES AND THERAPIST ORIENTATIONS

An important tenet of the RSM is to relationally and sensitively adapt engagement of SERT dynamics in psychotherapy to fit the worldview and treatment goals of specific clients, and this requires careful assessment and clinician self-awareness and flexibility. There is an empirical literature spanning about fifty years investigating client preferences and therapist orientations related to spiritual and religious issues in psychotherapy (Harris, Randolph, & Gordon, 2016; Worthington, Kurusu, McCullough, & Sandage, 1996). A review of this literature shows that a significant percentage of that research has been with students in university settings (sometimes utilizing therapy analogue study designs with students watching a video of counseling rather than directly sampling actual psychotherapy clients) and was often conducted in predominantly Christian contexts in the United States. To date, the available research fits findings at our clinic (see Chapter 1) suggesting that the majority of clients would like to engage spiritual and religious issues in their treatment, and the percentage increases for existential issues. It is not surprising that these effects tend to be much stronger among spiritually and religiously committed clients; however, there are exceptions to this pattern, including clients who may want to process problematic or even traumatic aspects of their spiritual and religious backgrounds. Clients who identify as nonspiritual and nonreligious also often value engagement with existential issues. Yet there is a need for more practice-based research in a variety of clinical contexts exploring clients' differing preferences about engaging SERT issues in treatment, as well as ways these preferences interact with therapists' differing orientations to SERT issues. Most of the prior research is quantitative, and qualitative studies could help reveal thicker and more contextual understandings of clients' SERT preferences. Key research directions in this area include the following:

1. *How do differing therapist orientations to SERT issues interact with differing client preferences over time?* This is clearly a central part of any approach to spiritually integrative psychotherapy. Do client preferences change over the course of treatment (including sometimes wanting more engagement with SERT issues, in other cases less, during different phases of treatment), and does this interact with therapist factors?

2. *How might differing clinical contexts impact client expectations and preferences and therapist orientations to SERT issues?* For example, does it seem to make a difference if a clinic or a specific provider explicitly identifies with a particular spiritual or religious orientation or tradition? How does this impact clients who recognize they differ from that clinic or clinician? What are the differing ways clinics and clinicians navigate spiritual and religious diversity among clients?

3. *How do therapists' orientations to SERT dynamics in psychotherapy interact with and/or differ from various dimensions of the therapeutic alliance?* For example, is sensitivity to clients' SERT perspectives and preferences a unique predictor of clients' ratings of treatment over and above other aspects of the working alliance (e.g., task, goal, bond; Hatcher & Gillaspy, 2006) or embedded within certain aspects of the working alliance? How do therapists negotiate engagement with SERT dynamics in treatment, and then renegotiate these issues following ruptures? Some therapists may be more effective than others in this regard, and so therapist effects may need to be statistically accounted for in examining these questions. Also, can the differentiation-based model presented in Chapter 6 drawing on intercultural and interreligious competence models be used to investigate the impact of differing therapist–client pairings (e.g., therapist in minimization paired with a client in adaptation) on clinical processes and outcomes?

CLINICAL TRAINING AND CONSULTATION

As noted in Chapter 11, the research and applied literature on spirituality and religion in clinical training is very modest and largely originates in Christian-affiliated training programs. The relational and therapist formation emphases in our pluralistic RSM approach to training and consultation leads us to several sets of research questions:

1. *Which training and consultation experiences, resources, and practices prove most helpful to clinicians for growing in capacities for effective, spiritually and religiously competent practice?* How does this differ over the course of a career journey? And how do these issues differ for clinicians from dominant and nondominant groups across various diversity factors? Qualitative and longitudinal designs could be particularly helpful for moving forward understandings of these issues. There are also promising online training resources (Pearce, Pargament, Oxhandler, Vieten, & Wong, 2019) and assessment tools (Oxhandler, 2019) available for training research on spiritual and religious competence.

2. *What are the unique training and consultation needs of experienced clinicians for (a) growing in spiritual and religious competence and (b) avoiding risks for burnout and declining effectiveness over time?* Relatedly, what percentage of licensed clinicians are in regular consultation groups that involve processing the existential and/or spiritual impact of providing clinical services? What factors differentiate consultation groups that prove to be helpful for therapist formation and clinical effectiveness from those that do not? How do these factors interface with the emerging deliberate practice literature (see Chapter 11)?

3. *Is spiritual and religious competence empirically distinct from other clinical capacities, such as cultural humility and multicultural/intercultural competence?* In theory, it seems like there can be unique challenges and strengths in differing diversity domains, so a clinician might be more competent in some areas than others. At the same time, certain relational development capacities may prove foundational to various areas of diversity competence.

4. *Does the finding hold up across various contexts that how clinicians engage spiritual and religious issues in therapy parallels how those issues were approached in their own experiences of psychotherapy?* Sorenson (1994, 1997a) found advanced doctoral students in clinical psychology at a Christian training program tended to approach spiritual and religious issues in their clinical work in ways that paralleled how they reported those issues were engaged in their own personal therapies. This finding makes sense from a relational development perspective, although there are also important possibilities for differentiation in clinician development. This would be a valuable area for further research from an RSM perspective in different contexts.

5. *Can trainee clinicians be clinically effective in relational, depth-oriented psychotherapies (such as the RSM), or do they, as some have suggested, need more highly structured and manualized approaches to treatment?* An initial practice-based study of

trainee cases at our relational psychodynamic clinic found clients tended to improve across a range of symptom and psychosocial functioning outcomes (Paine et al., 2019), and there is also a broader (but limited) literature on the clinical effectiveness of trainees (see Hilsenroth & Diener, 2017; Hilsenroth, Kivlighan, & Slavin-Mulford, 2015; Owen, Wampold, Kopta, Rousmaniere, & Miller, 2016). Trainee effectiveness with spiritual and religious dynamics in various treatment approaches needs further investigation.

RELATIONAL ECOLOGIES OF PSYCHOTHERAPY

The attention to the relational ecologies of psychotherapy in our RSM (Chapters 2 and 11) leads us to numerous questions about the impact of relational and systemic dynamics at multiple levels, and our initial research suggesting clients' alliance dynamics with administrative staff may impact clinical outcomes (Sandage, Moon, et al., 2017) needs further investigation. Numerous other research questions can also be considered in future work, such as

1. *What is the impact of various relational ecology dynamics in clinics and organizations on therapist well-being, burnout, and overall effectiveness?* Does this differ across levels of therapist experience?

2. *Can certain formation-based resources and practices buffer the negative impact of dysfunctional relational ecologies on therapist and client outcomes?* For example, how do administrative and clinical staff work together to repair certain ecological ruptures with clients (e.g., billing or insurance coverage mistakes)?

3. *What are the dynamics and practices of exemplar clinical relational ecologies?* Are such systems particularly good at engaging the relational development systems of focus in the RSM for the sake of effective collaboration and organizational well-being? Can relational ecologies of excellence prevent burnout in a health care environment that at times impedes mental health care resources? What is the relationship between therapist actions promoting a more just mental health care environments and therapist well-being?

4. *Is it more difficult to integrate healthy relational ecology dynamics with explicit engagement of SERT issues in highly spiritually diverse clinical contexts as compared to more spiritually homogenous settings?* Or does this depend upon the differentiation and diversity competence within the organization?

CONCLUSION

We have provided a summary of 10 key sets of ideas from the RSM in application to psychotherapy. This version of the RSM has evolved from earlier versions, and we will continue to develop the model through dialogue with other scholars, clinicians, and clients. We have also outlined what we consider some important future research directions related to the RSM, spiritual and religious competence, and spiritually integrative psychotherapy. We are encouraged by the growing clinical attention and sophistication of research on SERT dynamics in psychotherapy in recent years, and we hope in the years ahead to see clinical scholars and practitioners of various theoretical orientations continue to reflectively engage SERT considerations in ways that ultimately help to heal suffering and promote growth.

REFERENCES

Aarons, G. A. (2004). Mental health provider attitudes toward adoption of evidence-based practice: The Evidence-Based Practice Attitude Scale (EBPAS). *Mental Health Services Research, 6,* 61–74. http://dx.doi.org/10.1023/B:MHSR.0000024351.12294.65

Aarons, G. A., Hurlburt, M., & Horwitz, S. M. (2011). Advancing a conceptual model of evidence-based practice implementation in public service sectors. *Administration and Policy in Mental Health and Mental Health Services Research, 38,* 4–23. http://dx.doi.org/10.1007/s10488-010-0327-7

Abu-Raiya, H., Pargament, K. I., Krause, N., & Ironson, G. (2015). Robust links between religious/spiritual struggles, psychological distress, and well-being in a national sample of American adults. *American Journal of Orthopsychiatry, 85,* 565–575. http://dx.doi.org/10.1037/ort0000084

Ainsworth, M., & Eichberg, C. (1991). Effects on infant-mother attachment of mother's unresolved loss of an attachment figure, or other traumatic experience. In M. Parkes (Ed.), *Attachment across the life cycle* (pp. 160–183). New York, NY: Routledge.

Akhtar, S. (2014). Three pillars of therapeutic attitude. In G. Stavros & S. J. Sandage (Eds.), *The skillful soul of the psychotherapist: The link between spirituality and clinical excellence* (pp. 105–120). Lanham, MD: Rowman & Littlefield.

Albright, C. R. (2006). Spiritual growth, cognition, complexity: Faith as a dynamic process. In J. D. Koss-Choino & P. Hefner (Eds.), *Spiritual transformation and healing: Anthropological, theological, neuroscientific, and clinical perspectives* (pp. 168–186). Lanham, MD: AltaMira.

Al-Haddād, I. (2010). *Counsels of religion.* Louisville, KY: Fons Vitae.

Al-Karam, C. Y. (2018). *Islamically integrated psychotherapy: Uniting faith and professional practice.* West Conshohocken, PA: Templeton Press.

Allen, J. G. (2013). *Restoring mentalizing in attachment relationships: Treating trauma with plain old therapy.* Arlington, VA: American Psychiatric Publishing.

Allen, J. G., Fonagy, P., & Bateman, A. W. (2008). *Mentalizing in clinical practice*. Washington, DC: American Psychiatric Publishing.

Allport, G. W. (1960). *The individual and his religion: A psychological interpretation*. New York, NY: Macmillan.

Almagor, M. (2011). *The functional dialectic system approach to therapy for individuals, couples, and families*. Minneapolis: University of Minnesota Press. http://dx.doi.org/10.5749/minnesota/9780816669554.001.0001

Alperin, R. (2001). Barriers to intimacy: An object relations perspective. *Psychoanalytic Psychology, 18*, 137–156. http://dx.doi.org/10.1037/0736-9735.18.1.137

Amanelahi, A., Tardast, K., & Aslani, K. (2016). Prediction of love trauma syndrome based on the attachment styles and differentiation of self among Ahwaz universities females students whit love breakup experience. *Journal of Psychology, 20*, 310–327.

American Psychiatric Association. (2013). *Diagnostic and statistical manual of mental disorders* (5th ed.). Arlington, VA: Author.

American Psychological Association. (2017). *Ethical principles of psychologists and code of conduct* (2002, Amended June 1, 2010 and January 1, 2017). Retrieved from http://www.apa.org/ethics/code/index.aspx

Ammerman, N. (2013). *Sacred stories, spiritual tribes: Finding religion in everyday life*. New York, NY: Oxford University Press. http://dx.doi.org/10.1093/acprof:oso/9780199896448.001.0001

Aponte, H., & Kissil, K. (2014). If I can grapple with this I can truly be of use in the therapy room: Using the therapist's own emotional struggles to facilitate effective therapy. *Journal of Marital & Family Therapy, 40*, 152–164.

Armstrong, K. (1993). *A history of God: The 4000-year quest of Judaism, Christianity, and Islam*. New York, NY: Alfred A. Knopf.

Aron, L. (2004). God's influence on my psychoanalytic vision and values. *Psychoanalytic Psychology, 21*, 442–451. http://dx.doi.org/10.1037/0736-9735.21.3.442

Aron, L. (2018). Core competency four: Relational dynamic: The there and then and the here and now. In R. E. Barsness (Ed.), *Core competencies of relational psychoanalysis: A guide to practice, study, and research* (pp. 121–141). New York, NY: Routledge.

Aten, J. D., McMinn, M. R., & Worthington, E. L., Jr. (2011). *Spiritually oriented interventions for counseling and psychotherapy*. Washington, DC: American Psychological Association. http://dx.doi.org/10.1037/12313-000

Auerbach, J. S., & Blatt, S. J. (2001). Self-reflexivity, intersubjectivity, and therapeutic change. *Psychoanalytic Psychology, 18*, 427–450. http://dx.doi.org/10.1037/0736-9735.18.3.427

Augustyn, B. D., Hall, T. W., Wang, D. C., & Hill, P. C. (2017). Relational spirituality: An attachment-based model of spiritual development and psychological well-being [Supplemental material]. *Psychology of Religion and Spirituality, 9*, 197–208. http://dx.doi.org/10.1037/rel0000100

Aviv, A. (2010). Where intersubjectivity and group analysis meet. *International Journal of Group Psychotherapy, 60*, 91–109. http://dx.doi.org/10.1521/ijgp.2010.60.1.91

Azari, N. P., Missimer, J., & Seitz, R. J. (2005). Religious experience and emotion: Evidence for distinctive cognitive neural patterns. *International Journal for the Psychology of Religion, 15*, 263–281. http://dx.doi.org/10.1207/s15327582ijpr1504_1

Bailey, K. L., Jones, B. D., Hall, T. W., Wang, D. C., McMartin, J., & Fujikawa, A. M. (2016). Spirituality at a crossroads: A grounded theory of Christian emerging adults [Supplemental material]. *Psychology of Religion and Spirituality, 8,* 99–109. http://dx.doi.org/10.1037/rel0000059

Baird, P. (2016). Spiritual care intervention. In B. Ferrell (Ed.), *Spiritual, religious, and cultural aspects of care* (pp. 29–45). Oxford, England: Oxford University Press.

Bakan, D. (1966). *The duality of human existence: Isolation and communion in Western man.* Boston, MA: Beacon.

Balint, M. (1979). *The basic fault: Therapeutic aspects of regression.* London, England: Tavistock.

Baltes, P. B., & Smith, J. (2008). The fascination of wisdom: Its nature, ontogeny, and function. *Perspectives on Psychological Science, 3,* 56–64. http://dx.doi.org/10.1111/j.1745-6916.2008.00062.x

Barlow, D. H. (2002). *Anxiety and its disorders: The nature and treatment of anxiety and panic* (2nd ed.). New York, NY: Guilford Press.

Barlow, D. H., & Farchione, T. J. (2018). *Applications of the unified protocol for trans-diagnostic treatment of emotional disorders.* New York, NY: Oxford University Press.

Barsness, R. E. (Ed.). (2018). *Core competencies of relational psychoanalysis: A guide to practice, study and research.* New York, NY: Routledge.

Barsness, R. E., & Sorenson, A. (2018). Self-care: Staying connected when things fall apart: The personal and professional life of the analyst. In R. E. Barsness (Ed.), *Core competencies of relational psychoanalysis: A guide to practice, study, and research* (pp. 302–317). New York, NY: Routledge.

Barsness, R. E., & Strawn, B. (2018). Core competency seven: Courageous speech/disciplined spontaneity. In R. E. Barsness (Ed.), *Core competencies of relational psychoanalysis: A guide to practice, study, and research* (pp. 179–200). New York, NY: Routledge.

Bartoli, E. (2007). Religious and spiritual issues in psychotherapy practice: Training the trainer. *Psychotherapy, 44,* 54–65. http://dx.doi.org/10.1037/0033-3204.44.1.54

Basseches, M., & Mascolo, M. (2010). *Psychotherapy as a developmental process.* New York, NY: Routledge.

Bateman, A., & Fonagy, P. (2019). *Handbook of mentalizing in mental health practice* (2nd ed.). Washington, DC: American Psychiatric Publishing.

Bateson, G. (2000). *Steps to an ecology of mind.* Chicago, IL: University of Chicago Press.

Bearse, J. L., McMinn, M. R., Seegobin, W., & Free, K. (2013). Barriers to psychologists seeking mental health care. *Professional Psychology: Research and Practice, 44,* 150–157. http://dx.doi.org/10.1037/a0031182

Beck, R. (2006). Defensive versus existential religion: Is religious defensiveness predictive of worldview defense? *Journal of Psychology and Theology, 34,* 142–153. http://dx.doi.org/10.1177/009164710603400204

Becker, E. (1973). *The denial of death.* New York, NY: Free Press.

Beebe, B. (2004). Faces in relation: A case study. *Psychoanalytic Dialogues, 14,* 1–51. http://dx.doi.org/10.1080/10481881409348771

Beebe, B. (2010). Mother–infant research informs mother–infant treatment. *Clinical Social Work Journal, 38,* 17–36. http://dx.doi.org/10.1007/s10615-009-0256-7

Beebe, B., Knoblauch, S. H., Rustin, J., & Sorter, D. (2003). Introduction: A systems view. *Psychoanalytic Dialogues, 13,* 743–775.

Beebe, B., & Lachmann, F. M. (1994). Representation and internalization in infancy: Three principles of salience. *Psychoanalytic Psychology, 11,* 127–165. http://dx.doi.org/10.1037/h0079530

Beebe, B., Rustin, J., Sorter, D., & Knoblauch, S. (2003). An expanded view of intersubjectivity in infancy and its application to psychoanalysis. *Psychoanalytic Dialogues, 13*, 805–841. http://dx.doi.org/10.1080/10481881309348769

Beebe, B., Sorter, D., Rustin, J., & Knoblauch, S. (2003). A comparison of Meltzoff, Trevarthen, and Stern. *Psychoanalytic Dialogues, 13*, 777–804. http://dx.doi.org/10.1080/10481881309348768

Beidas, K., Edmunds, J., Cannuscio, C., Gallagher, M., Downey, M., & Kendall, P. (2013). Therapist perspectives on the effective elements of consultation following training. *Administration and Policy in Mental Health and Mental Health Services Research, 40*, 507–517.

Bell, C. A., Jankowski, P. J., & Sandage, S. J. (2018). Early treatment narcissism associated with later social and sexual functioning among psychotherapy clients. *Counselling & Psychotherapy Research*. Advance online publication. Retrieved from https://onlinelibrary.wiley.com/doi/10.1002/capr.12199

Benjamin, J. (2004). Beyond doer and done to: An intersubjective view of thirdness. *The Psychoanalytic Quarterly, 73*, 5–46. http://dx.doi.org/10.1002/j.2167-4086.2004.tb00151.x

Benjamin, J. (2018). *Beyond doer and done to: Recognition theory, intersubjectivity, and the Third*. New York, NY: Routledge.

Bennett, M. J. (2004). Becoming interculturally competent. In J. Wurzel (Ed.), *Toward multiculturalism: A reader in multicultural education* (2nd ed., pp. 62–77). Newton, MA: Intercultural Resource Corporation.

Berman, A. (2014). Post-traumatic victimhood and group analytic therapy: Intersubjectivity, empathic witnessing and otherness. *Group Analysis, 47*, 242–256. http://dx.doi.org/10.1177/0533316414545843

Berman, S. L., Weems, C. F., & Stickle, T. R. (2006). Existential anxiety in adolescents: Prevalence, structure, association with psychological symptoms and identity development. *Journal of Youth and Adolescence, 35*, 303–310. http://dx.doi.org/10.1007/s10964-006-9032-y

Berry, K., & Danquah, A. (2015). Attachment-informed psychotherapy for adults: Toward a unifying perspective on practice. *Psychology and Psychotherapy: Theory, Research and Practice, 89*, 15–32. http://dx.doi.org/10.1111/papt.12063

Blaustein, M. E., & Kinniburgh, K. M. (2010). *Treating traumatic stress in children and adolescents: How to foster resilience through attachment, self-regulation, and competency*. New York, NY: Guilford Press.

Bloom, S. (2010). Bridging the black hole of trauma: The evolutionary significance of the arts. *Psychotherapy and Politics International, 8*, 198–212. http://dx.doi.org/10.1002/ppi.223

Boettscher, H. T., Sandage, S. J., Latin, H. M., & Barlow, D. H. (2019). Transdiagnostic treatment for enhancing positive affect and well-being. In J. Gruber (Ed.), *Positive emotion and psychopathology* (pp. 525–538). New York, NY: Oxford University Press.

Bonab, B., Miner, M., & Proctor, M. (2013). Attachment to God in Islamic spirituality. *Journal of Muslim Mental Health, 7*, 1–28.

Boston Change Process Study Group. (2013). Enactment and the emergence of new relational organization. *Journal of the American Psychoanalytic Association, 61*, 727–749. http://dx.doi.org/10.1177/0003065113496636

Bowen, M. (1978). *Family therapy in clinical practice*. New York, NY: Jason Aronson.

Bowlby, J. (1980). *Attachment and loss: Loss, sadness and depression* (Vol. 3). New York, NY: Basic Books.

Bowlby, J. (1982). *Attachment and loss* (Vol. 1). New York, NY: Basic Books. (Original work published 1969)

Bowlby, J. (1988a). Developmental psychiatry comes of age. *The American Journal of Psychiatry, 145*(1), 1–10. http://dx.doi.org/10.1176/ajp.145.1.1

Bowlby, J. (1988b). *A secure base: Parent-child attachment and healthy human development.* New York, NY: Basic Books.

Boyd-Franklin, N. (2010). Incorporating spirituality and religion into the treatment of African-American clients. *The Counseling Psychologist, 38,* 976–1000. http://dx.doi.org/10.1177/0011000010374881

Brattland, H., Koksvik, J. M., Burkeland, O., Gråwe, R. W., Klöckner, C., Linaker, O. M., . . . Iversen, V. C. (2018). The effects of routine outcome monitoring (ROM) on therapy outcomes in the course of an implementation process: A randomized clinical trial. *Journal of Counseling Psychology, 65,* 1–11. http://dx.doi.org/10.1037/cou0000286

Bravo, A. J., Pearson, M. R., & Stevens, L. E. (2016). Making religiosity person-centered: A latent profile analysis of religiosity and psychological health outcomes. *Personality and Individual Differences, 88,* 160–169. http://dx.doi.org/10.1016/j.paid.2015.08.049

Bregman, L. (2014). *The ecology of spirituality: Meanings, virtues, and practices in a post-religious age.* Waco, TX: Baylor University Press.

Bretherton, I., & Main, M. (2000). Mary Dinsmore Salter Ainsworth (1913–1999): Obituary. *American Psychologist, 55,* 1148–1149. http://dx.doi.org/10.1037/0003-066X.55.10.1148

Bromberg, P. M. (2003). Something wicked this way comes. Trauma, dissociation, and conflict: The space where psychoanalysis, cognitive science and neuroscience overlap. *Psychoanalytic Psychology, 20,* 558–574. http://dx.doi.org/10.1037/0736-9735.20.3.558

Bromberg, P. M. (2006). *Awakening the dreamer: Clinical journeys.* New York, NY: Analytic Press.

Bromberg, P. M. (2009). Truth, human relatedness, and the analytic process: An interpersonal/relational perspective. *The International Journal of Psychoanalysis, 90,* 347–361. http://dx.doi.org/10.1111/j.1745-8315.2009.00137.x

Bromberg, P. M. (2011). *The shadow of the tsunami: Trauma and the growth of the relational mind.* New York, NY: Routledge.

Bronfenbrenner, U. (1979). *The ecology of human development: Experiments by nature and design.* Cambridge, MA: Harvard University Press.

Brown, D., Rodgers, Y. H., & Kapadia, K. (2008). Multicultural considerations for the application of attachment theory. *American Journal of Psychotherapy, 62,* 353–363. http://dx.doi.org/10.1176/appi.psychotherapy.2008.62.4.353

Brugué, M. S., & Burriel, M. P. (2016). Outlining the windows of achievement of intersubjective milestones in typically developing toddlers. *Infant Mental Health Journal, 37,* 356–371. http://dx.doi.org/10.1002/imhj.21576

Bryant, A. N., & Astin, H. S. (2008). The correlates of spiritual struggle during the college years. *Journal of Higher Education, 79,* 1–27. http://dx.doi.org/10.1353/jhe.2008.0000

Bucci, W. (2002). The referential process, consciousness, and the sense of self. *Psychoanalytic Inquiry, 22,* 766–793. http://dx.doi.org/10.1080/07351692209349017

Burke, B., Martens, A., & Faucher, E. (2010). Two decades of terror management theory: A meta-analysis of mortality salience research. *Personality and Social Psychology Review, 14,* 155–195. http://dx.doi.org/10.1177/1088868309352321

Burlingame, G. M., Strauss, B., & Joyce, A. S. (2013). Small group treatment: Evidence for effectiveness and mechanisms of change. In M. J. Lambert (Ed.), *Bergin & Garfield's handbook of psychotherapy and behavior change* (6th ed., pp. 640–689). New York, NY: Wiley.

Buser, J. K., & Gibson, S. (2014). Differentiation and eating disorder symptoms among males. *The Family Journal, 22,* 17–25. http://dx.doi.org/10.1177/1066480713504903

Captari, L. E., Hook, J. N., Hoyt, W., Davis, D. E., McElroy-Heltzel, S. E., & Worthington, E. L., Jr. (2018). Integrating clients' religion and spirituality within psychotherapy: A comprehensive meta-analysis. *Journal of Clinical Psychology, 74,* 1938–1951. http://dx.doi.org/10.1002/jclp.22681

Cashwell, C. S., Myers, J. E., & Shurts, W. M. (2004). Using the developmental counseling and therapy model to work with a client in spiritual bypass: Some preliminary considerations. *Journal of Counseling & Development, 82,* 403–409. http://dx.doi.org/10.1002/j.1556-6678.2004.tb00327.x

Cashwell, C. S., & Young, J. S. (Eds.). (2014). *Integrating spirituality and religion into counseling: A guide to competent practice* (2nd ed.). Alexandria, VA: American Counseling Association.

Cassell, E. (2004). *The nature of suffering and the goals of medicine.* New York, NY: Oxford University Press. http://dx.doi.org/10.1093/acprof:oso/9780195156164.001.0001

Castonguay, L. G. (2013). Psychotherapy outcome: An issue worth re-revisiting 50 years later. *Psychotherapy, 50,* 52–67. http://dx.doi.org/10.1037/a0030898

Castonguay, L. G., & Muran, J. C. (Eds.). (2016). *Practice-oriented research in psychotherapy: Building partnerships between clinicians and researchers.* New York, NY: Routledge.

Cernero, J., Strawn, B. D., & Abernethy, A. D. (2017). Embodied grief and primary metaphor: Towards a new paradigm for integrative bereavement groups. *Journal of Psychology and Christianity, 36,* 325–333. Retrieved from http://search.ebscohost.com.ezproxy.bu.edu/login.aspx?direct=true&db=psyh&AN=2018-15699-006&site=ehost-live&scope=site

Chang, S. H. (2018). Testing a model of codependency for college students in Taiwan based on Bowen's concept of differentiation. *International Journal of Psychology, 53,* 107–116. http://dx.doi.org/10.1002/ijop.12271

Chazan, L. (2015). "Teaching" the therapeutic alliance Part 2. Treating patients, supporting trainees: Towards a broader view of psychotherapy training. *Australasian Psychiatry, 23,* 581–583. http://dx.doi.org/10.1177/1039856215593398

Cheston, S. E., Piedmont, R. L., Eanes, B., & Lavin, L. P. (2003). Changes in clients' images of God over the course of outpatient therapy. *Counseling and Values, 47,* 96–108. http://dx.doi.org/10.1002/j.2161-007X.2003.tb00227.x

Choi, H. (2015). *A postcolonial self: Korean immigrant theology and church.* Albany: SUNY Press.

Chow, D. L., Miller, S. D., Seidel, J. A., Kane, R. T., Thornton, J. A., & Andrews, W. P. (2015). The role of deliberate practice in the development of highly effective psychotherapists. *Psychotherapy, 52,* 337–345. http://dx.doi.org/10.1037/pst0000015

Chung, M. C., Chung, C., & Easthope, Y. (2000). Traumatic stress and death anxiety among community residents exposed to an aircraft crash. *Death Studies, 24,* 689–704. http://dx.doi.org/10.1080/074811800750036578

Clay, R. A. (2018, February). Are you burned out? Here are signs and what you can do about them. *Monitor on Psychology, 49,* 30.

Cloitre, M., Garvert, D. W., Weiss, B., Carlson, E. B., & Bryant, R. A. (2014). Distinguishing PTSD, complex PTSD, and borderline personality disorder: A latent class analysis. *European Journal of Psychotraumatology, 5*, article 25097. Advance online publication. http://dx.doi.org/10.3402/ejpt.v5.25097

Cohen, A. B., Hall, D. E., Koenig, H. G., & Meador, K. G. (2005). Social versus individual motivation: Implications for normative definitions of religious orientation. *Personality and Social Psychology Review, 9*, 48–61. http://dx.doi.org/10.1207/s15327957pspr0901_4

Cohen, A. B., & Hill, P. C. (2007). Religion as culture: Religious individualism and collectivism among American Catholics, Jews, and Protestants. *Journal of Personality, 75*, 709–742. http://dx.doi.org/10.1111/j.1467-6494.2007.00454.x

Cohen, A. B., & Johnson, K. A. (2017). The relation between religion and well-being. *Applied Research in Quality of Life, 12*, 533–547. http://dx.doi.org/10.1007/s11482-016-9475-6

Cohen, B. D. (2000). Intersubjectivity and narcissism in group psychotherapy: How feedback works. *International Journal of Group Psychotherapy, 50*, 163–179. http://dx.doi.org/10.1080/00207284.2000.11490996

Cook, K. V., Kimball, C. N., Leonard, K. C., & Boyatzis, C. J. (2014). The complexity of quest in emerging adults' religiosity, well-being, and identity. *Journal for the Scientific Study of Religion, 53*, 73–89. http://dx.doi.org/10.1111/jssr.12086

Cooper, J. A., & McNair, L. (2015). How to distinguish research from quality improvement. *Journal of Empirical Research on Human Research Ethics, 10*, 209–210. http://dx.doi.org/10.1177/1556264615575513

Cooper, S. H. (2000). *Objects of hope: Exploring possibility and limit in psychoanalysis.* Hillsdale, NJ: Analytic Press.

Cornish, M. A., & Wade, N. G. (2010). Spirituality and religion in group counseling: A literature review with practice guidelines. *Professional Psychology: Research and Practice, 41*, 398–404. http://dx.doi.org/10.1037/a0020179

Cornish, M. A., Wade, N. G., & Knight, M. A. (2013). Understanding group therapists' use of spiritual and religious interventions in group therapy. *International Journal of Group Psychotherapy, 63*, 572–591. http://dx.doi.org/10.1521/ijgp.2013.63.4.572

Correa, J., & Sandage, S. J. (2018). Relational spirituality as scaffolding for cognitive-behavioral therapy: A case study of spirituality in clinical practice. *Spirituality in Clinical Practice, 5*, 54–63. http://dx.doi.org/10.1037/scp0000155

Costello, P. C. (2013). *Attachment-based psychotherapy: Helping patients develop adaptive capacities.* Washington, DC: American Psychological Association.

Cozolino, L. (2017). *The neuroscience of psychotherapy: Healing the social brain.* New York, NY: W. W. Norton.

Cozolino, L. J., & Santos, E. N. (2014). Why we need therapy—and why it works: A neuroscientific perspective. *Smith College Studies in Social Work, 84*, 157–177. http://dx.doi.org/10.1080/00377317.2014.923630

Cragun, C. L., & Friedlander, M. L. (2012). Experiences of Christian clients in secular psychotherapy: A mixed-methods investigation. *Journal of Counseling Psychology, 59*, 379–391. http://dx.doi.org/10.1037/a0028283

Crittenden, P. M., Farnfield, S., Landini, A., & Grey, B. (2013). Assessing attachment for family court decision making. *Journal of Forensic Practice, 15*, 237–248. http://dx.doi.org/10.1108/JFP-08-2012-0002

Daly, K. D., & Mallinckrodt, B. (2009). Experienced therapists' approach to psychotherapy for adults with attachment avoidance or attachment anxiety. *Journal of Counseling Psychology, 56*, 549–563. http://dx.doi.org/10.1037/a0016695

Danziger, E. (2013). Conventional wisdom: Imagination, obedience and inter-subjectivity. *Language & Communication, 33,* 251–262. http://dx.doi.org/10.1016/j.langcom.2013.06.002

Davidsen, A. S., & Fosgerau, C. F. (2015). Grasping the process of implicit mentalization. *Theory & Psychology, 25,* 434–454. http://dx.doi.org/10.1177/0959354315580605

Davis, D. E., DeBlaere, C., Owen, J., Hook, J. N., Rivera, D. P., Choe, E., . . . Placeres, V. (2018). The multicultural orientation framework: A narrative review. *Psychotherapy, 55,* 89–100. http://dx.doi.org/10.1037/pst0000160

Davis, D. E., Hook, J. N., Van Tongeren, D. R., Gartner, A. L., & Worthington, E. L., Jr. (2012). Can religion promote virtue? A more stringent test of the model of relational spirituality and forgiveness. *The International Journal for the Psychology of Religion, 22,* 252–266. http://dx.doi.org/10.1080/10508619.2011.646229

Davis, D. E., Van Tongeren, D. R., Hook, J. N., Davis, E. B., Worthington, E. L., & Foxman, S. (2014). Relational spirituality and forgiveness: Appraisals that may hinder forgiveness. *Psychology of Religion and Spirituality, 6,* 102–112. http://dx.doi.org/10.1037/a0033638

Davis, E. B., Cuthbert, A. D., Hays, L. W., Aten, J. D., Van Tongeren, D. R., & Hook, J. N. . . . Boan, D. (2016). Using qualitative and mixed methods to study relational spirituality. *Psychology of Religion and Spirituality, 8,* 92–98. http://dx.doi.org/10.1037/rel0000046

Davis, E. B., Granqvist, P., & Sharp, C. (2018). Theistic relational spirituality: Development, dynamics, health, and transformation. *Psychology of Religion and Spirituality.* Advance online publication. http://dx.doi.org/10.1037/rel0000219

de Castro, J. M. (2017). A model of enlightened/mystical/awakened experience. *Psychology of Religion and Spirituality, 9,* 34–45. http://dx.doi.org/10.1037/rel0000037

Dein, S., Cook, C. C. H., & Koenig, H. (2012). Religion, spirituality, and mental health: Current controversies and future directions. *Journal of Nervous and Mental Disease, 200,* 852–855. http://dx.doi.org/10.1097/NMD.0b013e31826b6dle

Desrosiers, A., Kelley, B. S., & Miller, L. (2011). Parent and peer relationships and relational spirituality in adolescents and young adults. *Psychology of Religion and Spirituality, 3,* 39–54. http://dx.doi.org/10.1037/a0020037

Desrosiers, A., & Miller, L. (2007). Relational spirituality and depression in adolescent girls. *Journal of Clinical Psychology, 63,* 1021–1037. http://dx.doi.org/10.1002/jclp.20409

DeYoung, P. (2015). *Relational psychotherapy: A primer* (2nd ed.). New York, NY: Routledge. http://dx.doi.org/10.4324/9781315723709

Dimaggio, G. (2006). Changing the dialogue between self voices during psychotherapy. *Journal of Psychotherapy Integration, 16,* 313–345. http://dx.doi.org/10.1037/1053-0479.16.3.313

Doran, J. M. (2016). The working alliance: Where have we been, where are we going? *Psychotherapy Research, 26,* 146–163. http://dx.doi.org/10.1080/10503307.2014.954153

Doran, J. M., Safran, J. D., & Muran, J. C. (2016). The Alliance Negotiation Scale: A psychometric investigation. *Psychological Assessment, 28,* 885–897. http://dx.doi.org/10.1037/pas0000222

Doran, J. M., Safran, J. D., & Muran, J. C. (2017). An investigation of the relationship between the Alliance Negotiation Scale and psychotherapy process and outcome. *Journal of Clinical Psychology, 73*, 449–465. http://dx.doi.org/10.1002/jclp.22340

Douglas, A. N., Jimenez, S., Lin, H.-J., & Frisman, L. K. (2008). Ethnic differences in the effects of spiritual well-being on long-term psychological and behavioral outcomes within a sample of homeless women. *Cultural Diversity and Ethnic Minority Psychology, 14*, 344–352. http://dx.doi.org/10.1037/1099-9809.14.4.344

Dueck, A., & Reimer, K. (2009). *A peaceable psychology: Christian therapy in a world of many cultures.* Grand Rapids, MI: Brazos Press.

Dupré, L. (1989). Unio mystica: The state and the experience. In M. Idel & B. McGinn (Eds.), *Mystical union in Judaism, Christianity, and Islam: An ecumenical dialogue* (pp. 3–23). New York, NY: Continuum.

Duvall, N. D. (2000, October). *Unconscious theology and spirituality.* Presentation at the Institute for Spiritual Formation, Biola University, La Mirada, CA.

Eason, E. A. (2009). Diversity and group theory, practice, and research. *International Journal of Group Psychotherapy, 59*, 563–574. http://dx.doi.org/10.1521/ijgp.2009.59.4.563

Edwards, K., Hall, T., Slater, W., & Hill, J. (2011). The multidimensional structure of the quest construct. *Journal of Psychology and Theology, 39*, 87–110. http://dx.doi.org/10.1177/009164711103900201

Eliade, M. (1959). *The sacred and the profane: The nature of religion.* New York, NY: Harcourt, Brace & World.

Epstein, M. (2013). *The trauma of everyday life.* New York, NY: Penguin Press.

Erickson, P. (2008). *Ethnomedicine.* Long Grove, IL: Waveland Press.

Evans, W. R., Stanley, M. A., Barrera, T. L., Exline, J. J., Pargament, K. I., & Teng, E. J. (2018). Morally injurious events and psychological distress among veterans: Examining the mediating role of religious and spiritual struggles. *Psychological Trauma: Theory, Research, Practice and Policy, 10*, 360–367. http://dx.doi.org/10.1037/tra0000347

Exline, J. J., & Grubbs, J. (2011). "If I tell others about my anger toward God, how will they respond?" Predictors, associated behaviors, and outcomes in an adult sample. *Journal of Psychology and Theology, 39*, 304–315. http://dx.doi.org/10.1177/009164711103900402

Exline, J. J., Homolka, S. J., & Harriott, V. A. (2016). Divine struggles: Links with body image concerns, binging, and compensatory behaviours around eating. *Mental Health, Religion & Culture, 19*, 8–22. http://dx.doi.org/10.1080/13674676.2015.1087977

Exline, J. J., Pargament, K. I., Grubbs, J. B., & Yali, A. M. (2014). The religious and spiritual struggles scale: Development and initial validation. *Psychology of Religion and Spirituality, 6*, 208–222. http://dx.doi.org/10.1037/a0036465

Fadiman, A. (2012). *The spirit catches you and you fall down: A Hmong child, her American doctors, and the collision of two cultures.* New York, NY: Farrar, Straus and Giroux.

Falb, M. D., & Pargament, K. I. (2012). Relational mindfulness, spirituality, and the therapeutic bond. *Asian Journal of Psychiatry, 5*, 351–354. http://dx.doi.org/10.1016/j.ajp.2012.07.008

Fanon, F. (1963). *The wretched of the earth.* New York, NY: Grove Press.

Fanon, F. (1967). *Black skin, white masks.* New York, NY: Grove Press.

Farkas, C., Olhaberry, M., Santelices, M., & Cordella, P. (2017). Interculturality and early attachment: A comparison of urban/non-mapuche and rural/mapuche mother–baby dyads in chile. *Journal of Child and Family Studies, 26,* 205–216. http://dx.doi.org/10.1007/s10826-016-0530-6

Faver, C. A. (2004). Relational spirituality and social caregiving. *Social Work, 49,* 241–249. http://dx.doi.org/10.1093/sw/49.2.241

Fayek, A. (2004). Islam and its effect on my practice of psychoanalysis. *Psychoanalytic Psychology, 21,* 452–457. http://dx.doi.org/10.1037/0736-9735.21.3.452

Feder, A., Ahmad, S., Lee, E. J., Morgan, J. E., Singh, R., Smith, B. W., . . . Charney, D. S. (2013). Coping and PTSD symptoms in Pakistani earthquake survivors: Purpose in life, religious coping and social support. *Journal of Affective Disorders, 147,* 156–163. http://dx.doi.org/10.1016/j.jad.2012.10.027

Ferreira, L. C., Narciso, I., Novo, R. F., & Pereira, C. R. (2014). Predicting couple satisfaction: The role of differentiation of self, sexual desire and intimacy in heterosexual individuals. *Sexual and Relationship Therapy, 29,* 390–404. http://dx.doi.org/10.1080/14681994.2014.957498

Ferreira, L. C., Narciso, I., Novo, R. F., & Pereira, C. R. (2016). Partners' similarity in differentiation of self is associated with higher sexual desire: A quantitative dyadic study. *Journal of Sex & Marital Therapy, 42,* 635–647. http://dx.doi.org/10.1080/0092623X.2015.1113584

Firestone, R., Firestone, L., & Catlett, J. (2013). *The self under siege: A therapeutic model for differentiation.* New York, NY: Routledge.

Fishbane, M. (2008). *Sacred attunement: A Jewish theology.* Chicago, IL: University of Chicago Press. http://dx.doi.org/10.7208/chicago/9780226251745.001.0001

Flanagan, K. S., Pressley, J. D., Davis, E. B., Aten, J. D., Sanders, M., Carter, J. C., . . . Kent, J. (2013). Spiritual formation training in the Wheaton College PsyD Program: Nurturing the growth of servant-oriented practitioner-scholars. *Journal of Psychology and Christianity, 32,* 340–351.

Flores, P. J. (2010). Group psychotherapy and neuro-plasticity: An attachment theory perspective. *International Journal of Group Psychotherapy, 60,* 546–570. http://dx.doi.org/10.1521/ijgp.2010.60.4.546

Flores, P. J., & Porges, S. W. (2017). Group psychotherapy as a neural exercise: Bridging polyvagal theory and attachment theory. *International Journal of Group Psychotherapy, 67,* 202–222. http://dx.doi.org/10.1080/00207284.2016.1263544

Flückiger, C., Del Re, A. C., Wampold, B. E., & Horvath, A. O. (2018). The alliance in adult psychotherapy: A meta-analytic synthesis. *Psychotherapy, 55,* 316–340. Advance online publication. http://dx.doi.org/10.1037/pst0000172

Fonagy, P., & Allison, E. (2014). The role of mentalizing and epistemic trust in the therapeutic relationship. *Psychotherapy, 51,* 372–380. http://dx.doi.org/10.1037/a0036505

Fonagy, P., Campbell, C., & Luyten, P. (2017). Mentalizing. In S. N. Gold (Ed.), *APA handbook of trauma psychology: Foundations in knowledge* (pp. 373–388). Washington, DC: American Psychological Association. http://dx.doi.org/10.1037/0000019-019

Fonagy, P., Luyten, P., Allison, E., & Campbell, C. (2017). What we have changed our minds about: Part 2. Borderline personality disorder, epistemic trust and the developmental significance of social communication. *Borderline Personality Disorder and Emotion Dysregulation, 4,* article 9. http://dx.doi.org/10.1186/s40479-017-0062-8

Fossella, T. (2011, Spring). Human nature, Buddha nature: An interview with John Welwood. *Tricycle: The Buddhist Review, 20*(3), 43–47, 102–104.

Foucault, M. (1994). *The birth of the clinic: An archaeology of medical perception*. New York, NY: Vintage Books. (Original work published 1963)

Fowler, J. W. (1981). *Stages of faith: The psychology of human development and the quest for meaning*. San Francisco, CA: Harper & Row.

Fowler, J. W. (1995). *Will our children have faith?* Toronto, Ontario, Canada: John Westerhoff.

Fox, J., Cashwell, C. S., & Picciotto, G. (2017). The opiate of the masses: Measuring spiritual bypass and its relationship to spirituality, religion, mindfulness, psychological distress, and personality. *Spirituality in Clinical Practice, 4*, 274–287. http://dx.doi.org/10.1037/scp0000141

Frank, J. D., & Frank, J. B. (1993). *Persuasion and healing: A comparative study of psychotherapy* (3rd ed.). Baltimore, MD: Johns Hopkins University Press.

Fraley, R. C. (2019). Attachment in adulthood: Recent developments, emerging debates, and future directions. *Annual Review of Psychology, 70*, 401–422. http://dx.doi.org/10.1146/annurev-psych-010418-102813

Fraley, R. C., Hudson, N. W., Heffernan, M. E., & Segal, N. (2015). Are adult attachment styles categorical or dimensional? A taxometric analysis of general and relationship-specific attachment orientations. *Journal of Personality and Social Psychology, 109*, 354–368. http://dx.doi.org/10.1037/pspp0000027

Fraley, R. C., & Roisman, G. I. (2019). The development of adult attachment styles: Four lessons. *Current Opinion in Psychology, 25*, 26–30. http://dx.doi.org/10.1016/j.copsyc.2018.02.008

Frankel, E. (2003). *Sacred therapy: Jewish spiritual teachings on emotional healing and inner wholeness*. Boston, MA: Shambhala.

Frankfurt, S., Frazier, P., Syed, M., & Jung, K. R. (2016). Using group-based trajectory and growth mixture modeling to identify classes of change trajectories. *The Counseling Psychologist, 44*, 622–660. http://dx.doi.org/10.1177/0011000016658097

Frankl, V. (1959). *From death-camp to existentialism: A psychiatrist's path to a new therapy*. Boston, MA: Beacon Press.

Freedman, J., & Combs, G. (1996). *Narrative therapy: The social construction of preferred realities*. New York, NY: W. W. Norton.

Friedman, E. H. (1985). *Generation to generation: Family process in church and synagogue*. New York, NY: Guilford Press.

Fromm, E. (1941). *Escape from freedom*. New York, NY: Avon Books.

Gallagher, S. (2014). In your face: Transcendence in embodied interaction. *Frontiers in Human Neuroscience, 8*, 495. http://dx.doi.org/10.3389/fnhum.2014.00495

Geertz, C. (1973). *The interpretation of cultures: Selected essays*. New York, NY: Basic Books.

Gelo, O. C., & Salvatore, S. (2016). A dynamic systems approach to psychotherapy: A meta-theoretical framework for explaining psychotherapy change processes. *Journal of Counseling Psychology, 63*, 379–395. http://dx.doi.org/10.1037/cou0000150

Geniusas, S. (2013). On Nietzsche's genealogy and Husserl's genetic phenomenology. In C. Daigle & É. Boublil (Eds.), *Nietzsche and phenomenology: Power, life, subjectivity* (pp. 44–60). Bloomington: Indiana University Press.

Gergen, K. J. (2009). *Relational being: Beyond self and community*. Oxford, England: Oxford University Press.

Ghaemi, S. N. (2010). *The rise and fall of the Biopsychosocial Model: Reconciling art and science in psychiatry*. Baltimore, MD: Johns Hopkins University Press.

Giladi, L., & Bell, T. (2013). Protective factors for intergenerational transmission of trauma among second and third generation holocaust survivors. *Psychological Trauma: Theory, Research, Practice, and Policy, 5,* 384–391. http://dx.doi.org/10.1037/a0028455

Goldberg, S. B., Rousmaniere, T., Miller, S. D., Whipple, J., Nielsen, S. L., Hoyt, W. T., & Wampold, B. E. (2016). Do psychotherapists improve with time and experience? A longitudinal analysis of outcomes in a clinical setting. *Journal of Counseling Psychology, 63,* 1–11. http://dx.doi.org/10.1037/cou0000131

Gomez, R., & Fisher, J. W. (2003). Domains of spiritual well-being and development and validation of the Spiritual Well-Being Questionnaire. *Personality and Individual Differences, 35,* 1975–1991. http://dx.doi.org/10.1016/S0191-8869(03)00045-X

Gonsiorek, J. C., Richards, P. S., Pargament, K. I., & McMinn, M. R. (2009). Ethical challenges and opportunities at the edge: Incorporating spirituality and religion into psychotherapy. *Professional Psychology: Research and Practice, 40,* 385–395. http://dx.doi.org/10.1037/a0016488

Gottman, J. M. (2011). *The science of trust: Emotional attunement for couples.* New York, NY: W. W. Norton.

Grace, G. (1994). Urban education and the culture of contentment: The politics, culture and economics of inner-city schooling. In N. Stromquist (Ed.), *Education in urban areas: Cross-national dimensions* (pp. 45–59). Westport, CT: Praeger.

Granqvist, P., & Kirkpatrick, L. A. (2004). Religious conversion and perceived childhood attachment: A meta-analysis. *International Journal for the Psychology of Religion, 14,* 223–250. http://dx.doi.org/10.1207/s15327582ijpr1404_1

Granqvist, P., & Kirkpatrick, L. A. (2013). Religion, spirituality, and attachment. In K. I. Pargament, J. J. Exline, & J. W. Jones (Eds.), *APA handbook of psychology, religion, and spirituality: Vol. 1. Context, theory, and research* (pp. 139–155). Washington, DC: American Psychological Association.

Granqvist, P., & Kirkpatrick, L. A. (2016). Attachment and religious representations and behavior. In J. Cassidy & P. R. Shaver (Eds.), *Handbook of attachment: Theory, research, and clinical applications* (3rd ed., pp. 917–940). New York, NY: Guilford Press.

Granqvist, P., & Main, M. (2017). *The Religious Attachment Interview scoring and classification system.* Unpublished manuscript, Stockholm University and University of California, Berkeley.

Greenberg, L. S. (2012). Emotions, the great captains of our lives: Their role in the process of change in psychotherapy. *American Psychologist, 67,* 697–707. http://dx.doi.org/10.1037/a0029858

Griffith, J. L. (2011). *Religion that heals, religion that harms: A guide for clinical practice.* New York, NY: Guilford Press.

Groark, K. P. (2013). Toward a cultural phenomenology of intersubjectivity: The extended relational field of the Tzotzil Maya of highland Chiapas, Mexico. *Language & Communication, 33,* 278–291. http://dx.doi.org/10.1016/j.langcom.2011.10.003

Grosch, W. N., & Olsen, D. C. (2000). Clergy burnout: An integrative approach. *Journal of Clinical Psychology, 56,* 619–632. http://dx.doi.org/10.1002/(SICI)1097-4679(200005)56:5<619::AID-JCLP4>3.0.CO;2-2

Grossman, F. K., Spinazzola, J., Zucker, C., & Hopper, E. (2017). Treating adult survivors of childhood emotional abuse and neglect: A new framework. *American Journal of Orthopsychiatry, 87,* 86–93. http://dx.doi.org/10.1037/ort0000225

Guerin, P., Fogarty, T. F., Fay, L. F., & Kautoo, J. G. (1996). *Working with relationship triangles: The one-two-three of psychotherapy*. New York, NY: Guilford Press.

Hager, D. (1992). Chaos and growth. *Psychotherapy: Theory, Research, Practice, Training, 29*, 378–384. http://dx.doi.org/10.1037/h0088539

Hainlen, R., Jankowski, P. J., Paine, D. R., & Sandage, S. J. (2016). Adult attachment and well-being: Dimensions of differentiation of self as mediators. *Contemporary Family Therapy: An International Journal, 38*, 172–183. http://dx.doi.org/10.1007/s10591-015-9359-1

Hale-Smith, A., Park, C. L., & Edmondson, D. (2012). Measuring beliefs about suffering: Development of the views of suffering scale. *Psychological Assessment, 24*, 855–866. http://dx.doi.org/10.1037/a0027399

Halevi, E., & Idisis, Y. (2018). Who helps the helper? Differentiation of self as an indicator for resisting vicarious traumatization. *Psychological Trauma: Theory, Research, Practice, and Policy, 10*, 698–705. http://dx.doi.org/10.1037/tra0000318

Hall, T. W. (2004). Christian spirituality and mental health: A relational spirituality paradigm for empirical research. *Journal of Psychology and Christianity, 23*, 66–81.

Hall, T. W. (2007). Psychoanalysis, attachment, and spirituality Part I: The emergence of two relational traditions. *Journal of Psychology and Theology, 35*, 14–28. http://dx.doi.org/10.1177/009164710703500102

Hall, T. W. (2014). *Relational Spirituality Interview.* Unpublished semistructured interview, Biola University, La Mirada, CA.

Hall, T. W., & Edwards, K. J. (2002). The spiritual assessment inventory: A theistic model and measure for assessing spiritual development. *Journal for the Scientific Study of Religion, 41*, 341–357. http://dx.doi.org/10.1111/1468-5906.00121

Hall, T. W., & Fujikawa, A. M. (2013). God image and the sacred. In K. I. Pargament, J. J. Exline, & J. W. Jones (Eds.), *APA handbook of psychology, religion, and spirituality: Vol. 1. Context, theory, and research* (pp. 277–292). Washington, DC: American Psychological Association. http://dx.doi.org/10.1037/14045-015

Hall, T. W., Fujikawa, A., Halcrow, S. R., Hill, P. C., & Delaney, H. (2009). Attachment to God and implicit spirituality: Clarifying correspondence and compensation models. *Journal of Psychology and Theology, 37*, 227–244. http://dx.doi.org/10.1177/009164710903700401

Hamilton, N. G. (1990). *Self and others: Object relations theory in practice*. Lanham, MD: Jason Aronson.

Hammer, M. R. (2005). The Intercultural Conflict Style Inventory: A conceptual framework and measure of intercultural conflict resolution approaches. *International Journal of Intercultural Relations, 29*, 675–695. http://dx.doi.org/10.1016/j.ijintrel.2005.08.010

Hammer, M. R. (2011). Additional cross-cultural validity testing of the Intercultural Development Inventory. *International Journal of Intercultural Relations, 35*, 474–487. http://dx.doi.org/10.1016/j.ijintrel.2011.02.014

Hammermeister, J., Flint, M., Havens, J., & Peterson, M. (2001). Psychosocial and health-related characteristics of religious well-being. *Psychological Reports, 89*, 589–594. http://dx.doi.org/10.2466/pr0.2001.89.3.589

Hanh, T. N. (2001). *Anger: Wisdom for cooling the flames*. New York, NY: Riverhead Books.

Hanks, W. F. (2013). Counterparts: Co-presence and ritual intersubjectivity. *Language & Communication, 33*, 263–277. http://dx.doi.org/10.1016/j.langcom.2013.07.001

Hardy, K. V., & Laszloffy, T. (1995). The cultural genogram: Key to training culturally competent family therapists. *Journal of Marital and Family Therapy, 21,* 227–237. http://dx.doi.org/10.1111/j.1752-0606.1995.tb00158.x

Harris, J. I., Erbes, C. R., Engdahl, B. E., Ogden, H., Olson, R. H., Winskowski, A. M., . . . Mataas, S. (2012). Religious distress and coping with stressful life events: A longitudinal study. *Journal of Clinical Psychology, 68,* 1276–1286. http://dx.doi.org/10.1002/jclp.21900

Harris, K. A., Randolph, B. E., & Gordon, T. D. (2016). What do clients want? Assessing spiritual needs in counseling: A literature review. *Spirituality in Clinical Practice, 3,* 250–275. http://dx.doi.org/10.1037/scp0000108

Harris, T. (2004). Implications of attachment theory for working in psychoanalytic psychotherapy. *International Forum of Psychoanalysis, 13,* 147–156. http://dx.doi.org/10.1080/08037060410018462

Harrison, R. L., & Westwood, M. J. (2009). Preventing vicarious traumatization of mental health therapists: Identifying protective practices. *Psychotherapy: Theory, Research, Practice, Training, 46,* 203–219. http://dx.doi.org/10.1037/a0016081

Hatcher, R. L., & Gillaspy, J. A. (2006). Development and validation of a revised short version of the Working Alliance Inventory. *Psychotherapy Research, 16,* 12–25. http://dx.doi.org/10.1080/10503300500352500

Hathaway, W. L., Scott, S. Y., & Garver, S. A. (2004). Assessing religious/spiritual functioning: A neglected domain in clinical practice? *Professional Psychology: Research and Practice, 35,* 97–104. http://dx.doi.org/10.1037/0735-7028.35.1.97

Hay, D., Reich, K. H., & Utsch, M. (2006). Spiritual development: Intersections and divergence with religious development. In E. C. Roehlkepartain, P. E. King, L. Wagener, & P. L. Benson (Eds.), *The handbook of spiritual development in childhood and adolescence* (pp. 46–59). Thousand Oaks, CA: Sage. http://dx.doi.org/10.4135/9781412976657.n4

Hayes, A. M., Laurenceau, J. P., Feldman, G., Strauss, J. L., & Cardaciotto, L. (2007). Change is not always linear: The study of nonlinear and discontinuous patterns of change in psychotherapy. *Clinical Psychology Review, 27,* 715–723. http://dx.doi.org/10.1016/j.cpr.2007.01.008

Heiden-Rootes, K. M., Brimhall, A. S., Jankowski, P. J., & Reddick, G. T. (2017). Differentiation of self and clinicians' perceptions of client sexual behavior as "problematic." *Contemporary Family Therapy: An International Journal, 39,* 207–219. http://dx.doi.org/10.1007/s10591-017-9412-3

Heiden-Rootes, K. M., Jankowski, P. J., & Sandage, S. J. (2010). Bowen family systems theory and spirituality: Exploring the relationship between triangulation and religious questing. *Contemporary Family Therapy: An International Journal, 32,* 89–101. http://dx.doi.org/10.1007/s10591-009-9101-y

Helms, J. E., Nicolas, G., & Green, C. E. (2012). Racism and ethnoviolence as trauma: Enhancing professional and research training. *Traumatology, 18,* 65–74. http://dx.doi.org/10.1177/1534765610396728

Herman, J. (2015). *Trauma and recovery: The aftermath of violence—From domestic abuse to political terror.* New York, NY: Basic Books.

Hesse, E., & Main, M. (1999). Second-generation effects of unresolved trauma in non-maltreating parents: Dissociated, frightened, and threatening parental behavior. *Psychoanalytic Inquiry, 19,* 481–540. http://dx.doi.org/10.1080/07351699909534265

Hill, C. E., Spiegel, S. B., Hoffman, M. A., Kivlighan, D. M., Jr., & Gelso, C. J. (2017). Therapist expertise in psychotherapy revisited. *The Consulting Psychologist, 45*(1), 7–53.

Hill, P. C., & Pargament, K. I. (2003). Advances in the conceptualization and measurement of religion and spirituality: Implications for physical and mental health research. *American Psychologist, 58*, 64–74. http://dx.doi.org/10.1037/0003-066X.58.1.64

Hill, P. C., Pargament, K. I., Hood, R. W., McCullough, M. E., Swyers, J. P., Larson, D. B., & Zinnbauer, B. J. (2000). Conceptualizing religion and spirituality: Points of commonality, points of departure. *Journal for the Theory of Social Behaviour, 30*, 51–77. http://dx.doi.org/10.1111/1468-5914.00119

Hilsenroth, M. J., & Diener, M. J. (2017). Some effective strategies for the supervision of psychodynamic psychotherapy. In T. Rousmaniere, R. K. Goodyear, S. D. Miller, & B. E. Wampold (Eds.), *The cycle of excellence: Using deliberate practice to improve supervision and training* (pp. 161–188). Hoboken, NJ: Wiley-Blackwell. http://dx.doi.org/10.1002/9781119165590.ch8

Hilsenroth, M. J., Kivlighan, D. M., Jr., & Slavin-Mulford, J. (2015). Structured supervision of graduate clinicians in psychodynamic psychotherapy: Alliance and technique. *Journal of Counseling Psychology, 62*, 173–183. http://dx.doi.org/10.1037/cou0000058

Hodge, D. R. (2001). Spiritual genograms: A generational approach to assessing spirituality. *Families in Society, 82*, 35–48. http://dx.doi.org/10.1606/1044-3894.220

Hodge, D. R. (2005). Spiritual ecograms: A new assessment instrument for identifying clients' strengths in space and across time. *Families in Society, 86*, 287–296. http://dx.doi.org/10.1606/1044-3894.2467

Hoffman, M. T. (2011). *Toward mutual recognition: Relational psychoanalysis and the Christian narrative*. New York, NY: Routledge. http://dx.doi.org/10.4324/9780203881279

Holmes, J. (2001). *The search for the secure base: Attachment theory and psychotherapy*. Philadelphia, PA: Taylor & Francis.

Hood, R., Hill, P., & Spilka, B. (2018). *The psychology of religion: An empirical approach* (5th ed.). New York, NY: Guilford Press.

Hook, J. N., Davis, D., Owen, J., & DeBlaere, C. (2017). *Cultural humility: Engaging diverse identities in therapy*. Washington, DC: American Psychological Association. http://dx.doi.org/10.1037/0000037-000

Hook, J. N., Davis, D. E., Owen, J., Worthington, E. L., & Utsey, S. O. (2013). Cultural humility: Measuring openness to culturally diverse clients. *Journal of Counseling Psychology, 60*, 353–366. http://dx.doi.org/10.1037/a0032595

Hook, J. N., Worthington, E. L., & Davis, D. E. (2012). Religion and spirituality in counseling. In N. A. Fouad, J. A. Carter, & L. M. Subich (Eds.), *APA handbook of counseling psychology: Vol. 2. Practice, interventions, and applications* (pp. 417–432). Washington, DC: American Psychological Association. http://dx.doi.org/10.1037/13755-017

hooks, b. (1989). *Talking back: Thinking feminist, thinking Black*. Boston, MA: South End Press.

hooks, b. (1990). *Yearning: Race, gender and cultural politics*. Boston, MA: South End Press.

Huang, T. C., Hill, C. E., Strauss, N., Heyman, M., & Hussain, M. (2016). Corrective relational experiences in psychodynamic-interpersonal psychotherapy: Antecedents, types, and consequences. *Journal of Counseling Psychology, 63,* 183–197. http://dx.doi.org/10.1037/cou0000132

Ibn Arabi, M. (2004). *Divine sayings: Mishkat al-anwar* (S. Hirtenstein & M. Notcutt, Trans.) Oxford, England: Anqa Publishing.

Işik, E., & Bulduk, S. (2015). Psychometric properties of the Differentiation of Self Inventory—Revised in Turkish adults. *Journal of Marital and Family Therapy, 41,* 102–112. http://dx.doi.org/10.1111/jmft.12022

Jack, D., & Ali, A. (2010). *Silencing the self across cultures: Depression and gender in the social world.* Oxford, England: Oxford University Press. http://dx.doi.org/10.1093/acprof:oso/9780195398090.001.0001

Jackson, R., & Makransky, J. (2000). *Buddhist theology: Critical reflections by contemporary Buddhist scholars.* London, England: Routledge Curzon.

Jacobson, H. L., Hall, M. L., Anderson, T. L., & Willingham, M. M. (2016). Temple or prison: Religious beliefs and attitudes toward the body. *Journal of Religion and Health, 55,* 2154–2173. http://dx.doi.org/10.1007/s10943-016-0266-z

James, W. (1958). *Varieties of religious experience: A study in human nature.* New York, NY: Modern Library. (Original work published 1902)

Jankowski, P. J., Hooper, L. M., Sandage, S. J., & Hannah, N. J. (2013). Parentification and mental health symptoms: Mediating effects of perceived unfairness and differentiation of self. *Journal of Family Therapy, 35,* 43–65. http://dx.doi.org/10.1111/j.1467-6427.2011.00574.x

Jankowski, P. J., & Sandage, S. J. (2011). Meditative prayer, hope, adult attachment, and forgiveness: A proposed model. *Psychology of Religion and Spirituality, 3,* 115–131. http://dx.doi.org/10.1037/a0021601

Jankowski, P. J., & Sandage, S. J. (2014). Meditative prayer and intercultural competence: Empirical test of a differentiation-based model. *Mindfulness, 5,* 360–372. http://dx.doi.org/10.1007/s12671-012-0189-z

Jankowski, P. J., Sandage, S. J., Bell, C. A., Ruffing, E. G., & Adams, C. (2018). Humility and well-being: Testing a relational spirituality model among religious leaders. *Journal of Religion and Health.* http://dx.doi.org/10.1007/s10943-018-0580-8

Jankowski, P. J., Sandage, S. J., Bell, C. A., Rupert, D., Bronstein, M., & Stavros, G. S. (2019). Latent trajectories of change for clients at a psychodynamic training clinic. *Journal of Clinical Psychology, 75,* 1147–1168. http://dx.doi.org/10.1002/jclp.22769

Jankowski, P. J., Sandage, S. J., & Hill, P. C. (2013). Differentiation-based models of forgivingness, mental health and social justice commitment: Mediator effects for differentiation of self and humility. *The Journal of Positive Psychology, 8,* 412–424. http://dx.doi.org/10.1080/17439760.2013.820337

Jankowski, P. J., & Vaughn, M. (2009). Differentiation of self and spirituality: Empirical explorations. *Counseling and Values, 53,* 82–96. http://dx.doi.org/10.1002/j.2161-007X.2009.tb00116.x

Janoff-Bulman, R. (2002). *Shattered assumptions: Towards a new psychology of trauma.* New York, NY: Free Press.

Jarrett, L. M. (2003). *The nature of appreciation: The psychological experience of appreciating human cultural diversity* (Unpublished doctoral dissertation). University of Minnesota, Minneapolis.

Jaspers, K. (1970). *Philosophy: Vol. 2.* Chicago, IL: University of Chicago Press.

Jennings, P. (2010). *Mixing minds: The power of relationship in psychoanalysis and Buddhism*. Boston, MA: Wisdom.

Johnson, R. (2013). *Spirituality in counseling and psychotherapy: An integrative approach that empowers clients*. Hoboken, NJ: John Wiley & Sons.

Johnson, S. M. (2019). *Attachment theory in practice: Emotionally focused therapy (EFT) with individuals, couples, and families*. New York, NY: Guilford Press.

Johnson, W. B., Barnett, J. E., Elman, N. S., Forrest, L., Schwartz-Mette, R., & Kaslow, N. J. (2014). Preparing trainees for lifelong competence: Creating a communitarian training culture. *Training and Education in Professional Psychology, 8*, 211–220. http://dx.doi.org/10.1037/tep0000048

Jones, J. W. (2002). *Terror and transformation: The ambiguity of religion in psychoanalytic perspective*. New York, NY: Brunner-Routledge.

Jordan, J. (2018). *Relational-cultural therapy* (2nd ed.). Washington, DC: American Psychological Association. http://dx.doi.org/10.1037/0000063-000

Jung, C. G. (1953). *Psychology and alchemy* (2nd ed.; R. F. C. Hull, Trans.). Princeton, NJ: Princeton University Press. (Original work published 1944)

Jung, C. G., & Foote, M. (1976). *The visions seminars: From the complete notes of Mary Foote*. Zürich, Switzerland: Spring.

Kashdan, T. B., & Rottenberg, J. (2010). Psychological flexibility as a fundamental aspect of health. *Clinical Psychology Review, 30*, 865–878. http://dx.doi.org/10.1016/j.cpr.2010.03.001

Keating, L., Tasca, G. A., Gick, M., Ritchie, K., Balfour, L., & Bissada, H. (2014). Change in attachment to the therapy group generalizes to change in individual attachment among women with binge eating disorder. *Psychotherapy, 51*, 78–87. http://dx.doi.org/10.1037/a0031099

Kegan, R. (1980). There the dance is: Religious dimensions of a developmental framework. In C. Brusselmans, J. O'Donohoe, J. Fowler & A. Vergote (Eds.), *Toward moral and religious maturity: The first International Conference on Moral and Religious Development* (pp. 403–440). Morristown, NJ: Silver Burdett.

Kegan, R. (1982). *The evolving self: Problem and process in human development*. Cambridge, MA: Harvard University Press.

Kegan, R. (1994). *In over our heads: The mental demands of modern life*. Cambridge, MA: Harvard University Press.

Kegan, R., & Lahey, L. L. (2009). *Immunity to change: How to overcome it and unlock the potential in yourself and your organization*. Cambridge, MA: Harvard Business Review Press.

Kehoe, L. E., Hassen, S. C., & Sandage, S. J. (2016). Relational ecologies of psychotherapy: The influence of administrative attachment on therapeutic alliance. *Psychodynamic Practice: Groups and Organizations, 22*, 6–21. http://dx.doi.org/10.1080/14753634.2015.1124596

Kerig, P. K., & Becker, S. P. (2010). From internalizing to externalizing: Theoretical models of the processes linking PTSD to juvenile delinquency. In S. J. Egan (Ed.), *Posttraumatic stress disorder (PTSD): Causes, symptoms and treatment*. (pp. 1–46). Hauppauge, NY: Nova Science.

Kernberg, O. F. (2012). *The inseparable nature of love and aggression: Clinical and theoretical perspectives*. Arlington, VA: American Psychiatric Publishing.

Kerr, M. E. (2019). *Bowen theory's secrets: Revealing the hidden life of families*. New York, NY: W. W. Norton.

Kerr, M. E., & Bowen, M. (1988). *Family evaluation*. New York, NY: W. W. Norton.

Kierkegaard, S. (1980a). *The concept of anxiety: A simple psychologically orienting deliberation on the dogmatic issue of hereditary sin* (H. V. Hong & E. H. Hong, Trans. & Eds.). Princeton, NJ: Princeton University Press. (Original work published 1844)

Kierkegaard, S. (1980b). *The sickness unto death: A Christian psychological exploration for upbuilding and awakening* (H. V. Hong & E. H. Hong, Trans. & Eds.). Princeton, NJ: Princeton University Press. (Original work published 1849)

Kiesler, D. (2000). *Beyond the disease model of mental disorders*. Westport, CT: Praeger.

Kim, S., Miles-Mason, E., Kim, C., & Esquivel, G. B. (2013). Religiosity/spirituality and life satisfaction in Korean American adolescents. *Psychology of Religion and Spirituality, 5*, 33–40. http://dx.doi.org/10.1037/a0030628

Kimball, C. N., Cook, K. V., Boyatzis, C. J., & Leonard, K. C. (2016). Exploring emerging adults' relational spirituality: A longitudinal, mixed-methods analysis. *Psychology of Religion and Spirituality, 8*, 110–118. http://dx.doi.org/10.1037/rel0000049

King, P. E., Carr, D., & Boitor, C. (2011). Religion, spirituality, positive youth development, and thriving. *Advances in Child Development and Behavior, 41*, 161–195. http://dx.doi.org/10.1016/B978-0-12-386492-5.00007-5

Kirkpatrick, L. A. (2005). *Attachment, evolution, and the psychology of religion*. New York, NY: Guilford Press.

Kissil, K., & Niño, A. (2017). Does the person-of-the-therapist training (POTT) promote self-care? Personal gains of MFT trainees following POTT: A retrospective thematic analysis. *Journal of Marital and Family Therapy, 43*, 526–536. http://dx.doi.org/10.1111/jmft.12213

Kleinman, A. (1988). *The illness narratives: Suffering, healing, and the human condition*. New York, NY: Basic Books.

Knox, J. (2013). 'Feeling for' and 'feeling with': Developmental and neuroscientific perspectives on intersubjectivity and empathy. *The Journal of Analytical Psychology, 58*, 491–509. http://dx.doi.org/10.1111/1468-5922.12029

Koenig, H. G. (2018). *Religion and mental health: Research and clinical applications*. London, England: Academic Press.

Kohut, H. (1971). *The analysis of the self: A systematic approach to the psychoanalytic treatment of narcissistic personality disorders*. New York, NY: International Universities Press.

Kohut, H. (1972). Thoughts on narcissism and narcissistic rage. *The Psychoanalytic Study of the Child, 27*, 360–400. http://dx.doi.org/10.1080/00797308.1972.11822721

Kohut, H. (1977). *The restoration of the self*. Chicago, IL: University of Chicago Press.

Kohut, H., & Ornstein, P. H. (Eds.). (2011). *The search for the self: Selected writings of Heinz Kohut: 1950–1978* (Vol. 1). London, England: Karnac Books.

Krauss, S. W., & Flaherty, R. W. (2001). The effects of tragedies and contradictions on religion as a quest. *Journal for the Scientific Study of Religion, 40*, 113–122. http://dx.doi.org/10.1111/0021-8294.00042

Kwee, M. (2010). *New horizons in Buddhist psychology: Relational Buddhism for collaborative practices*. Chagrin Falls, OH: Taos Institute.

Lahood, G. (2010a). Relational spirituality, Part 1. Paradise unbound: Cosmic hybridity and spiritual narcissism in the "One Truth" of New Age transpersonalism. *International Journal of Transpersonal Studies, 29*, 31–57. http://dx.doi.org/10.24972/ijts.2010.29.1.31

Lahood, G. (2010b). Relational spirituality, Part 2. The belief in others as a hindrance to enlightenment: Narcissism and the denigration of relationship within transpersonal psychology and the New Age. *International Journal of Transpersonal Studies, 29*, 58–78. http://dx.doi.org/10.24972/ijts.2010.29.1.58

Laird, L. D., Curtis, C. E., & Morgan, J. R. (2017). Finding spirits in spirituality: What are we measuring in spirituality and health research? *Journal of Religion and Health, 56*, 1–20. http://dx.doi.org/10.1007/s10943-016-0316-6

Lam, C. M., & Chan-So, P. C. (2015). Validation of the Chinese version of Differentiation of Self Inventory (C-DSI). *Journal of Marital and Family Therapy, 41*, 227–235. http://dx.doi.org/10.1111/jmft.12031

Lampis, J., & Cataudella, S. (2019). Adult attachment and differentiation of self-constructs: A possible dialogue? *Contemporary Family Therapy, 41*, 227–235. http://dx.doi.org/10.1007/s10591-019-09489-7

Lampis, J., Cataudella, S., Agus, M., Busonera, A., & Skowron, E. A. (2019). Differentiation of self and dyadic adjustment in couple relationships: A dyadic analysis using the actor-partner interdependence model. *Family Process, 58*, 698–715. Retrieved from https://www.ncbi.nlm.nih.gov/pubmed/29888447

Lawson, D. M., Barnes, A. D., Madkins, J. P., & Francois-Lamonte, B. M. (2006). Changes in male partner abuser attachment styles in group treatment. *Psychotherapy, 43*, 232–237. http://dx.doi.org/10.1037/0033-3204.43.2.232

Lee, H., & Johnson, R. W. (2017). Differentiation of self as a predictor of Asian-American immigrants' perceptions of cultural harmony. *Journal of Family Therapy, 39*, 151–168. http://dx.doi.org/10.1111/1467-6427.12154

Lepherd, L. (2015). Spirituality: Everyone has it, but what is it? *International Journal of Nursing Practice, 21*, 566–574. http://dx.doi.org/10.1111/ijn.12285

Levi, O., Liechtentritt, R., & Savaya, R. (2012). Posttraumatic stress disorder patients' experiences of hope. *Qualitative Health Research, 22*, 1672–1684. http://dx.doi.org/10.1177/1049732312458184

Levine, P. (2008). *Healing trauma: A pioneering program for restoring the wisdom of your body.* Boulder, CO: Sounds True.

Levitt, H. M., & Piazza-Bonin, E. (2017). The professionalization and training of psychologists: The place of clinical wisdom. *Psychotherapy Research, 27*, 127–142. http://dx.doi.org/10.1080/10503307.2015.1090034

Lewis, T., Amini, F., & Lannon, R. (2000). *A general theory of love.* New York, NY: Vintage.

Liljenfors, R., & Lundh, L. (2015). Mentalization and intersubjectivity: Towards a theoretical integration. *Psychoanalytic Psychology, 32*, 36–60. http://dx.doi.org/10.1037/a0037129

Linehan, M. M. (1993). *Cognitive-behavioral treatment of borderline personality disorder.* New York, NY: Guilford Press.

Linehan, M. M. (2015). *DBT skills training manual.* New York, NY: Guilford Press.

Lingiardi, V., Holmqvist, R., & Safran, J. D. (2016). Relational turn and psychotherapy research. *Contemporary Psychoanalysis, 52*, 275–312. http://dx.doi.org/10.1080/00107530.2015.1137177

Liu, W. M. (2017). White male power and privilege: The relationship between White supremacy and social class. *Journal of Counseling Psychology, 64*, 349–358. http://dx.doi.org/10.1037/cou0000227

Loder, J. E. (1989). *The transforming moment.* Colorado Springs, CO: Helmers & Howard.

Lord, S. A. (2010). Meditative dialogue: Cultivating sacred space in psychotherapy— An intersubjective fourth? *Smith College Studies in Social Work, 80*, 269–285. http://dx.doi.org/10.1080/00377311003754187

Luckhurst, R. (2008). *The trauma question.* London, England: Routledge.

Lyons-Ruth, K. (1999). The two-person unconscious: Intersubjective dialogue, enactive relational representation, and the emergence of new forms of relational organization. *Psychoanalytic Inquiry, 19*, 576–617. http://dx.doi.org/10.1080/07351699909534267

Lyons-Ruth, K. (2007). The interface between attachment and intersubjectivity: Perspective from the longitudinal study of disorganized attachment. *Psychoanalytic Inquiry, 26*, 595–616. http://dx.doi.org/10.1080/07351690701310656

MacKenzie, T., Gifford, A. H., Sabadosa, K. A., Quinton, H. B., Knapp, E. A., Goss, C. H., & Marshall, B. C. (2014). Longevity of patients with cystic fibrosis in 2000 to 2010 and beyond: Survival analysis of the Cystic Fibrosis Foundation patient registry. *Annals of Internal Medicine, 161*(4), 233–241. http://dx.doi.org/10.7326/M13-0636

Maddock, J. W., & Larson, N. R. (1995). *Incestuous families: An ecological approach to understanding and treatment.* New York, NY: W. W. Norton.

Maddock, J. W., & Larson, N. R. (2004). The ecological approach to incestuous families. In D. R. Catherall (Ed.), *Handbook of stress, trauma, and the family* (pp. 367–391). New York, NY: Brunner-Routledge.

Maddux, J., & Winstead, B. (Eds.). (2015). *Psychopathology: Foundations for a contemporary understanding* (4th ed.). New York, NY: Routledge.

Maercker, A., & Perkonigg, A. (2013). Applying an international perspective in defining PTSD and related disorders: Comment on Friedman (2013). *Journal of Traumatic Stress, 26*, 560–562. http://dx.doi.org/10.1002/jts.21852

Mahoney, A. (2013). The spirituality of us: Relational spirituality in the context of family relationships. In K. I. Pargament, J. J. Exline, & J. W. Jones (Eds.), *APA handbook of psychology, religion, and spirituality: Vol. 1. Context, theory, and research* (pp. 365–389). Washington, DC: American Psychological Association. http://dx.doi.org/10.1037/14045-020

Mahoney, A., & Cano, A. (2014). Introduction to the special section on religion and spirituality in family life: Delving into relational spirituality for couples. *Journal of Family Psychology, 28*, 583–586. http://dx.doi.org/10.1037/fam0000030

Main, M. (1995). Recent studies in attachment: Overview, with implications for clinical work. In S. Goldberg, R. Muir, & J. Kerr (Eds.), *Attachment theory: Social, developmental and clinical perspectives* (pp. 407–474). Hillsdale, NJ: Analytic Press.

Main, M., & Goldwyn, R. (1994). *Adult attachment scoring and classification system.* Unpublished manuscript, University of California at Berkeley.

Mallinckrodt, B. (2015, May). *Attachment theory and the psychotherapy relationship: Summarizing what we know.* Retrieved from www.societyforpsychotherapy.org/attachment-theory-and-the-psychotherapyrelationship-summarizing-what-we-know.

Marmarosh, C. L., Markin, R. D., & Spiegel, E. B. (2013). *Attachment in group psychotherapy.* Washington, DC: American Psychological Association. http://dx.doi.org/10.1037/14186-000

Maroda, K. (2018). Repetition and working through. In R. E. Barsness (Ed.), *Core competencies of relational psychoanalysis: A guide to practice, study and research* (pp. 158–178). New York, NY: Routledge.

Maunder, B., & Hunter, J. (2015). *Love, fear, and health: How our attachments to others shape health and health care.* Toronto, Ontario, Canada: University of Toronto Press. http://dx.doi.org/10.3138/9781442668409

Maxwell, H., Tasca, G. A., Ritchie, K., Balfour, L., & Bissada, H. (2014). Change in attachment insecurity is related to improved outcomes 1-year post group therapy in women with binge eating disorder. *Psychotherapy, 51*, 57–65. http://dx.doi.org/10.1037/a0031100

McAdams, D. P. (1993). *The stories we live by: Personal myths and the making of the self.* New York, NY: Guilford Press.

McAdams, D. P. (2006). *The redemptive self: Stories Americans live by.* New York, NY: Oxford University Press. http://dx.doi.org/10.1093/acprof:oso/9780195176933.001.0001

McArdle, P. (2008). *Relational health care: A practical theology of personhood.* Saarbrücken, Germany: VDM Verlag.

McCoy, S. K., Pyszczynski, T., Solomon, S., & Greenberg, J. (2000). Transcending the self: A terror management perspective on successful aging. In A. Tomer (Ed.), *Death attitudes and the older adult: Theories, concepts, and applications* (pp. 37–63). New York, NY: Brunner-Routledge.

McCullough, M. E., Kimeldorf, M. B., & Cohen, A. D. (2008). An adaptation for altruism? The social causes, social effects, and social evolution of gratitude. *Current Directions in Psychological Science, 17*, 281–285. http://dx.doi.org/10.1111/j.1467-8721.2008.00590.x

McGoldrick, M., Gerson, R., & Petry, S. (2008). *Genograms in family assessment.* New York, NY: W. W. Norton.

McGoldrick, M., & Hardy, K. V. (Eds.). (2019). *Re-visioning family therapy: Addressing diversity in clinical practice* (3rd ed.). New York, NY: Guilford Press.

McMinn, M. R., & Campbell, C. D. (2007). *Integrative psychotherapy: Toward a comprehensive Christian approach.* Downers Grove, IL: InterVarsity Press.

McWilliams, N. (2011). *Psychoanalytic diagnosis.* New York, NY: Guilford Press.

McWilliams, N. (2014). Reflections on the effects of a Protestant girlhood. In G. Stavros & S. J. Sandage (Eds.), *The skillful soul of the psychotherapist: The link between spirituality and clinical excellence* (pp. 17–29). Lanham, MD: Rowman & Littlefield.

Meltzoff, A. N., Kuhl, P. K., Movellan, J., & Sejnowski, T. J. (2009). Foundations for a new science of learning. *Science, 325*, 284–288. http://dx.doi.org/10.1126/science.1175626

Mesman, J., van IJzendoorn, M. H., & Bakermans-Kranenburg, M. J. (2009). The many faces of the still-face paradigm: A review and meta-analysis. *Developmental Review, 29*, 120–162. http://dx.doi.org/10.1016/j.dr.2009.02.001

Mesman, J., van IJzendoorn, M. H., & Sagi-Schwartz, A. (2016). Cross-cultural patterns of attachment: Universal and contextual dimensions. In J. Cassidy & P. R. Shaver (Eds.), *Handbook of attachment: Theory, research, and clinical applications* (3rd ed., pp. 852–877). New York, NY: Guilford Press.

Mikulincer, M., & Shaver, P. R. (2016). *Attachment in adulthood: Structure, dynamics, and change* (2nd ed.). New York, NY: Guilford Press.

Mikulincer, M., Shaver, P. R., & Berant, E. (2013). An attachment perspective on therapeutic processes and outcomes. *Journal of Personality, 81*, 606–616. http://dx.doi.org/10.1111/j.1467-6494.2012.00806.x

Miller, L. (2015). *The spiritual child: The new science on parenting for health and lifelong thriving.* New York, NY: Picador.

Miller, L. (2016). Reflections on the special section "qualitative and mixed methods research on relational spirituality." *Psychology of Religion and Spirituality, 8*, 131–133. http://dx.doi.org/10.1037/rel0000072

Miller, M. M., Korinek, A. W., & Ivey, D. C. (2006). Integrating spirituality into training: The spiritual issues in supervision scale. *The American Journal of Family Therapy, 34*, 355–372. http://dx.doi.org/10.1080/01926180600553811

Miller, W. R., & C'de Baca, J. (2001). *Quantum change: When epiphanies and sudden insights transform ordinary lives*. New York, NY: Guilford Press.

Miller-Bottome, M., Talia, A., Safran, J. D., & Muran, J. C. (2017, July 6). Resolving alliance ruptures from an attachment-informed perspective. *Psychoanalytic Psychology*. Advance online publication. Retrieved from https://www.ncbi.nlm.nih.gov/pubmed/29651196

Mitchell, S. A. (2000). *Relationality: From attachment to intersubjectivity*. New York, NY: The Analytic Press.

Mitchell, S. A. (2002). *Can love last?: The fate of romance over time*. New York, NY: W. W. Norton.

Mitchell, S. A., & Aron, L. (2013). *Relational psychoanalysis: Vol. 1. The emergence of a tradition*. New York, NY: Routledge.

Montgomery, B., Oord, T. J., & Winslow, K. (Eds.). (2012). *Relational theology: A contemporary introduction*. Eugene, OR: Wipf & Stock.

Moon, S. H., & Sandage, S. J. (2019). Cultural humility for people of color: Critique of current theory and practice. *Journal of Psychology and Theology, 47*, 76–86. Advance online publication. http://dx.doi.org/10.1177/0091647119842407

Moore, R. L. (2001). *The archetype of initiation: Sacred space, ritual process, and personal transformation*. Bloomington, IN: Xlibris.

Morgan, J., & Sandage, S. J. (2016). A developmental model of interreligious competence. *Archiv für Religionspsychologie [Archive for the Psychology of Religion], 38*, 129–158. http://dx.doi.org/10.1163/15736121-12341325

Morton, M. (2016). We can work it out: The importance of rupture and repair processes in infancy and adult life for flourishing. *Health Care Analysis, 24*, 119–132. http://dx.doi.org/10.1007/s10728-016-0319-1

Muran, J. C., Safran, J. D., Gorman, B. S., Samstag, L. W., Eubanks-Carter, C., & Winston, A. (2009). The relationship of early alliance ruptures and their resolution to process and outcome in three time-limited psychotherapies for personality disorders. *Psychotherapy, 46*, 233–248. http://dx.doi.org/10.1037/a0016085

Murdock, G. (1980). *Theories of illness: A world survey*. Pittsburgh, PA: University of Pittsburgh Press.

Napier, A. Y., & Whitaker, C. A. (1978). *The family crucible*. New York, NY: Harper & Row.

Neville, R. (2006). *On the scope and truth of theology: Theology as symbolic engagement*. New York, NY: T & T Clark.

Neville, R. (2013). *Ultimates: Philosophical theology*. Albany: State University of New York Press.

Neville, R. (2014). *Existence: Philosophical theology*. Albany: State University of New York Press.

Newell, J. M., & MacNeil, G. A. (2010). Professional burnout, vicarious trauma, secondary traumatic stress, and compassion fatigue: A review of theoretical terms, risk factors, and preventive methods for clinicians and researchers. *Best Practices in Mental Health: An International Journal, 6*, 57–68.

Ng, Y. T. (2014). Spirituality and differentiation of self of parents living in the "city of sadness." *Mental Health, Religion & Culture, 17*, 655–664. http://dx.doi.org/10.1080/13674676.2014.894008

Nielsen, M. E. (1998). An assessment of religious conflicts and their resolutions. *Journal for the Scientific Study of Religion, 37*, 181–190. http://dx.doi.org/10.2307/1388036

Nietzsche, F. (1964). *The joyful wisdom* (T. Common, Trans.). New York, NY: Russell & Russell. (Original work published 1887)

Norcross, J. C., & Lambert, M. J. (2018). Psychotherapy relationships that work III. *Psychotherapy, 55*, 303–315. http://dx.doi.org/10.1037/pst0000193

Norenzayan, A. (2013). *Big gods: How religion transformed cooperation and conflict.* Princeton, NJ: Princeton University Press. http://dx.doi.org/10.2307/j.ctt32bbp0

Ochs, C. (1997). *Women and spirituality* (2nd ed.). Totowa, NJ: Rowman & Allanheld.

Ogden, P., & Fisher, J. (2015). *Sensorimotor psychotherapy: Interventions for trauma and attachment.* New York, NY: W. W. Norton.

Okado, Y., & Azar, S. T. (2011). The impact of extreme emotional distance in the mother-child relationship on the offspring's future risk of maltreatment perpetration. *Journal of Family Violence, 26*, 439–452. http://dx.doi.org/10.1007/s10896-011-9378-0

Olsen, D. C., & Devor, N. G. (2015). *Saying no to say yes: Everyday boundaries and pastoral excellence.* Lanham, MD: Rowman & Littlefield.

Olson, C. G. (2011). Relational spirituality among adult students in nontraditional programs. *Christian Higher Education, 10*, 276–295. http://dx.doi.org/10.1080/15363759.2011.576216

Orange, D. M. (2009). Intersubjective systems theory: A fallibilist's journey. *Annals of the New York Academy of Sciences, 1159*, 237–248. http://dx.doi.org/10.1111/j.1749-6632.2008.04347.x

Orange, D. M. (2011). *The suffering stranger: Hermeneutics for everyday clinical practice.* New York, NY: Routledge. http://dx.doi.org/10.4324/9780203863633

Orange, D. M., Atwood, G. E., & Stolorow, R. D. (1997). *Working intersubjectively: Contextualism in psychoanalytic practice.* Hillsdale, NJ: The Analytic Press.

Owen, J., Adelson, J., Budge, S., Wampold, B., Kopta, M., Minami, T., & Miller, S. (2015). Trajectories of change in psychotherapy. *Journal of Clinical Psychology, 71*, 817–827. http://dx.doi.org/10.1002/jclp.22191

Owen, J., & Hilsenroth, M. J. (2014). Treatment adherence: The importance of therapist flexibility in relation to therapy outcomes. *Journal of Counseling Psychology, 61*, 280–288. http://dx.doi.org/10.1037/a0035753

Owen, J., Tao, K. W., Drinane, J. M., Hook, J., Davis, D. E., & Kune, N. F. (2016). Client perceptions of therapists' multicultural orientation: Cultural (missed) opportunities and cultural humility. *Professional Psychology: Research and Practice, 47*, 30–37. http://dx.doi.org/10.1037/pro0000046

Owen, J., Wampold, B. E., Kopta, M., Rousmaniere, T., & Miller, S. D. (2016). As good as it gets? Therapy outcomes of trainees over time. *Journal of Counseling Psychology, 63*, 12–19. http://dx.doi.org/10.1037/cou0000112

Oxhandler, H. K. (2019). Revalidating the Religious/Spiritually Integrated Practice Assessment Scale with five helping professions. *Research on Social Work Practice, 29*, 223–233. http://dx.doi.org/10.1177/1049731516669592

Paine, D. R., Bell, C. A., Sandage, S. J., Rupert, D., Bronstein, M., O'Rourke, C. G., . . . Kehoe, L. E. (2019). Trainee psychotherapy effectiveness at a psychodynamic training clinic: A practice-based study. *Psychoanalytic Psychotherapy, 33*, 20–33. Advance online publication. http://dx.doi.org/10.1080/02668734.2019.1582084

Paine, D. R., Jankowski, P. J., & Sandage, S. J. (2016). Humility as a predictor of intercultural competence: Mediator effects for differentiation-of-self. *The Family Journal, 24*, 15–22. http://dx.doi.org/10.1177/1066480715615667

Paine, D. R., Moon, S. H., Sandage, S. J., Langford, R., Patel, S., Hollingsworth, A., . . . Salimi, B. (2017). Group therapy for loss: Intersubjectivity and attachment in healing. *International Journal of Group Psychotherapy, 67,* 565–589. http://dx.doi.org/10.1080/00207284.2016.1278172

Paine, D. R., & Sandage, S. J. (2015). More prayer, less hope: Empirical findings on spirituality instability. *Journal of Spirituality in Mental Health, 17,* 223–238. http://dx.doi.org/10.1080/19349637.2015.1026429

Paine, D. R., Sandage, S. J., Ruffing, E. G., & Hill, P. C. (2018). Religious and spiritual salience, well-being, and psychosocial functioning among psychotherapy clients: Moderator effects for humility. *Journal of Religion and Health, 57,* 2398–2415. http://dx.doi.org/10.1007/s10943-018-0612-4

Paine, D. R., Sandage, S. J., Rupert, D., Devor, N. G., & Bronstein, M. (2015). Humility as a psychotherapeutic virtue: Spiritual, philosophical, and psychological foundations. *Journal of Spirituality in Mental Health, 17,* 3–25. http://dx.doi.org/10.1080/19349637.2015.957611

Panksepp, J., & Biven, L. (2012). *The archaeology of mind: Neuroevolutionary origins of human emotions.* New York, NY: W. W. Norton.

Pargament, K. I. (2007). *Spiritually integrated psychotherapy: Understanding and addressing the Sacred.* New York, NY: Guilford Press.

Pargament, K. I., Koenig, H. G., Tarakeshwar, N., & Hahn, J. (2001). Religious struggle as a predictor of mortality among medically ill elderly patients: A 2-year longitudinal study. *Archives of Internal Medicine, 161,* 1881–1885. http://dx.doi.org/10.1001/archinte.161.15.1881

Pargament, K. I., Magyar, G. M., Benore, E., & Mahoney, A. (2005). Sacrilege: A study of sacred loss and desecration and their implications for health and well-being in a community sample. *Journal for the Scientific Study of Religion, 44,* 59–78. http://dx.doi.org/10.1111/j.1468-5906.2005.00265.x

Pargament, K. I., Mahoney, A., Exline, J. J., Jones, J. W., & Shafranske, E. P. (2013). Envisioning an integrative paradigm for the psychology of religion and spirituality. In K. I. Pargament, J. J. Exline, & J. W. Jones (Eds.), *APA handbook of psychology, religion, and spirituality: Vol. 1. Context, theory, and research* (pp. 3–19). Washington, DC: American Psychological Association. http://dx.doi.org/10.1037/14045-001

Pargament, K. I., Mahoney, A., & Shafranske, E. P. (2013). From research to practice: Toward an applied psychology of religion and spirituality. In K. I. Pargament, A. Mahoney, & E. P. Shafranske (Eds.), *APA handbook of psychology, religion, and spirituality: Vol. 2. An applied psychology of religion and spirituality* (pp. 3–22). Washington, DC: American Psychological Association. http://dx.doi.org/10.1037/14046-000

Pargament, K. I., Murray-Swank, N. A., Magyar, G. M., & Ano, G. G. (2005). Spiritual struggle: A phenomenon of interest to psychology and religion. In W. Miller & H. Delaney (Eds.), *Judeo–Christian perspectives on psychology: Human nature, motivation, and change* (pp. 245–268). Washington, DC: American Psychological Association. http://dx.doi.org/10.1037/10859-013

Pargament, K. I., & Saunders, S. M. (2007). Introduction to the special issue on spirituality and psychotherapy. *Journal of Clinical Psychology, 63,* 903–907. http://dx.doi.org/10.1002/jclp.20405

Paris, P. (1995). *The spirituality of African peoples: The search for a common moral discourse.* Minneapolis, MN: Fortress Press.

Park, C. L., Currier, J. M., Harris, J. I., & Slattery, J. M. (2017). *Trauma, meaning, and spirituality: Translating research into clinical practice.* Washington, DC: American Psychological Association. http://dx.doi.org/10.1037/15961-000

Patsiopoulos, A. T., & Buchanan, M. J. (2011). The practice of self-compassion in counseling: A narrative inquiry. *Professional Psychology: Research and Practice, 42*, 301–307. http://dx.doi.org/10.1037/a0024482

Patton, M. J., Connor, G. E., & Scott, K. J. (1982). Kohut's psychology of the self: Theory and measures of counseling outcome. *Journal of Counseling Psychology, 29*, 268–282. http://dx.doi.org/10.1037/0022-0167.29.3.268

Pearce, M. J., Pargament, K. I., Oxhandler, H. K., Vieten, C., & Wong, S. (2019). A novel training program for mental health providers in religious and spiritual competencies. *Spirituality in Clinical Practice, 6*, 73–82. http://dx.doi.org/10.1037/scp0000195

Peleg, O. (2014). The relationships between stressful life events during childhood and differentiation of self and intergenerational triangulation in adulthood. *International Journal of Psychology, 49*, 462–470. http://dx.doi.org/10.1002/ijop.12054

Peleg, O., & Arnon, T. (2013). Are differentiation levels associated with schizophrenia? *Deviant Behavior, 34*, 321–338. http://dx.doi.org/10.1080/01639625.2012.726176

Peleg, O., & Messerschmidt-Grandi, C. (2018). Differentiation of self and trait anxiety: A cross-cultural perspective. *International Journal of Psychology*. Advance online publication. http://dx.doi.org/10.1002/ijop.12535

Peteet, J. R. (2010). *Depression and the soul: A guide to spiritually integrated treatment.* New York, NY: Routledge.

Pew Research Center. (2017). *More Americans now say they're spiritual but not religious.* Retrieved from http://pewrsr.ch/2xP0Y8w

Pieper, J. (1986). *On hope.* San Francisco, CA: Ignatius Press.

Pitman, R. K., & Orr, S. P. (1990). The black hole of trauma. *Biological Psychiatry, 27*, 469–471. http://dx.doi.org/10.1016/0006-3223(90)90437-7

Piven, J. (2004). *Death and delusion: A Freudian analysis of mortal terror.* Greenwich, CT: Information Age.

Porter, S. L., Sandage, S. J., Wang, D. C., & Hill, P. C. (2019). Measuring the spiritual, character, and moral formation of seminarians: In search of a meta-theory of spiritual change. *Journal of Spiritual Formation and Soul Care, 12*, 5–24. http://dx.doi.org/10.1177/1939790918797481

Post, B. C., & Wade, N. G. (2009). Religion and spirituality in psychotherapy: A practice-friendly review of research. *Journal of Clinical Psychology, 65*, 131–146. http://dx.doi.org/10.1002/jclp.20563

powell, j. a. (2012). *Racing to justice: Transforming our conceptions of self and other to build an inclusive society.* Bloomington: Indiana University Press.

Prochaska, J. O., Norcross, J. C., & DiClemente, C. C. (2007). *Changing for good: A revolutionary six-stage program for overcoming bad habits and moving your life positively forward.* New York, NY: HarperCollins.

Punzi, E. (2015). 'These are the things I may never learn from books'. Clinical psychology students' experiences of their development of practical wisdom. *Reflective Practice, 16*, 347–360. http://dx.doi.org/10.1080/14623943.2015.1023280

Pyszczynski, T., Greenberg, J., & Solomon, S. (1999). A dual-process model of defense against conscious and unconscious death-related thoughts: An extension of terror management theory. *Psychological Review, 106*, 835–845.

Raia, F., & Deng, M. (2015). *Relational medicine: Personalizing modern healthcare.* New Jersey: World Scientific.

Rambo, S. (2010). *Spirit and trauma: A theology of remaining*. Louisville, KY: Westminster John Knox Press.

Rank, O. (1941). *Beyond psychology*. New York, NY: Dover.

Rank, O. (1978). *Will therapy*. New York, NY: Norton.

Ratcliffe, M. (2008). *Feelings of being: Phenomenology, psychiatry and the sense of reality*. Oxford, England: Oxford University Press. http://dx.doi.org/10.1093/med/9780199206469.001.0001

Reginster, B. (2009). *The affirmation of life: Nietzsche on overcoming nihilism*. Cambridge, MA: Harvard University Press.

Reynolds, N. L., Rupert, D., & Sandage, S. J. (2019). Therapeutic progress and symptom elevation in treating dismissive attachment: A case study. *Psychodynamic Practice: Individuals, Groups and Organisations, 25*, 5–19. Advance online publication. http://dx.doi.org/10.1080/14753634.2018.1562363

Richards, P. S., & Bergin, A. E. (2005). *A spiritual strategy for counseling and psychotherapy* (2nd ed.). Washington, DC: American Psychological Association. http://dx.doi.org/10.1037/11214-000

Richards, P. S., & Bergin, A. E. (Eds.). (2014). *Handbook of psychotherapy and religious diversity* (2nd ed.). Washington, DC: American Psychological Association. http://dx.doi.org/10.1037/14371-000

Ricoeur, P. (1967). *The symbolism of evil* (E. Buchanan, Trans.). New York, NY: Harper & Row.

Ringstrom, P. A. (2010). Meeting Mitchell's challenge: A comparison of relational psychoanalysis and intersubjective systems theory. *Psychoanalytic Dialogues, 20*, 196–218. http://dx.doi.org/10.1080/10481881003716289

Rizzuto, A. M. (1979). *Birth of the living God: A psychoanalytic study*. Chicago, IL: University of Chicago Press.

Rizzuto, A. M. (2004). Roman Catholic background and psychoanalysis. *Psychoanalytic Psychology, 21*, 436–441. http://dx.doi.org/10.1037/0736-9735.21.3.436

Rizzuto, A. M., & Shafranske, E. P. (2013). Addressing religion and spirituality in treatment from a psychodynamic perspective. In K. I. Pargament, A. Mahoney, & E. P. Shafranske (Eds.), *APA handbook of psychology, religion, and spirituality: Vol. 2. An applied psychology of religion and spirituality* (pp. 125–146). Washington, DC: American Psychological Association. http://dx.doi.org/10.1037/14046-006

Rodríguez-Gonzáles, M., Schweer-Collins, M., Skowron, E. A., Jódar, R., Cagigal, V., & Major, S. O. (2018). Stressful life events and physical and psychological health: Mediating effects of differentiation of self in a Spanish sample. *Journal of Marital and Family Therapy*. http://dx.doi.org/10.1111/jmft.12358

Rodríguez-González, M., Skowron, E. A., & Jódar Anchía, R. (2015). Spanish adaptation of the Differentiation of Self Inventory—Revised (DSI–R). *Terapia Psicológica, 33*, 47–58. http://dx.doi.org/10.4067/S0718-48082015000100005

Rose, E. M., Westefeld, J. S., & Ansley, T. N. (2008). Spiritual issues in counseling: Clients' beliefs and preferences. *Psychology of Religion and Spirituality, S*(1), 18–33. http://dx.doi.org/10.1037/1941-1022.S.1.18

Rosmarin, D. H., Bigda-Peyton, J. S., Öngur, D., Pargament, K. I., & Björgvinsson, T. (2013). Religious coping among psychotic patients: Relevance to suicidality and treatment outcomes. *Psychiatry Research, 210*, 182–187. http://dx.doi.org/10.1016/j.psychres.2013.03.023

Rousmaniere, T. (2016). *Deliberate practice for psychotherapists: A guide for improving clinical effectiveness*. New York, NY: Routledge. http://dx.doi.org/10.4324/9781315472256

Rousmaniere, T. (2019). *Mastering the inner skills of psychotherapy: A deliberate practice manual*. Seattle, WA: Gold Lantern Books.

Routledge, C., & Vess, M. (Eds.). (2018). *Handbook of terror management theory*. London, England: Academic Press.

Rupert, D., Moon, S. H., & Sandage, S. J. (2018). Clinical training groups for spirituality and religion in psychotherapy. *Journal of Spirituality in Mental Health, 21*, 163–177. http://dx.doi.org/10.1080/19349637.2018.1465879.

Russell, J. A. (2003). Core affect and the psychological construction of emotion. *Psychological Review, 110*, 145–172. http://dx.doi.org/10.1037/0033-295X.110.1.145

Russell, S. R., & Yarhouse, M. A. (2006). Training in religion/spirituality within APA-accredited psychology postdoctoral internships. *Professional Psychology: Research & Practice, 37*, 430–436. http://dx.doi.org/10.1037/0735-7028.37.4.430

Ryan, R. M., Rigby, S., & King, K. (1993). Two types of religious internalization and their relations to religious orientations and mental health. *Journal of Personality and Social Psychology, 65*, 586–596. http://dx.doi.org/10.1037/0022-3514.65.3.586

Safran, J. D. (2016). Agency, surrender, and grace in psychoanalysis. *Psychoanalytic Psychology, 33*, 58–72. http://dx.doi.org/10.1037/a0038020

Safran, J. D., & Kraus, J. (2014). Alliance ruptures, impasses, and enactments: A relational perspective. *Psychotherapy, 51*, 381–387. http://dx.doi.org/10.1037/a0036815

Safran, J. D., & Muran, J. C. (2000). *Negotiating the therapeutic alliance: A relational treatment guide*. New York, NY: Guilford Press.

Safran, J. D., Muran, J. C., & Eubanks-Carter, C. (2011). Repairing alliance ruptures. *Psychotherapy, 48*, 80–87. http://dx.doi.org/10.1037/a0022140

Saint John of the Cross. (1990). *Dark night of the soul* (E. A. Peers, Trans. & Ed.). New York, NY: Image Books. (Original work published 1578)

Sameroff, A. (2010). A unified theory of development: A dialectic integration of nature and nurture. *Child Development, 81*, 6–22. http://dx.doi.org/10.1111/j.1467-8624.2009.01378.x

Sandage, S. J. (2010). Intergenerational suicide and family dynamics: A hermeneutic phenomenological case study. *Contemporary Family Therapy, 32*, 209–227. http://dx.doi.org/10.1007/s10591-009-9102-x

Sandage, S. J., Bell, C. A., Moon, S. H., & Ruffing, E. G. (2019). Religious and spiritual problems in couples. In L. Sperry, K. Helm, & J. Carlson (Eds.), *The disordered couple* (2nd ed., pp. 305–321). New York, NY: Routledge. http://dx.doi.org/10.4324/9781351264044-19

Sandage, S. J., & Brown, J. K. (2018). *Relational integration in psychology and Christian theology: Theory, research, and practice*. New York, NY: Routledge. http://dx.doi.org/10.4324/9781315671505

Sandage, S. J., Cook, K. V., Hill, P. C., Strawn, B. D., & Reimer, K. S. (2008). Hermeneutics and psychology: A review and dialectical model. *Review of General Psychology, 12*, 344–364. http://dx.doi.org/10.1037/1089-2680.12.4.344

Sandage, S. J., & Crabtree, S. (2012). Spiritual pathology and religious coping as predictors of forgiveness. *Mental Health, Religion & Culture, 15*, 689–707. http://dx.doi.org/10.1080/13674676.2011.613806

Sandage, S. J., Crabtree, S., & Schweer, M. (2014). Differentiation of self and social justice commitment mediated by hope. *Journal of Counseling & Development, 92*, 67–74. http://dx.doi.org/10.1002/j.1556-6676.2014.00131.x

Sandage, S. J., Dahl, C. M., & Harden, M. G. (2012). Psychology of religion, spirituality, and diversity. In P. C. Hill & B. Dik (Eds.), *Psychology of religion and workplace spirituality* (pp. 43–62). Charlotte, NC: Information Age.

Sandage, S. J., & Harden, M. G. (2011). Relational spirituality, differentiation of self, and virtue as predictors of intercultural development. *Mental Health, Religion & Culture, 14*, 819–838. http://dx.doi.org/10.1080/13674676.2010.527932

Sandage, S. J., Hill, P. C., & Vaubel, D. C. (2011). Generativity, relational spirituality, gratitude, and mental health: Relationships and pathways. *International Journal for the Psychology of Religion, 21*, 1–16. http://dx.doi.org/10.1080/10508619.2011.532439

Sandage, S. J., & Jankowski, P. J. (2013). Spirituality, social justice, and intercultural competence: Mediator effects for differentiation of self. *International Journal of Intercultural Relations, 37*, 366–374. http://dx.doi.org/10.1016/j.ijintrel.2012.11.003

Sandage, S. J., Jankowski, P. J., Bissonette, C. D., & Paine, D. R. (2017). Vulnerable narcissism, forgiveness, humility, and depression: Mediator effects for differentiation of self. *Psychoanalytic Psychology, 34*, 300–310. http://dx.doi.org/10.1037/pap0000042

Sandage, S. J., Jankowski, P. J., Crabtree, S., & Schweer, M. (2015). Attachment to God, adult attachment, and spiritual pathology: Mediator and moderator effects. *Mental Health, Religion & Culture, 18*, 795–808. http://dx.doi.org/10.1080/13674676.2015.1090965

Sandage, S. J., Jankowski, P. J., & Link, D. C. (2010). Quest and spiritual development moderated by spiritual transformation. *Journal of Psychology and Theology, 38*, 15–31. http://dx.doi.org/10.1177/009164711003800102

Sandage, S. J., & Jensen, M. L. (2013). Relational spiritual formation: Reflective practice and research on spiritual formation in a seminary context. *Reflective Practice: Formation and Supervision in Ministry, 33*, 95–109.

Sandage, S. J., Jensen, M. L., & Jass, D. (2008). Relational spirituality and transformation: Risking intimacy and alterity. *Journal of Spiritual Formation and Soul Care, 1*, 182–206. http://dx.doi.org/10.1177/193979090800100205

Sandage, S. J., Li, J., Jankowski, P. J., Frank, C., & Beilby, M. (2015). Spiritual predictors of change in intercultural competence in a multicultural counseling course. *Journal of Psychology and Christianity, 34*, 168–178.

Sandage, S. J., & Moe, S. P. (2011). Narcissism and spirituality. In W. K. Campbell & J. Miller (Eds.), *The handbook of narcissism and narcissistic personality disorder: Theoretical approaches, empirical findings, and treatment* (pp. 410–420). New York, NY: John Wiley & Sons.

Sandage, S. J., & Moe, S. (2013). Spiritual experience: Conversion and transformation. In K. I. Pargament, J. J. Exline, & J. W. Jones (Eds.), *APA handbook of psychology, religion, and spirituality: Vol. 1. Context, theory, and research* (pp. 407–422). Washington, DC: American Psychological Association.

Sandage, S. J., Moon, S. H., Rupert, D., Paine, D. R., Ruffing, E. G., Kehoe, L. E., . . . Hassen, S. C. (2017). Relational dynamics between psychotherapy clients and clinic administrative staff: A pilot study. *Psychodynamic Practice: Individuals, Groups and Organisations, 23*, 249–268. http://dx.doi.org/10.1080/14753634.2017.1335226

Sandage, S. J., & Morgan, J. (2014). Hope and positive religious coping as predictors of social justice commitment. *Mental Health, Religion & Culture, 17*, 557–567. http://dx.doi.org/10.1080/13674676.2013.864266

Sandage, S. J., Paine, D. R., & Morgan, J. (2019). Relational spirituality, differentiation, and mature alterity. In T. M. Crisp, S. L. Porter, & G. A. Van Tenselhof (Eds.), *Psychology and spiritual formation in dialogue: Moral and spiritual change in Christian perspective* (pp. 186–205). Downers Grove, IL: InterVarsity Press Academic.

Sandage, S. J., Paine, D. R., Ruffing, E. G., Moon, S. H., Rupert, D. R., Bronstein, M., . . . Jankowski, P. J. (2017, September). *Testing a relational spirituality model with adult psychotherapy clients: A pilot study.* Paper presentation at the Society of Psychotherapy Research conference sponsored by the UK and European Chapters, Oxford, England.

Sandage, S. J., & Shults, F. L. (2007). Relational spirituality and transformation: A relational integration model. *Journal of Psychology and Christianity, 26,* 261–269.

Saul, J. (2014). *Collective trauma, collective healing: Promoting community resilience in the aftermath of disaster.* New York, NY: Routledge.

Saunders, S. M., Petrik, M. L., & Miller, M. L. (2014). Psychology doctoral students' perspectives on addressing spirituality and religion with clients: Associations with personal preferences and training. *Psychology of Religion and Spirituality, 6,* 1–8. http://dx.doi.org/10.1037/a0035200

Schnarch, D. (1991). *Constructing the sexual crucible: An integration of sexual and marital therapy.* New York, NY: W. W. Norton.

Schnarch, D. (1997). *Passionate marriage: Keeping love and intimacy alive in committed relationships.* New York, NY: Henry Holt.

Schnarch, D. M. (2009). *Intimacy and desire: Awaken the passion in your relationship.* New York, NY: Beaufort Books.

Schnarch, D., & Regas, S. (2012). The crucible differentiation scale: Assessing differentiation in human relationships. *Journal of Marital and Family Therapy, 38,* 639–652. http://dx.doi.org/10.1111/j.1752-0606.2011.00259.x

Schnyder, U., Ehlers, A., Elbert, T., Foa, E. B., Gersons, B. P., Resick, P. A., . . . Cloitre, M. (2015). Psychotherapies for PTSD: What do they have in common? *European Journal of Psychotraumatology, 6,* article 28186. http://dx.doi.org/10.3402/ejpt.v6.28186

Schore, A. N. (2001). The effects of early relational trauma on right brain development, affect regulation, and infant mental health. *Infant Mental Health Journal, 22*(1–2), 201–269. http://dx.doi.org/10.1002/1097-0355(200101/04)22:1<201::AID-IMHJ8>3.0.CO;2-9

Schore, A. N. (2011). The right brain implicit self lies at the core of psychoanalysis. *Psychoanalytic Dialogues, 21,* 75–100. http://dx.doi.org/10.1080/10481885.2011.545329

Schore, A. N. (2012). *The science of the art of psychotherapy.* New York, NY: W. W. Norton.

Schore, A. N. (2017). Modern attachment theory. In S. N. Gold (Ed.), *APA handbook of trauma psychology: Foundations in knowledge* (pp. 389–406). Washington, DC: American Psychological Association. http://dx.doi.org/10.1037/0000019-020

Schore, A. N. (2018). The right brain and psychoanalysis. In R. E. Barsness (Ed.), *Core competencies of relational psychoanalysis: A guide to practice, study and research* (pp. 241–262). New York, NY: Routledge.

Schore, J. R., & Schore, A. N. (2014). Regulation theory and affect regulation psychotherapy: A clinical primer. *Smith College Studies in Social Work, 84,* 178–195. http://dx.doi.org/10.1080/00377317.2014.923719

Scott, B. G., & Weems, C. F. (2013). Natural disasters and existential concerns: A test of Tillich's theory of existential anxiety. *Journal of Humanistic Psychology, 53*, 114–128.

Sennett, R. (2012). *Together: The rituals, pleasures and politics of cooperation.* New Haven, CT: Yale University Press.

Shafranske, E. P. (2013). Addressing religiousness and spirituality in psychotherapy: Advancing evidence-based practice. In R. F. Paloutzian & C. L. Park (Eds.), *Handbook of the psychology of religion and spirituality* (2nd ed., pp. 595–616). New York, NY: Guilford Press.

Shaw, D. (2010). Enter ghosts: The loss of intersubjectivity in clinical work with adult children of pathological narcissists. *Psychoanalytic Dialogues, 20*, 46–59. http://dx.doi.org/10.1080/10481880903559120

Shechtman, Z., & Kiezel, A. (2016). Why do people prefer individual therapy over group therapy? *International Journal of Group Psychotherapy, 66*, 571–591. http://dx.doi.org/10.1080/00207284.2016.1180042

Sheppard, P. I. (2011). *Self, culture, and others in womanist practical theology.* New York, NY: Palgrave Macmillan. http://dx.doi.org/10.1057/9780230118027

Sheppard, P. I. (2014). Religion: "It's complicated!" The convergence of race, class, and sexuality in clinicians' reflection on religious experience. In G. Stavros & S. J. Sandage (Eds.), *The skillful soul of the psychotherapist: The link between spirituality and clinical excellence* (pp. 45–57). Lanham, MD: Rowman & Littlefield.

Shults, F. L. (2003). *Reforming theological anthropology: After the philosophical turn to relationality.* Grand Rapids, MI: W. B. Eerdmans.

Shults, F. L., & Sandage, S. J. (2003). *The faces of forgiveness: Searching for wholeness and salvation.* Grand Rapids, MI: Baker Academic.

Shults, F. L., & Sandage, S. J. (2006). *Transforming spirituality: Integrating theology and psychology.* Grand Rapids, MI: Baker Academic.

Siegel, D. J. (2007a). *The mindful brain: Reflections on attunement in the cultivation of well-being.* New York, NY: W. W. Norton.

Siegel, D. J. (2007b). Mindfulness training and neural integration: Differentiation of distinct streams of awareness and the cultivation of well-being. *Social Cognitive and Affective Neuroscience, 2*, 259–263. http://dx.doi.org/10.1093/scan/nsm034

Siegel, D. J., & Hartzell, M. (2013). *Parenting from the inside out: How a deeper self-understanding can help you raise kids who thrive* (10th anniv. ed.). New York, NY: Tarcher.

Silverman, G. S., Johnson, K. A., & Cohen, A. B. (2016). To believe or not to believe, that is not the question: The complexity of Jewish beliefs about God. *Psychology of Religion and Spirituality, 8*, 119–130. http://dx.doi.org/10.1037/rel0000065

Simpson, D. B., Newman, J. L., & Fuqua, D. R. (2008). Understanding the role of relational factors in Christian spirituality. *Journal of Psychology and Theology, 36*, 124–134. http://dx.doi.org/10.1177/009164710803600205

Singh, N. (2005). *The birth of the Khalsa: A feminist re-memory of Sikh identity.* Albany: State University of New York Press.

Skowron, E. (2004). Differentiation of self, personal adjustment, problem solving, and ethnic group belonging among persons of color. *Journal of Counseling & Development, 82*, 447–456. http://dx.doi.org/10.1002/j.1556-6678.2004.tb00333.x

Skowron, E. A., & Dendy, A. K. (2004). Differentiation of self and attachment in adulthood: Relational correlates of effortful control. *Contemporary Family*

Therapy: An International Journal, 26, 337–357. http://dx.doi.org/10.1023/B:COFT.0000037919.63750.9d

Skowron, E. A., Kozlowski, J. M., & Pincus, A. L. (2010). Differentiation, self–other representations, and rupture–repair processes: Predicting child maltreatment risk. *Journal of Counseling Psychology, 57,* 304–316. http://dx.doi.org/10.1037/a0020030

Skowron, E. A., & Schmitt, T. A. (2003). Assessing interpersonal fusion: Reliability and validity of a new DSI fusion with others subscale. *Journal of Marital and Family Therapy, 29,* 209–222. http://dx.doi.org/10.1111/j.1752-0606.2003.tb01201.x

Skowron, E. A., Van Epps, J. J., & Cipriano-Essel, E. A. (2014). Toward a greater understanding of differentiation of self in Bowen family systems theory: Empirical developments and future directions. In P. Titelman (Ed.), *Differentiation of self: Bowen family systems theory perspectives* (pp. 355–389). New York, NY: Routledge/Taylor & Francis.

Slade, A., & Holmes, J. (2019). Attachment in psychotherapy. *Current Opinion in Psychology, 25,* 152–156.

Sontag, S. (2001). *Illness as metaphor.* New York, NY: Picador USA.

Sorenson, R. L. (1994). Therapists' (and their therapists') God representations in clinical practice. *Journal of Psychology and Theology, 22,* 325–344. http://dx.doi.org/10.1177/009164719402200417

Sorenson, R. L. (1997a). Doctoral students' integration of psychology and Christianity: Perspectives via attachment theory and multidimensional scaling. *Journal for the Scientific Study of Religion, 36,* 530–548. http://dx.doi.org/10.2307/1387688

Sorenson, R. L. (1997b). Transcendence and intersubjectivity. In C. Spezzano & G. Gargiulo (Eds.), *Soul on the couch: Spirituality, religion and morality in contemporary psychoanalysis* (pp. 163–199). Mahwah, NJ: Analytic Press.

Sorenson, R. L. (2004a). Kenosis and alterity in Christian spirituality. *Psychoanalytic Psychology, 21,* 458–462. http://dx.doi.org/10.1037/0736-9735.21.3.458

Sorenson, R. L. (2004b). *Minding spirituality.* Hillsdale, NJ: The Analytic Press.

Sorenson, R. L., Derflinger, K. R., Bufford, R. K., & McMinn, M. R. (2004). National collaborative research on how students learn integration: Final report. *Journal of Psychology and Christianity, 23,* 355–365.

Sperry, L. (2012). *Spirituality in clinical practice: Theory and practice of spiritually oriented psychotherapy.* New York, NY: Taylor & Francis.

Starr, K. E. (2008). *Repair of the soul: Metaphors of transformation in Jewish mysticism and psychoanalysis.* New York, NY: Routledge.

Stavros, G., & Sandage, S. J. (Eds.). (2014). *The skillful soul of the psychotherapist: The Link between spirituality and clinical excellence.* Lanham, MD: Rowman & Littlefield.

Stephan, A. (2012). Emotions, existential feelings, and their regulation. *Emotion Review, 4,* 157–162. http://dx.doi.org/10.1177/1754073911430138

Stern, D. N. (1985). *The interpersonal world of the infant.* New York, NY: Basic Books.

Stern, D. N. (2004). *The present moment in psychotherapy and everyday life.* New York, NY: W. W. Norton.

Stern, D. N. (2005). Intersubjectivity. In E. S. Person, A. M. Cooper, & G. O. Gabbard (Eds.), *Textbook of psychoanalysis* (pp. 77–92). Washington, DC: American Psychiatric Publishing.

Stern, D. N., Bruschweiler-Stern, N., Harrison, A. M., Lyons-Ruth, K., Morgan, A. C., Nahum, J. P., . . . Tronick, E. Z. (1998). The process of therapeutic change involving implicit knowledge: Some implications of developmental observations for adult psychotherapy. *Infant Mental Health Journal, 19*, 300–308. http://dx.doi.org/10.1002/(SICI)1097-0355(199823)19:3<300::AID-IMHJ5>3.0.CO;2-P

Stiles, W. B., & Horvath, A. O. (2017). Appropriate responsiveness as a contribution to therapist effects. In L. G. Castonguay & C. E. Hill (Eds.), *How and why are some therapists better than others? Understanding therapist effects* (pp. 71–84). Washington, DC: American Psychological Association. http://dx.doi.org/10.1037/0000034-005

Stirman, S. W., Gutner, C. A., Langdon, K., & Graham, J. R. (2016). Bridging the gap between research and practice in mental health service settings: An overview of developments in implementation theory and research. *Behavior Therapy, 47*, 920–936. http://dx.doi.org/10.1016/j.beth.2015.12.001

Stolorow, R. D. (2016). Pain is not pathology. *Existential Analysis, 27*, 70–74.

Stolorow, R. D., & Atwood, G. E. (1992). *Contexts of being: The intersubjective foundations of psychological life*. Hillsdale, NJ: Analytic Press.

Stolorow, R. D., Atwood, G. E., & Orange, D. M. (2002). *Worlds of experience: Interweaving philosophical and clinical dimensions in psychoanalysis*. New York, NY: Basic Books.

Strawn, B. D., Wright, R. W., & Jones, P. (2014). Tradition-based integration: Illuminating the stories and practices that shape our integrative imagination. *Journal of Psychology and Christianity, 33*, 37–54.

Strunk, O., Jr. (1965). *Mature religion: A psychological study*. New York, NY: Abingdon Press.

Sue, D. W., & Sue, D. (2016). *Counseling the culturally diverse: Theory and practice* (7th ed.). Hoboken, NJ: John Wiley & Sons.

Sullivan, D. (2016). *Cultural–existential psychology: The role of culture in suffering and threat*. Cambridge, England: Cambridge University Press. http://dx.doi.org/10.1017/CBO9781316156605

Summers, F. (2005). *Self-creation: Psychoanalytic theory and the art of the possible*. Hillsdale, NJ: Analytic Press.

Sundararajan, K., & Mukerji, B. (1997). *Hindu spirituality II: Postclassical and modern*. New York, NY: Crossroad.

Surrey, J. L., & Kramer, G. (2013). Relational mindfulness. In C. K. Germer, R. D. Siegel, & P. R. Fulton (Eds.), *Mindfulness and psychotherapy* (2nd ed., pp. 94–111). New York, NY: Guilford Press.

Swenson, C. (2016). *DBT principles in action: Acceptance, change, and dialectics*. New York, NY: Guilford Press.

Tan, S.-Y. (1996). Religion in clinical practice: Implicit and explicit integration. In E. P. Shafranske (Ed.), *Religion and the clinical practice of psychology* (pp. 365–387). Washington, DC: American Psychological Association. http://dx.doi.org/10.1037/10199-013

Taylor, C. (2002). *Varieties of religion today: William James revisited*. Cambridge, MA: Harvard University Press.

Teyber, E., & Teyber, F. M. (2014). Working with the process dimension in relational therapies: Guidelines for clinical training. *Psychotherapy, 51*, 334–341. http://dx.doi.org/10.1037/a0036579

Thibodeau, P. H., & Boroditsky, L. (2013). Natural language metaphors covertly influence reasoning. *PLoS One, 8*, e52961. http://dx.doi.org/10.1371/journal.pone.0052961

Thurman, H., & Smith, L., Jr. (2006). *Howard Thurman: Essential writings*. Maryknoll, NY: Orbis Books.

Tillich, P. (1952). *The courage to be*. New Haven, CT: Yale University Press.

Tillich, P. (1973). *Systematic theology: Volume one*. Chicago, IL: University of Chicago Press. http://dx.doi.org/10.7208/chicago/9780226159997.001.0001

Tillman, D. R., Dinsmore, J. A., Hof, D. D., & Chasek, C. L. (2013). Becoming confident in addressing client spiritual or religious orientation in counseling: A grounded theory understanding. *Journal of Spirituality in Mental Health, 15,* 239–255. http://dx.doi.org/10.1080/19349637.2013.799411

Tisdale, T. C., Key, T. L., Edwards, K. J., Brokaw, B. F., Kemperman, S. R., Cloud, H., . . . Okamoto, T. (1997). Impact of treatment on God image and personal adjustment, and correlations of God image to personal adjustment and object relations development. *Journal of Psychology and Theology, 25,* 227–239. http://dx.doi.org/10.1177/009164719702500207

Titelman, P. (2008). *Triangles: Bowen family systems theory perspectives*. New York, NY: Haworth Press.

Titelman, P. (Ed.). (2014). *Differentiation of self: Bowen family systems theory perspectives*. London, England: Routledge. http://dx.doi.org/10.4324/9780203121627

Tomlinson, J., Glenn, E., Paine, D., & Sandage, S. (2016). What is the "relational" in relational spirituality? A review of definitions and research directions. *Journal of Spirituality in Mental Health, 18,* 55–75. http://dx.doi.org/10.1080/19349637.2015.1066736

Tracy, D. (2005). Comparative theology. In L. Jones, M. Eliade, & C. Adams (Eds.), *Encyclopedia of religion* (pp. 9125–9134). Detroit, MI: Macmillan Reference.

Trevarthen, C. (2011). What is it like to be a person who knows nothing? Defining the active intersubjective mind of a newborn human being. *Infant and Child Development, 20,* 119–135. http://dx.doi.org/10.1002/icd.689

Tuan, Y.-F. (1977). *Space and place: The perspective of experience*. Minneapolis: University of Minnesota Press.

Tummala-Narra, P. (2009). The relevance of a psychoanalytic perspective in exploring religious and spiritual identity in psychotherapy. *Psychoanalytic Psychology, 26,* 83–95. http://dx.doi.org/10.1037/a0014673

Tummala-Narra, P. (2015). Cultural competence as a core emphasis of psychoanalytic psychotherapy. *Psychoanalytic Psychology, 32,* 275–292. http://dx.doi.org/10.1037/a0034041

Tummala-Narra, P. (2016). *Psychoanalytic theory and cultural competence in psychotherapy*. Washington, DC: American Psychological Association. http://dx.doi.org/10.1037/14800-000

Tung, E. S., Ruffing, E. G., Paine, D. R., Jankowski, P. J., & Sandage, S. J. (2018). Attachment to God as a mediator of the relationship between God representations and mental health. *Journal of Spirituality in Mental Health, 20,* 95–113. http://dx.doi.org/10.1080/19349637.2017.1396197

Turner, V. W. (1969). *The ritual process: Structure and anti-structure*. Ithaca, NY: Cornell University Press.

Unruh, A. M., Versnel, J., & Kerr, N. (2002). Spirituality unplugged: A review of commonalities and contentions, and a resolution. *Canadian Journal of Occupational Therapy, 69*(1), 5–19. http://dx.doi.org/10.1177/000841740206900101

Unterrainer, H.-F., Ladenhauf, K. H., Wallner-Liebmann, S. J., & Fink, A. (2011). Different types of religious/spiritual well-being in relation to personality and subjective well-being. *International Journal for the Psychology of Religion, 21,* 115–126.

Vaillant, G. (1996). John Bowlby, 1907–1990. *The American Journal of Psychiatry, 153,* 1483. http://dx.doi.org/10.1176/ajp.153.11.1483

van der Kolk, B. (2005). Developmental trauma disorder: Toward a rational diagnosis for children with complex trauma histories. *Psychiatric Annals, 35,* 401–408. http://dx.doi.org/10.3928/00485713-20050501-06

van der Kolk, B. (2014). *The body keeps the score: Brain, mind, and body in the healing of trauma.* New York, NY: Viking.

van der Kolk, B., & McFarlane, A. C. (2007). The black hole of trauma. In B. van der Kolk, A. McFarlane, & L. Weisaeth (Eds.), *Traumatic stress: The effects of overwhelming experience on mind, body, and society* (pp. 3–23). New York, NY: Guilford Press.

Van Deusen, S., & Courtois, C. A. (2015). Spirituality, religion, and complex developmental trauma. In D. Walker, C. Courtois, & J. Aten (Eds.), *Spiritually oriented psychotherapy for trauma* (pp. 29–54). Washington, DC: American Psychological Association. http://dx.doi.org/10.1037/14500-003

Van Tongeren, D. R., Davis, D. E., Hook, J. N., & Johnson, K. A. (2016). Security versus growth: Existential tradeoffs of various religious perspectives. *Psychology of Religion and Spirituality, 8,* 77–88. http://dx.doi.org/10.1037/rel0000050

Van Tongeren, D. R., Hakim, S., Hook, J. N., Johnson, K. A., Green, J. D., Hulsey, T. L., & Davis, D. E. (2016). Toward an understanding of religious tolerance: Quest religiousness and positive attitudes toward religiously dissimilar others. *International Journal for the Psychology of Religion, 26,* 212–224. http://dx.doi.org/10.1080/10508619.2015.1039417

Vereen, L., Wines, L., Lemberger-Truelove, T., Hannon, M., Howard, N., & Burt, I. (2017). Black existentialism: Extending the discourse on meaning and existence. *The Journal of Humanistic Counseling, 56,* 72–84. http://dx.doi.org/10.1002/johc.12045

Vieten, C., Scammell, S., Pierce, A., Pilato, R., Ammondson, I., Pargament, K. I., & Lukoff, D. (2016). Competencies for psychologists in the domains of religion and spirituality. *Spirituality in Clinical Practice, 3,* 92–114. http://dx.doi.org/10.1037/scp0000078

Vieten, C., Scammell, S., Pilato, R., Ammondson, I., Pargament, K. I., & Lukoff, D. (2013). Spiritual and religious competencies for psychologists. *Psychology of Religion and Spirituality, 5,* 129–144. http://dx.doi.org/10.1037/a0032699

Vogel, M. J., McMinn, M. R., Peterson, M. A., & Gathercoal, K. A. (2013). Examining religion and spirituality as diversity training: A multidimensional look at training in the American Psychological Association. *Professional Psychology: Research and Practice, 44,* 158–167. http://dx.doi.org/10.1037/a0032472

Wade, N. G., Cornish, M. A., Tucker, J. R., Worthington, E. L., Sandage, S. J., & Rye, M. S. (2018). Promoting forgiveness: Characteristics of the treatment, the clients, and their interaction. *Journal of Counseling Psychology, 65,* 358–371. http://dx.doi.org/10.1037/cou0000260

Wade, N. G., Post, B. C., Cornish, M. A., Vogel, D. L., & Runyon-Weaver, D. (2014). Religion and spirituality in group psychotherapy: Clinical application and case example. *Spirituality in Clinical Practice, 1,* 133–144. http://dx.doi.org/10.1037/scp0000013

Waldman, K., & Rubalcava, L. (2005). Psychotherapy with intercultural couples: A contemporary psychodynamic approach. *American Journal of Psychotherapy, 59,* 227–245. http://dx.doi.org/10.1176/appi.psychotherapy.2005.59.3.227

Wallin, D. J. (2007). *Attachment in psychotherapy.* New York, NY: Guilford Press.

Wallin, D. J. (2014). A therapist's psycho-spiritual autobiography with clinical implications. In G. S. Stavros & S. J. Sandage (Eds.), *The skillful soul of the psychotherapist: The link between spirituality and clinical excellence* (pp. 59–75). Lanham, MD: Rowman & Littlefield.

Walsh, F. (Ed.). (2010). *Spiritual resources in family therapy* (2nd ed.). New York, NY: Guilford Press.

Walsh, F. (2013). Religion and spirituality: A family systems perspective in clinical practice. In K. I. Pargament (Ed.), *APA handbook of psychology, religion, and spirituality: Vol. 2. An applied psychology of religion and spirituality* (pp. 189–205). Washington, DC: American Psychological Association. http://dx.doi.org/10.1037/14046-009

Walter, T. (1997). The ideology and organization of spiritual care: Three approaches. *Palliative Medicine, 11,* 21–30. http://dx.doi.org/10.1177/026921639701100103

Wampold, B. E., & Imel, Z. E. (2015). *The great psychotherapy debate: The evidence for what makes psychotherapy work* (2nd ed.). New York, NY: Routledge. http://dx.doi.org/10.4324/9780203582015

Ware, K. (2002). *The Orthodox way.* Crestwood, NY: St. Vladimir's Seminary Press.

Watkins, C. E., & Hook, J. N. (2016). On a culturally humble psychoanalytic supervision perspective: Creating the cultural third. *Psychoanalytic Psychology, 33,* 418–517. http://dx.doi.org/10.1037/pap0000044

Weber, S. R., & Pargament, K. I. (2014). The role of religion and spirituality in mental health. *Current Opinion in Psychiatry, 27,* 358–363. http://dx.doi.org/10.1097/YCO.0000000000000080

Weems, C. F., Costa, N. M., Dehon, C., & Berman, S. L. (2004). Paul Tillich's theory of existential anxiety: A preliminary conceptual and empirical examination. *Anxiety, Stress, and Coping: An International Journal, 17,* 383–399. http://dx.doi.org/10.1080/10615800412331318616

Weems, C. F., Russell, J. D., Neill, E. L., Berman, S. L., & Scott, B. G. (2016). Existential anxiety among adolescents exposed to disaster: Linkages among level of exposure, PTSD, and depression symptoms. *Journal of Traumatic Stress, 29,* 466–473. http://dx.doi.org/10.1002/jts.22128

Weiss, J. (1993). *How psychotherapy works.* New York, NY: Guilford Press.

Welwood, J. (2000). *Toward a psychology of awakening: Buddhism, psychotherapy, and the path of personal and spiritual transformation.* Boston, MA: Shambhala.

West, C. (2004). *Democracy matters: Winning the fight against imperialism.* New York, NY: Penguin Group.

Wildman, W. J. (2010). An introduction to relational ontology. In J. Polkinghorne & J. Zizioulas (Eds.), *The Trinity and an entangled world: Relationality in physical science and theology* (pp. 55–73). Grand Rapids, MI: Eerdmans.

Wildman, W. J. (2017). *In our own image: Anthropomorphism, apophaticism, and ultimacy.* Oxford, England: Oxford University Press. http://dx.doi.org/10.1093/oso/9780198815990.001.0001

Wildman, W. J. (2018). *Effing the ineffable: Existential mumblings at the limits of language.* Albany: State University of New York Press.

Williamson, I. T., & Sandage, S. J. (2009). Longitudinal analyses of religious and spiritual development among seminary students. *Mental Health, Religion & Culture, 12,* 787–801. http://dx.doi.org/10.1080/13674670902956604

Williamson, I. T., Sandage, S. J., & Lee, R. M. (2007). How social connectedness affects guilt and shame: Mediated by hope and differentiation of self. *Personality and Individual Differences, 43,* 2159–2170. http://dx.doi.org/10.1016/j.paid.2007.06.026

Wilt, J., Grubbs, J., Exline, J., & Pargament, K. (2016). Personality, religious and spiritual struggles, and well-being. *Psychology of Religion and Spirituality, 8,* 341–351. http://dx.doi.org/10.1037/rel0000054

Wolfson, R. (2013). *Relational Judaism: Using the power of relationships to transform the Jewish community.* Woodstock, VT: Jewish Lights.

Wong, P. T. P. (2011). Positive psychology 2.0: Toward a balanced interactive model of the good life. *Canadian Psychology, 52,* 69–81. http://dx.doi.org/10.1037/a0022511

Worthington, E. L., Jr., Hook, J. N., Davis, D. E., & McDaniel, M. A. (2011). Religion and spirituality. *Journal of Clinical Psychology, 67,* 204–214. http://dx.doi.org/10.1002/jclp.20760

Worthington, E. L., Jr., Kurusu, T. A., McCullough, M. E., & Sandage, S. J. (1996). Empirical research on religion and psychotherapeutic processes and outcomes: A 10-year review and research prospectus. *Psychological Bulletin, 119,* 448–487. http://dx.doi.org/10.1037/0033-2909.119.3.448

Worthington, E. L., Jr., & Sandage, S. J. (2016). *Forgiveness and spirituality in psychotherapy: A relational approach.* Washington, DC: American Psychological Association. http://dx.doi.org/10.1037/14712-000

Wortmann, J. H., Park, C. L., & Edmondson, D. (2011). Trauma and PTSD symptoms: Does spiritual struggle mediate the link? *Psychological Trauma: Theory, Research, Practice, and Policy, 3,* 442–452. http://dx.doi.org/10.1037/a0021413

Wright, R., Jones, P., & Strawn, B. D. (2014). Tradition-based integration. In E. D. Bland & B. D. Strawn (Eds.), *Christianity and psychoanalysis: A new conversation* (pp. 37–54). Downers Grove, IL: InterVarsity Press. Retrieved from http://search.ebscohost.com.ezproxy.bu.edu/login.aspx?direct=true&db=psyh&AN=2014-12218-002&site=ehost-live&scope=site

Wulff, D. (1997). *Psychology of religion: Classic and contemporary.* New York, NY: John Wiley & Sons.

Wuthnow, R. (1998). *After heaven: Spirituality in America since the 1950s.* Berkeley: University of California Press. http://dx.doi.org/10.1525/california/9780520213968.001.0001

Xavier, J., Magnat, J., Sherman, A., Gauthier, S., Cohen, D., & Chaby, L. (2016). A developmental and clinical perspective of rhythmic interpersonal coordination: From mimicry toward the interconnection of minds. *Journal of Physiology–Paris, 110*(4, Part B), 420–426. http://dx.doi.org/10.1016/j.jphysparis.2017.06.001

Xue, Y., Xu, Z. Y., Zaroff, C., Chi, P., Du, H., Ungvari, G. S., . . . Xiang, Y. T. (2018). Associations of differentiation of self and adult attachment in individuals with anxiety-related disorders. *Perspectives in Psychiatric Care, 54,* 54–63. http://dx.doi.org/10.1111/ppc.12200

Yalom, I. D. (1980). *Existential psychotherapy.* New York, NY: Basic Books.

Yalom, I. D., & Leszcz, M. (2005). *The theory and practice of group psychotherapy* (5th ed.). New York, NY: Basic Books.

Yang, Q., Liu, S., Sullivan, D., & Pan, S. (2016). Interpreting suffering from illness: The role of culture and repressive suffering construal. *Social Science & Medicine, 160,* 67–74. http://dx.doi.org/10.1016/j.socscimed.2016.05.022

Yansen, J. (2016). *Daughter Zion's trauma: Reading lamentations with insights from trauma studies* (Unpublished doctoral dissertation). Boston University, Boston, MA.

Yeomans, F. E., Levy, K. N., & Caligor, E. (2013). Transference-focused psychotherapy. *Psychotherapy, 50,* 449–453. http://dx.doi.org/10.1037/a0033417

INDEX

ABOUT THE AUTHORS

Steven J. Sandage, PhD, LP, is Albert and Jessie Danielsen Professor of Psychology of Religion with a joint appointment in the School of Theology and the Department of Psychological and Brain Sciences at Boston University. He is director of research and senior staff psychologist at the Danielsen Institute and visiting faculty in psychology of religion at MF Norwegian School of Theology in Oslo. His books include *To Forgive Is Human: How to Put Your Past in the Past*; *The Faces of Forgiveness: Searching for Wholeness and Salvation*; *Transforming Spirituality: Integrating Theology and Psychology*; *The Skillful Soul of the Psychotherapist: The Link Between Spirituality and Clinical Excellence*; *Forgiveness and Spirituality in Psychotherapy: A Relational Approach*; and *Relational Integration of Psychology and Christian Theology: Theory, Research, and Practice*. Dr. Sandage practices as a licensed psychologist with clinical specializations that include couple and family therapy, multicultural therapy, and spiritually integrative therapy. The American Psychological Association produced a clinical demonstration video with Dr. Sandage, *Forgiveness in Couple Therapy*, in 2018.

David Rupert, PsyD, LP, is the director of training at the Danielsen Institute, Boston University, and a licensed psychologist in private practice. He has a doctorate in clinical psychology and master's degrees in psychology and theology from Fuller Seminary. Dr. Rupert has been in full-time clinical practice since 1996. His areas of research interest and clinical specialization are relational approaches to psychotherapy; spiritual, religious, and existential issues; cultural competence/humility and social justice; and formative approaches to training for psychotherapists.

George Stavros, MDiv, PhD, LP, is the executive director of the Danielsen Institute and clinical associate professor of pastoral psychology at Boston University. His teaching and research interests are in religion and spirituality in clinical practice and training, psychotherapy process and outcomes, and clergy and clergy family wellness. He is a licensed psychologist and holds a master of divinity from Holy Cross Greek Orthodox School of Theology. He is coeditor of *The Skillful Soul of the Psychotherapist: The Link Between Spirituality and Clinical Excellence*.

Nancy G. Devor, MDiv, PhD, LP, is the former training and executive director of the Danielsen Institute and currently a senior staff psychologist. Dr. Devor has divided her career between the Danielsen Institute at Boston University and working with the Solihten Institute, a national network of counseling centers that have integrated faith, spirituality, and mental health care over the last 60 years. A licensed psychologist with a doctoral degree from Boston University, she received a master of divinity degree from Yale Divinity School and is ordained in the United Church of Christ. She is the coauthor of *Saying No to Say Yes: Everyday Boundaries and Pastoral Excellence*.